Homoeopathic Remedies

Douglas M. Gibson
MB, BS (Lond.), FRCS (Edin.), FFHom

Edited for publication by
Marianne Harling
BA, BM, BCh, FFHom
and
Brian Kaplan
MB, BCh, MFHom

BEACONSFIELD PUBLISHERS LTD
Beaconsfield, Bucks, England

First published in 1987
Reprinted 1991, 1994, 1996, 2000

British Library Cataloguing in Publication Data
Gibson, Douglas, M.
    Studies in homoeopathic remedies –
    (The Beaconsfield Homoeopathic Library; No. 7)
    1. Homoeopathy – Materia medica and therapeutics
    I. Title   II. Harling, Marianne   III. Kaplan, Brian
    615.5'32   RX601
    ISBN 0–906584–17–5

Phototypeset by Gem Graphics, Trenance, Mawgan Porth, Cornwall
in 9½ on 12 point Times.
Printed in Great Britain at The Bath Press, Bath.

Preface

Dr Douglas Gibson was born in 1888 and educated at Cheltenham College. He studied medicine at St Thomas' Hospital, later taking the Edinburgh FRCS. Twenty-seven years as a medical missionary in China was brought to a sudden end by the Second World War, and he then worked for four years at a large tuberculosis hospital in Canada.

He was introduced to homoeopathy in 1936, and in 1946 came to study it at the Royal London Homoeopathic Hospital, where he became first a Member and then a Fellow of the Faculty of Homoeopathy, and joined the Outpatients staff of the hospital. He also had a private practice. In 1972 he retired to Canada, where he died in 1977, two weeks before his eighty-ninth birthday.

Dr Gibson was a remarkable person, with strong convictions and a lively sense of humour. His many interests ranged from music and literature through natural history to Rugby football and cricket. He was a prolific writer, and contributed the series of Studies in Materia Medica to the British Homoeopathic Journal in forty-seven instalments between 1963 and 1977. In this he was strongly encouraged by Dr Ralph Twentyman, the Editor throughout that period, and to whom therefore is due the credit of being midwife to this remarkable offspring.

The studies appeared in groups of two, or occasionally three, connected through their action or source (for example Belladonna, Hyoscyamus, Stramonium). For the reader's convenience we have rearranged them in alphabetical order, but a list of the original groups, in the order in which they were published, appears as an Appendix.

Each remedy is described under a number of different headings:

1) The *Source* gives the origin and nature of the remedy, whether animal, vegetable or mineral; a description of it and of its ecology, not only with regard to the physical world, but also in myth, literature and history. Dr Gibson devotes more attention to this aspect than the authors of previous materia medicas. Sometimes he draws a parallel between the external manifestations of a plant, mineral or animal, and the mental and physical symptoms which make up the drug picture of the remedy. He

iii

does not however suggest a causal relationship nor invoke any philosophical principle.

A world of nature and symbolism is concentrated into each homoeopathic remedy. This is significant, and cannot lightly be dismissed by quoting Hahnemann's warning against the Doctrine of Signatures. Dr Gibson says: 'These parallels and correspondences are sufficiently numerous and striking to deserve mention, as well as being an aid to the understanding and memorising of the materia medica picture of each remedy.'

2) *Pharmacology*. describes the gross chemical effects produced by the remedy in its natural state before potentisation.

3) *Proving*. A reference has been inserted here to the earliest published proving of the remedy.

The above three headings relate to the remedy itself, whereas the remainder are devoted to its effect upon the patient.

4) The general physical *Appearance* is described, together with mannerisms, gait, and so on. It is not suggested that a remedy will give rise to particular physical characteristics; rather that people of a certain build and temperament have been found to be sensitive to some remedies, and that they respond well to those remedies in a clinical situation.

5) *Psychology* includes the mental and emotional symptoms which are so important in homoeopathic prescribing. They can range from traits of personality, such as the untidiness and argumentativeness of Sulphur, to symptoms of toxic psychosis, for example, mania in Belladonna poisoning.

6) *Physiology* refers to the general symptoms such as patterns of sleep, food likes and dislikes, reactions to climate, and so on.

7) *Symptomatology* describes particular symptoms relating to the different systems of the body, listed in the order adopted by homoeopaths. *Modalities* have been included at the end of this section.

8) Finally, *Clinical Notes* covers details of dosage and treatment, relationships of remedies, and otherwise unclassifiable items of interest.

We have added remedy pictures of four nosodes – Medorrhinum, Syphilinum, Tuberculinum and Carcinosin – which we feel to be so important that they should not be left out of any practical materia medica.

M.E.H., B.K.

Contents

Contents

Aconitum Napellus

Aconitum napellus, monk's-hood, wolf's-bane, is a member of the Ranunculaceae, a family which also includes such remedies as Cimicifuga, Helleborus, Hydrastis, Paeonia and Ranunculus.

This is a very striking plant; its tall, upright, 4 to 5 foot stem is resplendent at the top with a thick cluster of deep blue sombre-hued flowers arranged in a spike. The leaves are deeply cleft. The root, a dark conical tuber, is whitish on section and has a bitter taste, associated with tingling and numbness in the mouth if eaten. The root has on occasion been mistaken for horseradish and eaten with disastrous results.

The habitat of the plant shows a preference for damp shady spots in hilly or mountainous country, but it is the flowers that are remarkable. These blooms, shaped like a monk's cowl, are no longer radially symmetrical like those of the spring Ranunculaceae – anemones, aquilegia, paeonia – but are isobilateral. They have given up the radiate flower form and attained a higher form of symmetry suggestive of the animal kingdom. The higher invertebrates as well as all vertebrates possess bilateral symmetry as their fundamental morphological concept.

Figuratively speaking, the flowers of the plant reach out into the sphere of animal life, and the extremely poisonous nature of the whole plant may be connected with this fact. From the root upwards all parts of the plant contain the aconitine alkaloids; the whole plant is used in the preparation of the mother tincture.

It is of interest that *Aconitum napellus* is in polar contrast to *Helleborus niger*, the Christmas rose, which is the most ancient member of the Ranunculaceae. *Aconitum* is a more recent representative of this very primitive family of plants. It shows much more advanced structures, in the specialized upper sepal which forms a protective covering for the other parts of the flower, in the deep blue colour of the flowers, and in the arrangement of the blossoms, not on single stems but in an inflorescence.

Seasonally also the plant is at the opposite pole to the Christmas rose. Instead of pushing its way up through the snows of winter it springs vigorously upwards to burst into bloom at the peak of summer. Thus instead of torpor, the characteristic of *Helleborus*, there is here a suggestion of terror. Instead of the sluggishness of winter growth this upstanding summer-flowering plant betokens swift, sudden, strenous activity.

PHARMACOLOGY

There is something rather sinister and suggestive of death about this plant, its forbidding appearance, its rather menacing hue, its fondness for 'hiding away in damp woods and shady hedgerows'. It is said, indeed, to be Britain's most poisonous plant.

Down the ages the poisonous proclivities of the plant have been widely known. Plutarch gives an account of Mark Antony's army being in want of food, grubbing up some of these roots, which they devoured, with the result that 'every man died in a paroxysm'. The root was formerly known as 'kill-panther'; the sorceress Hecate was said to have discovered its properties and passed on the knowledge to her lethally-minded daughters Circe and Medea.

The plant was the chief ingredient of the deadly draught employed on the island of Ceos for the liquidation of 'senile persons of no value to the state'. It has been used as an arrow poison, and even in recent times murders have been committed with an infusion of the leaves, or by means of the chief of the poisonous alkaloids in the plant, namely aconitine.

This swiftly-acting alkaloid is deadly in its effects; three milligrams are sufficient to kill a horse. The symptoms of acute poisoning by the plant have been observed in numberless instances. The sequence is as follows:

Within a few minutes to half an hour the mouth and throat begin to burn and tingle. The tingling spreads over the whole body and causes the victim great distress. It is perhaps the most characteristic symptom. The hands seem to be 'made of fur and enclosed in a glove'.

Cold sweats and shivering are followed by generalized numbness with a peculiar feeling of deathly chill over the whole body, as if the veins contained iced water instead of blood.

Agonizing pains are felt in head, neck, back and in the cardiac region. The face becomes grey, cheeks sunken, and in a half to three hours death ensues as the result of total circulatory failure, respiratory paralysis and cardiac arrest.

The pulse is at first slowed, then becomes irregular and finally imperceptible. The embarrassment of the circulation with consequent anoxia of tissues gives rise to a feeling of intense terror and fear of imminent death, tending to complete panic, not lessened by acute palpitation and suffocative dyspnoea.

Towards the end the mind becomes clouded, with total inability to formulate an idea (cerebral anoxia). Hearing becomes disturbed, also vision – glistening white objects are seen as yellowish-green in colour. A rapid onset of blindness precedes death. The pupils, however, are unaffected unless actual convulsions occur, when they tend to dilate.

The drug has a two-fold action on the heart. In the first place the heartbeat is slowed in rate by stimulation of the inhibitory vagus centre in the medulla; secondly, a direct action on the organ itself involving the bundle of His leads to an increased rate of beat, followed by irregularity of rhythm.

There is an action on the peripheral nervous system with stimulation of the terminal organs of the sensory nerves in the skin, producing prickling and tingling sensations. In the mucosa of the mouth the tingling sensation is accompanied by profuse salivation.

A special affinity is noted with the trigeminal nerve, leading to severe facial neuralgia.

PROVING

Aconite was proved by Hahnemann, and appears in the first volume of *Materia Medica Pura*.

APPEARANCE

Aconite is most likely to be indicated in robust, thick-set persons rather than in the weak and debilitated.

A red countenance is probable, or possibly a unilateral flush. The expression is often scared, even terrified.

Piteous wailing may occur with a child.

The skin is hot and dry. Temperature is apt to reach a peak at 9 p.m. The pupils remain small.

A marked feature is great restlessness with incessant tossing and turning to and fro.

PSYCHOLOGY

The chief characteristic of the Aconite mentality is fear, a most acute anxiety, a horrible fear leading to panic and frantic impatience.

There may be fear of the dark, of ghosts, of crowds, of crossing the road or even going out on the street. Sometimes it is a fear of imminent death, with actual naming of the hour of decease, or perhaps an intangible but very real fear of 'doesn't really know what'.

There is great intolerance of pain, which becomes unbearable, also of noise and even music. The sufferer tends to become quite inappeasable, 'beside himself', demanding that 'something must be done, and done quickly!'

The subject is very easily startled. Children are apt to be alert and alarmed. On the other hand there may be confusion of mind, thoughts and ideas chasing each other in a confused riot.

One feature is a marked aversion to being touched or uncovered, probably due to hypersensitivity of the skin.

Obviously the Aconite picture may be precipitated by any situation or experience which holds a threat, real or imaginary, and which is thus liable to induce fear.

PHYSIOLOGY

The Aconite subject is alternately cold and hot, vasomotor control being badly off poise and the distribution of bloodflow correspondingly irregular.

Thirst is usually intense, for large quantities of cold water.

There is a tendency to drowsiness during the day, but sleep may depart at night, with a liability to excessive yawning; or sleep may be disturbed by a plethora of dreams or even nightmares. Restless insomnia in old age may respond to Aconite.

Sweating may occur on covered parts, with relief of symptoms; cool clammy sweat may be present on the palms.

SYMPTOMATOLOGY

General

Typical is a sudden onset of high fever with burning head but the rest of the body cold. This acute onset may occur within a few hours of exposure to the causal factor; it is likened by one writer to 'the storm which sweeps the mountain heights where the *Aconitum* plant grows'. The high temperature is usually preceded by a severe chill. Hence the advice to take a dose of Aconite 'at the first shiver'. Pains are particularly severe and unbearable, driving the sufferer to desperation, so that he 'screams with pain' which is described as burning, stinging, cutting or stabbing. Moreover the pains are likely to be accompanied by numbness, tingling, formication and, possibly, sudden flashes of heat. The severity of the pain experienced is probably due to hyperalgesia, a lowering of the pain threshold, the result of interference with bloodflow inducing anoxia of the sensory nerves. Another Aconite feature is haemorrhage, sudden severe bleeding of bright blood from nose, uterus, rectum or other site, and associated with acute mental turmoil and alarm.

Head
Giddiness is a prominent symptom, with 'everything twirling and whirling'. It is especially noticed on rising from a recumbent posture, or it may come on suddenly as the result of some frightening or upsetting experience. Headache is sudden and severe with pains described as shooting, pinching or squeezing, and a burning hot head; the headache is made worse by movement, by talking, by attempts to sit up, even by the act of taking a drink. It is somewhat relieved in the open air. Neuralgic pains are described affecting the face, like 'hot wires piercing the tissues', associated with formication and, perhaps, a sensation as if 'iced water were poured along the nerves'.

Eyes
Eye symptoms are very acute, out of the blue, with heat, redness and lachrymation, photophobia, and possibly sudden dimness of vision. There is not usually much discharge, but on separating the lids there may be a gush of hot watery fluid. Opening the lids may be quite difficult owing to the extreme swelling. It is worthy of note that the remedy is of special value in relation to eye injuries, and Aconite has been described as 'the Arnica of the eye'.

Ears
Acute pain of throbbing, cutting intensity may come on suddenly after being out in severe cold; it is accompanied by hypersensitivity to noise, and music is unbearable.

Respiratory System
Smell is acute and especially sensitive to unpleasant odours. Coryza is brought on by exposure to cold winds; the discharge is fluent, especially in the morning, with dripping or dropping of clear hot water. The condition is aggravated by talking; it is relieved in the open air. Sore throat is accompanied by dryness, numbness and tingling, with a feeling of constriction and pain on swallowing. A hoarse, croaky, convulsive cough is easily intensified by eating or drinking, by lying down, by attempting to talk, by contact with tobacco smoke, as the result of emotional upset, and at night. Various shooting or stitching pains are felt

in the chest. Suffocative asthmatic attacks occur, associated with great anxiety. The child may wake in the first half of the night, after exposure to cold, with violent croupy, choking cough. Aconite is indicated in first stage pneumonia with sudden onset, great pain in chest, of shooting, tearing, burning type, especially affecting the upper half of the left lung; it is only possible to lie on the back; there is a hard dry cough and cherry-red sputum.

Alimentary System
Numbness and tingling is noticed in lips and tongue. Taste is affected, everything tasting bitter except water. The mouth is excessively dry. Toothache is caused by exposure to cold wind; the teeth are very sensitive to cold in any form.

Hiccough, belching, waterbrash, bilious vomiting may occur, as also a sensation of fullness, tension and weight in the epigastrium or lower left chest. Stomach upsets of sudden onset are accompanied by intense craving for water – just 'cannot get enough to drink'. Pinchings, burnings, cuttings are felt in the belly, associated with great tenderness to touch and intolerance of movement. Sudden onset of acute diarrhoea may occur in summer, with cholera-like stools, collapse, deathly anxiety and great restlessness. Stools may look like chopped spinach. Intussusception may occur.

Cardiovascular System
Sudden violent attacks of palpitation are accompanied by intense fear and anxiety; the sufferer sits bolt upright and can hardly get a breath. Shooting or squeezing pains are felt in the chest, aggravated by going up stairs or by walking fast.

Urinary System
Sudden acute onset of urinary distress with cutting, tearing pains. Urine is hot, dark, reddish, even bloody. Acute retention from shock; retention in the newly born.

Genital System
Sudden orchitis due to exposure to cold, violent in nature. Gynaecological complaints prominently associated with nervous upset or actual fear.

Nervous System
Numbness and weakness are noticed in the limbs, especially the left arm. Tremors occur in the hands. Creeping pains are felt in the fingers. Palms

of hands are hot while the feet are as cold as ice. Varied stitches, twitches, paraesthesias and pareses occur in limbs or back.

Locomotor System

Acute inflammation of joints. Special mention is made of pain in the hip-joint which forces a cry at every step. Weakness and instability is felt at both knee and hip. Limbs feel heavy, bruised, numb.

Skin

In addition to the paraesthesias mentioned already, a purpuric or morbilliform eruption may occur. Pruritus is associated with desquamation. The skin may be so sensitive that the least touch or contact is resented.

MODALITIES

Either extreme of temperature will aggravate symptoms; these also tend to be worse in a warm room, in direct sunlight, from taking wine or stimulants, if lying on the affected side, and at night, especially around midnight.

Relief is felt in the open air, as result of sleep, and after profuse sweating. Aconite may often be indicated when complaints are brought on with suddenness, either by bitter cold in winter or by excessive summer heat, i.e. dry cold or dry heat. Other factors which may precipitate an Aconite picture are bathing in cold water, surgical operation and associated shock.

CLINICAL NOTES

Aconite is a short-acting remedy of immense value in the early hours of acute illness. Its use in this way may abort a more serious condition, but if symptoms persist the use of a different remedy must be considered. If the skin has become moist and profuse sweating has occurred, the opportunity for Aconite has probably passed.

A condition calling for the remedy may, however, ensue at any moment during the course of an illness, in chronic disease, or after a surgical operation.

Aconite rivals Chamomilla and Coffea as a pain-reliever.

The remedy is followed well by Arnica, Belladonna, Bryonia, or Ipecacuanha, according to the symptom picture, and at times Sulphur will be called for to complete the cure.

Agaricus Muscarius

SOURCE

This remedy is prepared from that intriguing little toadstool *Amanita muscaria*, also known as fly agaric and scarlet cap. It was used in medieval times broken up in milk to stupefy flies. It has a most arresting scarlet or orange-red top on which are concentric circles of little white blobs; these are the remnants of the torn volva membrane; they are easily washed off by rain.

The cap is some five inches in diameter. The stem reaches a height of about seven inches; it is white or pinkish in colour, about an inch in cross section, ringed by a reflexed collar of membrane, and swollen at the base by rings of warty scales. The gills are crowded, distinct and white; the spores also are white.

The toadstools are found growing in clusters in the autumn in birch or pine woods, and favour northern climes in Scotland, northern Europe and north-eastern Asia.

PHARMACOLOGY

The plant is not so much a lethal poison as an intoxicant and narcotic, though it has in rare cases caused death. The Vikings used it in order to 'go berserk'. In the prohibition era in the USA its use was said to be as effective as bootleg liquor, and less expensive. The usual method of taking the fungus is to roll it into a bolus and swallow it without chewing.

The desired effect ensues in one to two hours and is evidenced by giddiness, a flushed visage, cheerfulness of spirit, uncontrolled speech and behaviour, passing on occasion into complete loss of consciousness. Sometimes violent muscle spasms occur, or the effects are quite ludicrous; if a subject under the influence steps over a piece of straw or a small stick he takes a stride or a jump, as if clearing the trunk of a tree; a talkative type talks at random and may disclose secret matters; one fond of music constantly bursts into song.

Three alkaloids have been isolated from the fungus, muscarine, muscaridine and choline. The second seems to be responsible for toxic effects on the central nervous system, causing excitation of the myoneural and glanduloneural receptor organs; this induces muscle spasms and twitchings, increased salivation, secretion of tears and alimentary juices. Muscarine produces the curious illusion related to size – objects appearing inordinately large, or a crack in the ground looking like a chasm requiring to be leapt over.

PROVING

Agaricus was proved by Hahnemann and his colleagues, and the pathogenesy published in *Chronic Diseases*; there have been several re-provings since.

APPEARANCE

Mentioned features are light hair, lax skin and musculature, and pallor of face. Speech is apt to be jerky and indistinct. Muscular twitchings, jerkings, tremblings cease during sleep. Movements tend to be clumsy – drops things.

PSYCHOLOGY

Subject is peevish, indifferent, averse to making any effort, even that of talking. There may be wild delirium – a mixture of violence and hilarity. Complains of feeling pricked or stabbed by 'ice-needles'.

PHYSIOLOGY

A chilly individual; hugs the fire. Easily tired mentally; child is mentally retarded.

SYMPTOMATOLOGY

General

May complain of a widespread bruised sensation associated with shifting neuralgic pains. These are worse when at rest and eased when becoming warm in bed. The pains may have a diagonal distribution, e.g. right arm and left knee.

Head

Giddiness occurs in the morning, in bright sunlight, when walking in open air, on turning the head rapidly. Shooting headache in frontal region extending to the root of the nose, worse after study and accompanied by heaviness in the occipital region and a tendency to fall backwards. Headache localized to small spots. Perhaps a sensation as if a

9

chunk of ice was resting on the head. Headaches in drunkards. Headaches associated with chorea, or with spinal trouble. Head constantly in motion. Facial neuralgia with 'splinter pains'.

Eyes

Oscillating movements of eyeballs. Twitching of eyelids. Reading interfered with by tendency of type to move or swim. Double vision. Lids itch, burn and agglutinate. Redness of inner canthi.

Ears

Become red, burn and itch as if frostbitten.

Respiratory System

Clear water drops from nose, quite apart from 'cold in the head'. Itching of nose both internal and external, spasmodic sneezing. Nosebleed in the elderly. Sensation of stitches along the pharyngotympanic canal. Throat feels dry, contracted and swallowing is difficult. Coughs up small solid balls of phlegm. Violent paroxysmal cough is associated with much sneezing. Sputum is purulent or composed of small hard lumps of mucus. Chest feels 'too narrow'. Chest symptoms are eased by deep breathing and when walking.

Alimentary System

Trembling of the tongue makes speech difficult. Oral aphthae and ulceration. Herpes on lips. Lips burn and smart. Splinter pains felt in tongue. Sweet taste in mouth 'like apples'. Liability to hiccough. Flatulent distension of stomach and abdomen. Borborygmi, colicky pains, passage of inodorous flatus. Burning in stomach about three hours after a meal, changing to a dull pressure. Stitching pains in liver and below ribs on left side. Violent but ineffective urge to stool. Diarrhoea with passage of horribly offensive flatus and stool followed by tenesmus.

Cardiovascular System

Irregular, tumultuous palpitation, possibly associated with tobacco. Pulse liable to be intermittent and irregular. May complain of a sense of constriction in the cardiac region.

Urinary System

Stitches are felt in the urethra. Sudden and violent urging to urinate. Frequency of micturition.

Genital System

Severe bearing-down pains occur in women as if all the pelvic organs were prolapsed. Leucorrhoea is profuse, burning, blood-stained and excoriating. Itching and tearing pains in genitals.

Locomotor System

Muscular twitchings, tremors or convulsions, which cease during sleep. Stiffness all over. Rheumatic pains are relieved by movement. Cramp occurs in soles of feet. Weakness, trembling, even paralysis of lower limbs. There is great sensitivity of the spine to touch, associated with paraspinal pain; every movement, every turn of the body causes pain in the spine, but continued movement may afford relief, especially in the sacral region.

Skin

Burning, itching and redness of areas of skin. Scratching of pruritic areas gives some relief, but parts scratched become icy cold and itching spreads to other areas. Fiery chilblains are made worse by heat, especially heat of fire. Miliary eruptions occur, accompanied by intolerable itching and burning. Possible angioneurotic oedema or rosacea.

MODALITIES

Aggravation results from mental exertion; from exposure to cold air; from draughts; from thunder; when walking out of doors; after taking a meal; before the menstrual period; after coitus.

Tends to feel better during the evening and when warm in bed.

CLINICAL NOTES

Indicated in mental retardation of children; convulsions; chorea; epilepsy; delirium tremens. Of value in conditions resulting from any form of excess, drunkenness or debauchery.

Can be considered in relation to nystagmus, facial tic, facial neuralgia, also uterine prolapse.

A special indication is in relation to chilblains in association with Tamus ointment applied locally.

Alumina

SOURCE

This remedy is a preparation of aluminium oxide or corundum, described as a mineral of extreme hardness, occurring in opaque and impure form as emery, and when coloured as ruby, sapphire, topaz, emerald or amethyst.

PHARMACOLOGY

There is affinity with skin and mucous membrane, inducing impaired secretory activity; this results in extreme dryness and a tendency to fissure formation.

There is also affinity with nervous tissue, causing paraesthesia and paresis, notably of involuntary muscle in gut and blood vessels.

PROVING

Alumina was proved by Hahnemann for the second edition of the *Chronic Diseases*.

APPEARANCE

The subject is a spare, dark, tired, tottery individual presenting a dried-up appearance; is almost too weary to talk and makes long pauses before replying to a question.

The voice is husky or aphonic. The nose is apt to be sore and cracked at the tip. Tremors of head and limbs may be evident.

PSYCHOLOGY

A great variety of emotional and mental states may be met with. The mood may be mild and cheerful, peevish and fretful, or sad and constantly moaning.

Complains of a hurried feeling; time passes too slowly.

Feels incapable of coming to a decision or tackling a job.

Unease towards evening, with a feeling as if something untoward is going to happen.

Laughter and tears alternate; weeping often involuntary and without cause.

Subject to sudden urges with shuddering; impulse to kill on sight of knife or other lethal weapon; impulse to suicide but afraid of death.

Sense of duality, as if what he is saying is being spoken by someone else or what he is looking at is seen by another person, not by himself.

Sense of great lassitude; intolerable ennui; entire lack of enthusiasm for any kind of effort; impelling desire to lie down, but recumbency only increases the feeling of fatigue; frequent desire to stretch the limbs when sitting down.

Complains of dazed feeling; makes mistakes in writing and speaking.

Cannot bear the sight of blood or of sharp instruments.

Illusions of largeness, smoothness, numbness.

All mental symptoms are worse in the morning and tend to improve as the day goes on.

PHYSIOLOGY

A chilly person, often of advanced years.

May complain of no appetite, or may have a craving for all sorts of indigestible things – earth, chalk, clay, charcoal, cloves, coffee grounds, tea leaves and such.

Aversion to potatoes and beer; may show intolerance of potatoes, salt, vinegar, onions, tobacco. The least amount of alcohol intoxicates.

Rabid hunger alternates with loathing of all food; everything eaten tastes like straw or wood-shavings.

Sleep very disturbed; keeps waking up; awakes shouting or crying.

Seems unable to perspire.

SYMPTOMATOLOGY

General
Symptoms are often associated with chronic illness. There is extremely easy fatigue, even after a short walk or from the effort of talking. Symptoms may show periodicity; are often left-sided. The body may seem constricted by a tight cord.

Head
Vertigo – objects seem to turn in a circle. There is inability to walk upright in the dark or with eyes closed. Face feels as if 'covered with cobwebs', or as if 'white of egg has dried on the skin'.

Eyes

Eyelids feel dry, burn, smart, stick together on first waking in morning, become thickened. Lachrymation during daytime; chronic conjunctivitis. Ptosis of upper lids; strabismus; diplopia; may result from weakness of eye muscles. A yellow halo is seen round a light. Sensation of 'hairs in front of eyes'. Constant urge to rub the eyes.

Respiratory System

Nasal mucosa is dry and irritable; there is frequent sneezing. Post-nasal drip may be noticed. Loss of sense of smell. Chronic nasal catarrh with headache and thick yellow discharge. Great dryness of throat with constant desire to hawk and clear the throat. Chronic oedema of uvula. Sensation of 'fishbone in throat'. Difficulty in swallowing food. Cough in morning soon after waking. Wheezing or rattling respiration. Condiments induce fit of coughing. Chest feels constricted. Continual dry hacking cough with vomiting and choking.

Alimentary System

Sensation of constriction in oesophagus when swallowing just a morsel of food; passage of food is felt the whole length of the oesophagus. May complain of a crawling sensation at the pit of the stomach or in the rectum, as if from the presence of worms. Lack of rectal urge; is unable to pass stool despite much straining; lack of expulsive power results in great accumulation of faeces and inadequate emptying of colon. Stools are hard, dry, knotty; even a soft stool is passed with difficulty. Stools may be likened to sheep's dung or pipestems, and if soft may adhere to anal margin as passed. Passage of even a soft stool may cause bleeding at anus.

Urinary System

Weakness of muscle of bladder; considerable delay in starting urination; passage of loose stool when urinating; frequency in old age.

Genital System

In male, impotence; prostatic enlargement; prostatorrhoea when straining at stool. In female, menses scanty and pale, like coloured water. Profuse acrid vaginal discharge runs down to heels; relieved by cold bathing.

Nervous System

Impairment of tactile sensation, feels as if 'walking on cushions'. Paretic weakness and feebleness. Positive Romberg Sign. Girdle pains.

Locomotor System
Great heaviness in lower limbs, can hardly drag them along, worse toward evening; staggers and has to sit down. Even when sitting, lower limbs feel excessively weary. Burning pain felt in lumbar region, as if scorched by hot iron. Soles painful when walking.

Skin
Extreme dryness of skin. Absence of sweating. Skin of hands thickened. Formication and burning in back and lower limbs; itching between fingers and between toes. Intolerable itching, worse when warm in bed; scratches till draws blood. Liability to chapped hands; nails become brittle.

MODALITIES

There is aggravation from exposure to cold air, in winter, also in very dry weather. Is worse on alternate days or at certain periods; is worse when sitting still for any length of time; is worse first thing on waking in the morning; worse also at new and full moon.

Amelioration is induced by warmth, by warm food and drink, in warm, wet weather. Feels better when actually eating and, possibly, from a cold bath or cold shower.

CLINICAL NOTES

The action of this remedy is slow in developing.

It is an important remedy in constipation, especially at the extremes of life.

A variety of emotional and mental symptoms call for its consideration.

It is often indicated in old people who have a wrinkled, dried-up appearance.

Associated remedies in paretic conditions are Baryta Carb. and Causticum; in locomotor ataxia, Argentum Nit.; in constipation, Bryonia and Platina.

Ambra Grisea

SOURCE

Ambergris is a curious substance formed in the intestinal tract of the sperm whale. Fresh ambergris is soft in consistency, black in colour, and has an unpleasant odour. Exposed to sun, air and sea water the material hardens, the colour changes to ash grey and it develops a subtle and pleasing fragrance. Pieces of ambergris weighing usually only a few ounces are found on the beaches of a number of eastern countries, also in the Bahamas, Ireland, and other areas washed by tropical seas. The substance is of considerable value, being used commercially as the basis of a large variety of perfumes.

The chemical composition is not fully explored; it contains alkaloids, acids and a fatty element, ambrein.

PHARMACOLOGY

There is a definite affinity with the nervous system, leading to hypersensitivity both physical and psychological.

PROVING

Ambra Grisea was proved by Hahnemann, who reported on it in the sixth volume of the *Materia Medica Pura.*

APPEARANCE

The subject may be emaciated, withered, tremulous. Children appear prematurely old. Speech is flighty; gait is tottering.

PSYCHOLOGY

The subject is shy, blushes easily and shows aversion to strangers.

Violent tempers alternate with depression, even despair. There is a tendency to dwell on disagreeable things.

Is nervy, very easily upset, extremely sensitive to smells and sounds, finds music intolerable.

Becomes embarrassed in company and cannot pass a stool in the presence of other persons.

Sluggish mentally; must read something three or four times and even then cannot grasp the meaning fully. Is dreamy, forgetful, jumps from one topic to another.

May cross the street to avoid meeting people she formerly enjoyed talking to.

Is incredibly timid; may actually weep at the sound of music. Desires solitude.

PHYSIOLOGY

The subject is warm-blooded. Suffers from insomnia due to vexation; may be unable to stay in bed. Sleep is disturbed by hideous imaginations and visions.

Finds relief in cold air, when walking at a slow pace out of doors, from cold food and cold drinks; feels better after a meal.

SYMPTOMATOLOGY

General

Extreme sensitivity is met with, chiefly in children or in subjects enfeebled by old age, overwork or persistent insomnia.

Head

Vertigo may be extreme, forcing the sufferer to sit down or lie down until feeling better. A tearing pain is located in the upper half of the brain. Alopecia may occur.

Eyes

There is a sensation of pressure on the eyes. The lids may itch violently.

Respiratory System

Violent paroxysmal cough is accompanied by belching and huskiness of voice. There is much tickling in throat, larynx and trachea; chest feels oppressed; cough causes dyspnoea. Breathing may be asthmatic. Chokes when hawking up sputum. Cough is often worse on waking in morning.

Alimentary System

Belching is very persistent, accompanied by a cold feeling in the stomach. The belly becomes distended, especially after midnight. Eructations taste acid. Pains in the right hypochondrium are relieved by lying on the painful side. Constipation is associated with frequent but ineffectual urge to stool. The child especially is unable to pass a stool if anybody else is present, even its nurse.

Cardiovascular System
Palpitation is common, associated with hot flushes and a feeling of weight in the chest. There is awareness of throbbing and pulsations in the arteries.

Urinary System
Pain occurs simultaneously in bladder and rectum. Burning sensations are felt at the urethral orifice and anus. Urination is accompanied by burning and itching in the urethra. When not urinating there may be a feeling as if a few drops of urine were being passed. The urine is apt to be turbid and form a brown sediment.

Genital System
There is much itching of the scrotum. External genitalia feel numb. Erections may be violent and unaccompanied by libido. In women a loss of blood per vaginam between periods results from the least upset. Voluptuous itching occurs in the genital region; parts may be sore and swollen. Menses appear too early. Leucorrhoea is thick, mucoid and bluish in colour; it occurs mainly or solely at night.

Locomotor System
Cramps occur in hands and fingers, worse if grasping an object. Part goes numb if pressed on. Lower limbs feel heavy. Cramps may occur in calves at night.

Skin
Itching, soreness or numbness affects different sites.

MODALITIES

Is worse in a warm room, from taking warm drinks, in the presence of other people. Is worse when lying down, on waking from sleep, from reading aloud or talking, when listening to music.

CLINICAL NOTES

The remedy is of special value in excitable, asthenic children and young girls, also in old people with worn-out nerves.

Ammonium Carbonicum

SOURCE

The source of this remedy is ammonium carbonate, an alkaline salt. It is a main ingredient in 'smelling salts', also in 'sal volatile'. It gives off the pungent gas ammonia, NH_3, which is readily soluble in water.

PHARMACOLOGY

There is affinity with the respiratory mucous membrane, inducing acute irritation and profuse mucoid catarrh with resultant dyspnoea, even to the point of asphyxia. In the process of excretion in the form of urea, a diuretic effect is produced.

PROVING

A pathogenesis of Ammonium Carb. appeared in the first edition of Hahnemann's *Chronic Diseases*.

APPEARANCE

Face appears dusky and puffy, possibly with the presence of pimples. Skin looks mottled with a background of pallor, or shows a reddish flush all over.

Looks tired and weary. Tends to be overweight and uncleanly in habits.

Presence of tetters round mouth, often also of cracks at corners of mouth.

PSYCHOLOGY

There is a lack of docility; easily takes offence; of weepy disposition.

Is ill-humoured, especially in humid or stormy weather. May be depressed with a positive loathing of life – absolutely in despair – 'cannot go on like this'.

Is preoccupied with his or her health; is upset by too much talking or listening to other people talking.

PHYSIOLOGY

Is very sensitive to cold air. Has an aversion to water; hates being washed. May have a hot head with cold feet.

May have a voracious hunger yet become satisfied after a few mouthfuls. When feeling ill liable to frequent recourse to the bottle of 'smelling salts'; may also develop an unconquerable desire to eat sugar.

Is constantly drowsy during the day, but tends to be sleepless at night or sleep is disturbed by horrific dreams. May start awake, feeling as if strangled.

SYMPTOMATOLOGY

General

The subject feels weak, tired, asthenic, played out, as if 'bruised all over'. May complain of a sensation of heaviness in various organs. Is easily prostrated by trifles. There is a liability to haemorrhages of dark, almost black, fluid blood that does not clot. States of malignant toxaemia may develop, with grave prostration and extreme weakness. Symptoms tend to be right-sided.

Head

Chronic headache is accompanied by a feeling as if something was trying to burst out of the forehead, by pulsations and sensation of weight; it is worse in the morning. The remedy has been used in the early stages of cerebrospinal fever associated with cyanosis and coldness of the surface of the body.

Eyes

Eyes burn or feel unduly cold and there is aversion to light. May see 'sparks before the eyes'. Blepharitis may occur, with soreness at canthi and tendency to fissures. May be helpful in eyestrain.

Ears

Deafness is described, also itching in the external auditory meatus.

Respiratory System

Chronic coryza is associated with nasal symptoms, e.g. nostrils obstructed at night forcing the subject to sleep with the mouth open; epistaxis on washing face or hands, sometimes after taking a meal; intra-nasal itching, pustules, boils; burning watery catarrh; snuffles of children. Enlarged tonsils are associated with swollen lymph nodes in neck. Burning pain in throat. A tiresome cough is associated with constant tickle in throat, much dryness and a scraped sensation. The remedy to be considered in the presence of gangrenous ulceration of tonsils; also in diphtheria with definite nasal obstruction; laryngitis with hoarseness of voice.

Chest conditions in which the remedy may be indicated are numerous. Emphysema with oppressed breathing, worse after any effort and on entering a warm room or going up even a few steps. An irritating, incessant cough coming on at 3 a.m., associated with blood-streaked sputum, palpitations and prostration. The sputum is raised with difficulty or cannot be raised at all; this condition is aggravated in a warm room, almost to the point of suffocation. Pneumonia is accompanied by extreme prostration. Chronic bronchitis may be associated with pulmonary oedema. Asthma associated with hoarseness. Effects of poisoning by charcoal fumes.

Alimentary System
Mouth and lips tend to be extremely dry and excoriated. Gums are swollen, tender and bleed easily. Pressing teeth firmly together sends shocks through head, eyes and ears. Tongue may show a sore spot in the centre of the upper surface; vesicles occur on tongue associated with a sour, metallic taste. Acrid saliva causes cracks in the lips. The corners of the mouth are sore, cracked and burn. Jaws are apt to crack when chewing. Teeth ache as a result of weather changes or from alteration of mouth temperature.

Raw sensation and burning occur in the oesophagus after eating. There may be complaint of epigastric pain, heartburn, nausea, waterbrash and chilliness. Flatulent dyspepsia is associated with passage of foetid flatus. Stools tend to be hard and knotty and passed with difficulty. The skin round the anus becomes excoriated and pruritic. Haemorrhoids tend to bleed, especially during the menstrual period; protrude after stool; are better when lying down.

Cardiovascular System
Cardiac asthenia is accompanied by a rapid or imperceptible pulse. Dilatation of heart occurs with palpitation and dyspnoea, worse ascending stairs and in warm room. There may be violent audible pulsation, aggravated by the least movement. This may be accompanied by fear, cold sweat, lachrymation, aphonia, noisy respiration, and shaking hands.

21

Urinary System

There is frequency of urge; involuntary urination may occur at night. Urine may be copious, turbid and foetid, possibly containing blood. Uraemia is accompanied by drowsiness, rattling, bubbling respiration, picking at bedclothes, brown, dry tongue.

Genital System

Menstrual periods are early, profuse, especially during the night or when sitting; they tend to be preceded by pain in the teeth, by colic, and accompanied by sensation of tiredness, especially in the thighs. The blood is black with clots. Choleraic diarrhoea may occur on the first day of the period. Exhaustion is severe. Watery leucorrhoea is accompanied by burning and smarting, and associated with excoriation of vulva and pruritus.

Locomotor System

Tearing pains in the joints are relieved by warmth of bed. There is a desire to stretch the limbs. Cramps occur in calves and soles. Bones ache as if breaking. Heels hurt on standing.

Skin

Blisters burn and itch violently. Scarlatiniform rashes or miliary rashes may be present. Boils, pimples, red blotches are accompanied by severe pruritus.

MODALITIES

Is worse in cold or wet humid weather; as a result of washing or taking a bath, during or after a meal. Is worse also during the menstrual period and at about 3 a.m. when wakes in a cold sweat with dyspnoea, thready pulse and pale cold face; the actual respiratory distress is, however, relieved by a supply of cold air.

Is better when the weather is dry and warm; by lying in the prone position or on the side that is painful.

CLINICAL NOTES

The main indications for the remedy are chest conditions and the characteristic type of haemorrhage. It has been used with benefit in scarlet fever accompanied by drowsiness and poorly developed eruption. Erysipelas in the aged, and whitlow, are other mentioned indications. The remedy is incompatible with Lachesis. A frequent complementary remedy is Causticum.

Anacardium Orientale

SOURCE

The source of this remedy is the fruit of *Semecarpus anacardium*, the marking-nut tree. This tree-like shrub is quite lofty, has ash-coloured rough bark, numerous spreading, somewhat hairy branches, and huge oval dark green well-veined leaves on short stalks. The small star-shaped flowers of a dull greenish-yellow hue are found in terminal erect panicles. The fruit is a black, shiny, heart-shaped nut, sitting on a yellow receptacle.

Between the shell and the kernel of the fruit is a layer containing a corrosive resinous juice; this is a pale milky colour when fresh but soon turns black on exposure to air. Hence its use in the East Indies for marking cotton fabrics. It is this layer which is used in the preparation of the mother tincture.

PHARMACOLOGY

There is a marked irritant effect on the skin, similar to that produced by other members of the Sumach family, for instance *Rhus toxicodendron*. The reaction manifests erythema, vesication, oedema accompanied by severe burning and also fever.

An important affinity with the alimentary tract is evidenced by disturbance of gastric secretion and rhythm, and also by a notable feature, namely rectal inertia.

Affinity with the central nervous system results in disturbance of mental poise and impairment of memory. There is also a tendency to motor paralysis and disturbance of respiratory function.

PROVING

Anacardium was proved by Hahnemann, and published in the second edition of *Chronic Diseases*.

APPEARANCE

The patient usually looks tired and bored, with pale visage and dark rings round the eyes. Movements are apt to be clumsy, and behaviour verging on the silly. Eats hurriedly.

PSYCHOLOGY

There is considerable disturbance in this sphere as recorded in the literature. Nevertheless the remedy may be indicated in digestive disturbance apart from the following rather peculiar psychological features.

There may be sudden loss of memory; forgets everything, especially recent events. Loss of self-confidence, especially before an exam or some other ordeal, induces irresolution and a lack of ability to make decisions.

There is a curious condition of moral conflict. An irresistible desire to curse and swear, to do cruel, violent or malicious acts is countered by a conscious compunction to do right.

Strange and fixed ideas may obtrude – 'is two people'; 'no reality in anything'; 'seems in a dream'; 'as if mind and body were separate'; 'someone behind is in pursuit'; and the like. This may produce a state of mind that is suspicious of everyone or always expecting trouble. Is inclined to bluster, but is easily cowed.

An important and characteristic aberration of sensation is a feeling of pressure as if by a plug almost anywhere in the body, or else as if constricted by a hoop round limb or trunk. Other senses also may be disturbed; smells filth where none is present; hears voices in the distance.

There is a tendency to laugh when he ought to be serious and to remain solemn when others are laughing – the death's head at the feast. Depression may lead to the urge to suicide by shooting.

PHYSIOLOGY

Feels the cold excessively; with fever complains of an icy coldness creeping over the body.

Appetite is impaired; all food tastes insipid.

Thirst is constant, but may complain of a feeling of suffocation when drinking.

Drowsy during the day; at night sleep is disturbed by vivid dreams – of fire, dead bodies, steep places and so on, so that he wakes unrefreshed.

May sweat, especially in the evening and when sitting still, on head, belly and back. Night sweats occur.

SYMPTOMATOLOGY
General
Pains are made worse by movement and are better when at rest, but legs tend to become fidgety when sitting still for long. Pains may remit for a

few days, then return. Undue fatigue ensues on even slight exertion, accompanied by weakness and trembling in the limbs. The pains are pressive or plug-like. Symptoms tend to start on the right and spread to the left.

Head

Mental fatigue causes a confused type of headache, possibly associated with attacks of giddiness. It is aggravated by movement, especially by bending the head backwards, but taking food affords definite relief.

Eyes

Vision may be blurred. Muscae volitantes may be troublesome. A plug sensation is felt in the orbit. Mydriasis may be noticed in the left eye.

Respiratory System

Coryza with much sneezing and lachrymation is apt to become chronic. The sense of smell is interfered with, being either over-acute or perhaps lost. Olfactory illusions may be complained of, and may be persistent. A violent paroxysmal cough occurs, accompanied by a tickle and choking sensation in the throat and an oppressed feeling in the chest. The cough is aggravated by talking; taking food may either aggravate or alleviate the cough.

Alimentary System

This is, perhaps, the sphere of the remedy's special usefulness. The tongue feels swollen; is white and rough. Food tastes offensive. There is an unpleasant taste in the mouth apart from taking food. Is apt to gulp his food and fluids despite a tendency to choking, possibly as a result of so doing. May feel nauseated in the morning. Pain is felt in the stomach when the organ is empty, hunger pain – eating gives relief but the pain returns two to three hours later and persists till further food is taken. Warm food is preferred for relief. If cold drinks are taken to relieve thirst the pain is aggravated. There is a violent urge to stool, but when the attempt is made to defaecate the desire passes and the stool is retained. The rectum seems inert and feels 'plugged'. The expulsive power of the bowel is inadequate, even a soft stool is only passed with great difficulty. Piles, pruritus, perianal eczema, anal fissure may be present. All the alimentary symptoms are aggravated by emotional tension or upset.

Cardiovascular System

Palpitation accompanies quite slight ailments in old people, and is often associated with coryza. The remedy may be called for in rheumatic pericarditis characterized by sharp stitches coming on in pairs, one soon after the other, and then a long interval before the next pair.

Urinary System

There is frequency and urgency of urination, and nocturia.

Locomotor System

Cramps occur in calves when walking, also sometimes at night. Any part of the body which is left immobile for long tends to become numb – 'go to sleep'. Stitches and plug sensations are noticed in the pectoral region; these are worse when walking and better when resting. There may be seeming paresis of single parts. The knees especially are likely to be affected, feel as if bandaged tightly and so weak as to make walking difficult.

Skin

Among skin affections are described psychogenic eczema; pustular eruptions; intolerable itching; much burning; a vesicular rash of small pock-like blisters, which discharge yellowish serum and form crusts. There is a liability to warts, especially on the palms.

MODALITIES

There is aggravation from cold and cold draughts, from exertion, when the stomach is empty, from mental effort, from hot applications, and in the morning.

Feels better when at rest, in the evening and especially while eating. This last modality – relief from taking food – is a paramount indication for the selection of this remedy.

CLINICAL NOTES

Of value in peptic ulcer. Follows well after Lycopodium or Pulsatilla.

Antimonium Crudum

SOURCE

The remedy is prepared from black sulphide of antimony, a natural product occurring in the shape of black parallel needles having a metallic lustre; the ore contains twenty-eight parts of sulphur with one hundred parts of antimony.

PHARMACOLOGY

There is affinity with mucous membrane, especially that of the alimentary tract, giving rise to irritation; also with the skin, inducing the formation of pustular eruptions and hyperkeratotic lesions.

PROVING

The earliest pathogenesis of Antimonium Crudum was published in the *Arzneimittellehre* of Hartlaub and Trinks, and this formed a basis for the one published in the second edition of Hahnemann's *Chronic Diseases*.

APPEARANCE

Children have red cheeks, often chapped. Eyelids appear red and sore.
 There is a tendency to stoutness, possibly with dependent oedema.
 Cracks and ulceration may be present at the corners of the mouth and the naso-labial commissure.
 The skin is often scaly and rough with horny patches; nails tend to split.

PSYCHOLOGY

Children are averse to being touched, looked at or questioned.
 The subject is usually peevish, sulky and responds with anger to proffered kindness.
 Sadness is extreme to the point of loathing of life, frequent tears and absence of any desire to live. This may produce an impulse to suicide by drowning or by shooting.

There may be an irresistible desire to talk in rhyme or repeat verse. Mental symptoms are aggravated in moonlight.

Illness may derive from disappointed affection.

PHYSIOLOGY

The subject is chilly, extremely sensitive to cold, to breathing cold air or contact with cold water.

Appetite varies. There may be a greedy desire for pickles and acid things; or complete anorexia with a loathing for all food. There is intolerance for pork, pastry and bread, which give rise to nausea. Becomes very thirsty in the evening.

Copious, exhausting sweats follow quite slight exertion and also occur at night.

Drowsiness is a feature, especially in the forenoon.

SYMPTOMATOLOGY

General

Complaints are liable to be induced by cold bathing or by immersion in cold water. The stomach seems to take part in all complaints. Symptoms change from side to side with a preponderance on the left; or they move from one site to another. In fever there is chill without thirst, followed by hot spells accompanied by thirst and sweating. Debility and exhaustion are prominent features, especially in hot weather.

Head

Headache often accompanies other complaints; may result from river bathing, from stomach upset, from indulgence in alcohol, from taking a chill. The scalp may be itchy; alopecia may be evident.

Eyes

The eyes become sore, especially at the lateral canthus; are extremely sensitive to any bright glare. Itching may be intense, with inflamed lids which agglutinate at night.

Ears

Digging and shooting pains may be felt in the ears with heat and redness. Deafness may be present as if the ears were swathed in a bandage. Tinnitus may be constant with buzzing and roaring.

Respiratory System
The nose becomes blocked at night or on entering a hot room. The nostrils are apt to be sore, cracked and crusted.

Cough is associated with stitches, burning and oppression in chest, back and shoulder regions. The cough is peculiar: the first bout extremely severe, succeeding paroxysms diminishing in severity with each bout. The cough is liable to come on if entering a warm room.

Alimentary System
The lips are dry and cracked. A milky white coating covers the tongue on its upper surface, but the edges are sore and red. Gums are retracted and bleed easily. Toothache in a hollow tooth extends to the head; it is worse at night and aggravated by contact with cold water, by impact of the tongue and after eating. It is often better when walking in the open. Gastric symptoms are prominent. There is much nausea with retching, gagging and vomiting of food ingested. The stomach feels full all the time. There is a constant discharge of wind both upwards and downwards; no relief, however, is obtained from vomiting or the passage of flatus. Violent pains are felt in the abdomen with burning and great distension. The liver may be involved, with considerable pain in the organ with or without accompanying jaundice. Watery diarrhoea occurs, with undigested food particles in the stool; this condition is aggravated by becoming overheated, by taking vinegar or acids; it is also made worse by cold bathing and is especially troublesome at night and in the early morning. Diarrhoea alternates with constipation, when the stool is hard and only passed with great difficulty. The stool may be partly solid and partly fluid. Passage of stool is followed by tenesmus. Piles burn and protrude; they are aggravated by cold bathing, by taking sour food or wine. Smarting, pressure and throbbing are felt in the anal region.

Urinary System
Frequency may be accompanied by strangury and urethral discharge. Enuresis is apt to occur on coughing.

Genital System
There may be impairment of sexual function with atrophy of testes. Uterine prolapse is associated with a constant bearing down sensation, as if the organ was being extruded from the vagina. Ovarian tenderness is felt. Vaginal discharge is watery in type, with the presence of solid lumps; it may be associated with smarting down the thighs.

Locomotor System

Rheumatic pains are felt in muscles and joints, especially the finger joints. Gouty nodosities are common. Contractures may be present. There is much restless unease of the limbs due to tension and twitching of muscles anywhere in the body. Characteristic of the remedy is extreme tenderness of the soles of the feet and the heels, which makes walking painful; the feet also are often icy cold.

Skin

Bluish spots may be seen on thighs and shins. Fingernails become brittle, turn black and tend to split easily. Corns, very tender callosities, horny excrescences may develop; the latter if beneath the nail are very painful. Warts occur, especially on the hands. Pimples, pustules, furuncles, intertrigo may occur. There may be much itching in neck, chest, back and limbs. Prickly heat may be present, made worse by exercise, warmth and wine; better by rest and in cool air.

MODALITIES

Symptoms are aggravated by heat, but the patient is very sensitive to cold. Worse for cold bathing. Worse at night. Mental symptoms aggravated by moonlight. Worse for touch.

Better for rest, and lying down.

CLINICAL NOTES

The remedy is called for most frequently at the extremes of life. It can be given for prolonged periods in low potency, e.g. in relation to corns or callosities.

Antimonium Tartaricum

SOURCE

This remedy is prepared from tartar emetic, antimony-potassium tartrate, which may be in the form of a white powder or else colourless, transparent crystals. Much used formerly as an emetic it carried serious risks, being a highly poisonous substance when absorbed into the body. Its use medicinally was revived early in the present century for the treatment of kala-azar, the debilitating and often fatal disease associated with infection by the Protozoan *Leishmania donovani*. Intravenous injection of the drug produces severe vomiting; treatment had to be protracted. Other and less nauseating antimony preparations are now available.

The substance has been used for homicidal purposes, though much less frequently than arsenic. It produces symptoms very similar to those resulting from arsenic poisoning, but the symptoms are more rapid in onset and more grave in effect.

PHARMACOLOGY

The salt has affinity with a variety of tissues and organs, notably mucous membranes, leading to irritation and increased secretory activity. This is manifested in such conditions as gastro-enteritis and bronchial catarrh. Fatty degenerative changes are produced in the myocardium, liver and kidneys. The latter organs and the skin are also affected as the poison is being eliminated. A more direct action on the skin causes an erythema with formation of a papular or pustular eruption. An effect on the central nervous system is to produce profound depression of mind and impaired vitality of medullary centres.

The symptoms of acute poisoning are instructive. On swallowing a dose there is an immediate onset of symptoms – a metallic taste in the mouth, burning in throat and stomach, violent and incessant vomiting, severe purging and tenesmus. Profound depression follows with vertigo, extreme thirst, subnormal temperature, thready pulse, cyanosis, cramps, coma, collapse, and death in twelve to twenty-four hours. The skin is cold and covered in clammy sweat.

Chronic poisoning is characterized by anorexia, nausea, vomiting, diarrhoea, emaciation and great depression, associated with headache, giddiness, mental confusion, dimness of vision and drowsiness. Finally extreme exhaustion ends in death.

PROVING

Tartar emetic has no place in any of our classical collections of pathogenesy, but provings of it have been made from time to time, from Hahnemann onwards. These are collected, together with numerous poisonings, in the article on it in Allen's *Encyclopaedia*.

APPEARANCE

The seriously ill patient looks almost moribund. Cheeks are pale or cyanosed, there are dark rings round the sunken eyes. The nose looks pinched, with actively dilating nostrils; lips and nails are blue, or lips are pale and shrivelled.

There is a cold sweat on the forehead; hands and feet are cold as ice. There is constant twitching of the facial muscles and tremors are present, affecting head and hands.

Respiration is distressed with gasping and bubbling, and the sufferer is obliged to sit up in order to breathe. The child exhibits much pitiful whining and crying, associated with moaning respiration.

A horrible pungent odour is present in the sickroom – the smell of death.

PSYCHOLOGY

The child shows a great aversion to being touched or looked at, but likes to be carried and clings to those around.

The adult manifests irritability, restlessness, anxiety, does not want to be meddled with or bothered; everything is a burden. There is often a despair of recovery such as is met with under Arsenicum Alb., Natrum Sulph. and Psorinum.

PHYSIOLOGY

The Antimonium Tart. patient feels chilly but is averse to a stuffy hot atmosphere or to being too heavily wrapped up. This is especially so when there is much respiratory distress, accompanied by a desire for cool air and for the windows to be thrown wide open.

There may be a craving for apples, as also for acid drinks, which tend to disagree. There is aversion to and, indeed, intolerance of milk, which incites nausea and vomiting. In association with nausea there is often a deadly loathing of all forms of food.

Thirst may be conspicuously absent or, on the other hand, intense for sour drinks. These have to be swallowed in sips, as fluids are apt to be vomited soon after ingestion. The unthirsty patient will show annoyance when offered a drink, probably because of the fear of fresh vomiting.

Drowsiness is very pronounced, especially after a bout of vomiting. The child on waking seems stupid. The drowsiness may alternate with giddiness.

Cold sweats occur in association with pallor and prostration.

SYMPTOMATOLOGY

General

There is no sudden violent onset as is characteristic of Aconite, Belladonna and Ipecacuanha, but a gradual subsiding into a state of poor reactivity and prostration. There is only low fever, with general hypotonus, chilliness and cold sweats. Mucous membranes tend to become ulcerated, with resulting haemorrhage from nose or stomach. Jerkings, tremblings accompany great weariness, weakness and lassitude; there may be a generalized soreness and tenderness all over the body.

Head

A variety of stitches, shooting and other pains have been noted in the head, but the most characteristic condition is one of dullness, confusion and bewilderment accompanied by the drowsiness mentioned above.

Eyes

Eyes feel fatigued, bruised; wants to keep lids firmly closed. The eye symptoms accompanying measles, scarlet fever, smallpox and other exanthemata may call for this remedy.

Respiratory System

Fluent nasal catarrh is often accompanied by ulceration and uncontrollable epistaxis. Every change to wet weather tends to bring on a fresh catarrh of throat, and involve larynx, trachea and lungs. There is a great accumulation of mucus in the air passages, but cough is weak and feeble, and tends to be worse at 4 a.m. There is great difficulty in raising the sputum which is thick, ropy, white in colour and as sticky as glue. Respiration is consequently noisy with coarse rattling and bubbling. The cough is made worse by anger or annoyance. This is especially so in children, and eating also tends to aggravate the cough. The remedy may be called for in whooping-cough. It should also be considered when repeated attacks of bronchitis occur in children; no sooner is the child over one chesty cold than another is contracted, with the rattling respiration and concomitant weakness and debility. The remedy is of value in relation to pneumonia associated with hepatic congestion and jaundice, meteorism, nausea and vomiting, such as occurs in alcoholics. A further indication is in connection with recurrent attacks of bronchitis in old people, with much thick white phlegm, great dyspnoea, driving from bed or causing the sufferer to sit up and ask to be fanned. Asthma also may require this remedy, when there is aggravation at 3 a.m., causing the patient to sit up, with much wheezing, rattling and cyanosis. On falling asleep severe dyspnoea brings on fresh distress.

Alimentary System
Copious saliva accumulates in the mouth. The tongue may be heavily coated with white fur or streaked with red. Nausea is severe and very persistent, accompanied by great anxiety, much yawning, cold sweat on brow, prostration and trembling; it is, however, relieved by vomiting. There is much uneasy vomiting, gagging and retching, associated with tremors of hands and drowsiness. It may lead to actual fainting, and is sometimes eased by lying on the right side. Eructations taste like rotten eggs. The vomitus is watery, contains green bile, food and much slimy, ropy mucus. Gastric symptoms are accompanied by superficial tenderness in the epigastrium. There may be a sensation as if the 'belly was full of stones', which is aggravated while sitting and on stooping. Sometimes there is a complaint of an indescribable sinking feeling in the stomach. Sharp, cutting, colicky pains are associated with thin, slimy, offensive, grass-green stools. Combined vomiting and purging may induce a state of collapse suggestive of Veratrum Alb. With Antimonium Tart. there is more drowsiness, whereas with Veratrum Alb. there is more cold sweat on the forehead and the whole body is of marble coldness.

Cardiovascular System
General hypotonus may give rise to palpitations, often with a complaint of a warm or hot feeling in the heart region. Circulatory weakness may result in oedema.

Urinary System
A variety of bladder symptoms are described, among them burning in the urethra during and after urination; some blood may be passed in the

urine at end of the act, accompanied by violent pain in the bladder. Nocturnal frequency may occur, with burning thirst and scanty urine.

Locomotor System
Violent pain may occur in the lumbosacral region, and the slightest effort to move will cause retching and the outbreak of a cold, clammy sweat. A dragging, downward sensation may be felt, as of a heavy weight in the coccyx. Gouty infiltration and dropsical swellings of joints are associated with this remedy.

Skin
Pustular eruptions occur, tending to leave a bluish-red mark when healed. The remedy may be called for in impetigo or smallpox, also in chickenpox if the pustules are large and severe.

MODALITIES

Aggravation results from exposure to damp cold and from change in the weather, also from bathing in cold water. There is aggravation from lying down and in the evening.

Relief is obtained from cool air, by sitting erect, by belching, and by bringing up phlegm.

CLINICAL NOTES

The remedy is not usually indicated at the start of an illness but rather when weakness and lack of reactivity have supervened, unless the sufferer is already in a debilitated condition before the more obvious illness sets in.

It is of special value in both acute and chronic chest conditions, as described above. In chronic bronchitic patients the 6c potency can be given daily for considerable periods.

It is useful in relation to the ill effects of vaccination when Thuja has not given relief.

It is indicated in children suffering from suppressed eruptions, especially when there are associated head symptoms and dyspnoea in a desperately ill child.

It may be needed in sequence to Ipecacuanha in chest complaints in children.

Baryta Carb. is complementary to the remedy, notably in old people who have difficulty in raising sputum.

A rash resulting from Antimonium Tart. can be antidoted with Conium.

Apis Mellifica

The honey bee is the source of this remedy, the whole insect being used in the preparation of the mother tincture. It is interesting that in connection with suggested prophylactic desensitization for bee-keepers it is recommended that 'whole-insect extracts be used rather than venom-sac contents, since the antigen causing reactions is present throughout the insect's body'.

An enormous amount of brilliant observational research has been carried out in relation to the behaviour and life story of this fascinating insect and provider of natural food for man and animal, not to mention the African honey bird. Many of the features brought to light have most interesting correspondences with the mentality and the reactions of the Apis patient.

The honey bee is a highly sensitive creature, as witness its unerring sense of direction from and back to the hive in quest of nectar. It is also violently reactive, as witness the phenomenon of swarming and also the fury of onslaught en masse if interfered with or annoyed. It well behoves the honey-bear of Ceylon to protect itself with its long-haired thick fur. Moreover marauding wasps or robber bees from other hives, if they dare to intrude at the hive entrance, are summarily seized and executed on the spot by the worker bees on guard duty.

The bee is a restless being; it flits from place to place, never staying too long with one flower. The dreams of provers are said to be 'full of flying activities, of travelling from place to place, of taking great leaps, and also of business affairs, of care and toil'.

Again, the bee takes great care not to be overheated, using an ingenious system of bringing droplets of water to the top of the hive, where a group of worker bees are fanning ceaselessly with their wings to evaporate the water, thus cooling the air when it becomes too warm. Sensitivity to heat in any form is a most prominent feature of the Apis picture.

It has been shown that 'each individual in the hive goes through a number of functions in invariable sequence during its life, the functions being parallel to the phases of bodily development. The first day to the third is passed cleaning comb cells; the third to the fifth days feeding the riper larvae with pollen and honey brought in by the other bees; the sixth until the tenth days providing younger larvae with the 'milk' poured out from the salivary glands (which in the worker bee develop amazingly just at this time); the tenth to the eighteenth days taking over the pollen brought in by collectors, stamping it into the honeycomb, building up the comb and cleaning the hive. Then follow the carrying away of waste material and, from the eighteenth to the twentieth days, patrol service performed near the entrance. Finally from the twentieth day the collection of pollen and nectar begins, necessitating long journeys to visit flowers, an activity which continues until the last day of life.'

The above is quoted at some length because of the significance of the fact that all this amazing, necessary and efficiently performed activity is not the result of teaching, instruction, suggestion or compulsion by order and command. It is spontaneous and unquestioning, and not under any kind of voluntary control.

Such activities provide a most interesting analogy with allergic phenomena, reactions arising from inherent or acquired sensitivities, which are spontaneous and by no means under voluntary control.

PHARMACOLOGY

The chemical composition of bee venom remains obscure, although various fractions, such as histamine, hyaluronidase and a bradykinin have been identified. Bee venom is known to have haemolytic, haemorrhagic and neurotoxic effects in addition to its profound histamine activity.

In addition to haemolysis, coagulation of fibrinogen and increased permeability of capillaries, there is also a lowering of surface tension and membrane potential, which results in reduction of osmotic pressure and facilitates diffusion of fluids. All this adds up to oedema and effusion, the central effect of Apis, the key to the understanding of most of the symptoms and modalities associated with the drug.

The symptoms produced by bee venom are both local and systemic. The local reaction is the triple response of redness, flare and weal. In addition there is stinging and burning, great sensitivity to touch. The part feels enlarged, as if it would burst. Alternatively the sensation may be described as one of constriction, and a bruised soreness is noticed.

The systemic reactions are of varied intensity and consist of urticaria, oedema, constriction of the chest, wheezing and gastrointestinal upsets; also dyspnoea, dysphagia, hoarseness, confusion and a feeling of impending disaster. The most severe reaction is evidenced by collapse, cyanosis, hypotension, incontinence and unconsciousness.

It has been pointed out that the field of action of Apis as a drug is related to the great cavity system of the body, including also pathological cavities such as cysts, and particularly the enormous network of cavities, the interstitial or intracellular spaces spread throughout the body. Indeed, a slide of oedematous tissue, viewed through the microscope, reveals a network of cellules filled with fluid, having a marked resemblance to the honeycomb of the bee.

The regulation of disturbed distribution of fluid, from the ventricles of the brain to the intercellular space, appears to be the basis of the therapeutic function of the life-force pent up in *Apis mellifica.*

PROVING

Apis has been proved, both as a trituration of the whole bee, and as a solution of its venom, by the Central New York State Homoeopathic Society, and the results were published in its *Transactions.*

APPEARANCE

The face is red, of a rosy or livid hue, different from the blazing bright red visage of Belladonna.

Irregular raised patches appear in the skin, weals which come and go, and which are either erythematous or show a definite pallor owing to compression of the local blood vessels by the oedema.

A puffy oedema may be observed, especially affecting the face, ears, lips, tongue, throat, scrotum and anus. The oedema is of the soft type, pitting on pressure.

Restlessness is usually very obvious, with constant fidgets; also the gait is awkward and there is a tendency to clumsiness and to dropping plates and dishes.

Tremulousness may be present, or muscular twitching and jerking, especially affecting the right side. Stiffness of movement of the lower jaw and difficulty in protruding the tongue may be noticed, as also snapping of the teeth, perhaps in protest at the tight feeling in the jaws.

With intracranial involvement there is likely to be rolling of the head from side to side in sleep, whining and whimpering or a sudden loud cry or scream, either when asleep or on waking.

Other signs which may be present are squint, dorsiflexion of big toe, stiffening of the whole body if touched, and a pulse which intermits.

PSYCHOLOGY

The Apis sufferer is tearful, fearful, fidgety, suspicious, jealous, joyless; desires company but not affection; when disturbed becomes full of obdurate rage.

There is emotional instability and unpredictability, a tendency to flit from one idea to another, a liability to causeless tears or ill-timed laughter (breaks the crockery and thinks it a great joke).

Fear is prominent – fear of 'having a stroke', fear that 'something will burst' when coughing or straining. There may be a feeling of imminent dissolution – distinct from an actual fear of death, such as is associated with Aconite or Arsenicum Alb.

There is hypersensitivity to the least contact and aversion to any kind of constriction. The whole body or single parts may feel swollen or bruised, or a sensation of internal trembling may be experienced.

Complaints calling for Apis may be induced by emotional upset or stress.

PHYSIOLOGY

In fevers the Apis chill is prominent at 3 p.m.; this contrasts with the Natrum Mur. chill, which occurs at 10 a.m. The Apis chill seems to start in the belly, hands, chest or knees, but even during the chill there is a desire for cool air.

There may be a desire for milk. Thirst is surprisingly absent in the hot stage of fevers but is present during the cold stage. Thirst is absent also in the presence of dropsy; the oedematous patient being internally drowned in his own fluids has his reflex thirst stimulus inhibited.

Drowsiness, progressing to stupor or semi-coma may occur. The patient may utter cries during sleep and push off the bedcovers in search of coolness. Insomnia may occur from worrying thoughts or cerebral excitement.

Sweats affect chiefly the head region. The sweats may have a musk-like odour.

SYMPTOMATOLOGY

General

Complaints tend to start on the right side and spread to the left, as is also the case with Lycopodium. The illness is violent in onset and gets rapidly worse. Pains are stinging, burning, shooting and tend to shift and wander from one site to another. They may be described as if 'pierced by red hot needles', a symptom shared by Arsenicum Alb. Widespread swellings may occur, inflammatory and rosy or oedematous with a pale waxy look or a transparent appearance of the skin, possibly with a slight icteric tinge. The swelling is associated with a feeling of tension and stiffness. Sudden serous effusions may occur into joint or serous cavities, accompanying, for instance, meningitis, pleuritis, pericarditis or peritonitis. This remedy lacks the immobility and aggravation by movement associated with Bryonia, another remedy often called for in serous effusions. Apis may be indicated in severe adynamic illness such as malignant scarlet fever, diphtheria and typhoid.

Head Region
There may be sudden onset of stupor or coma as the result of acute mental shock, or in relation to a suppressed eruption in connection with measles or other exanthem. Vertigo is worse when lying down and closing the eyes, and is better when walking about. With headache, the head feels on fire, swollen and throbbing, and the least jolt or jar is resented. It is worse in a warm room and there is a desire to have the head uncovered. A muzzy dull type of headache is noted also, relieved somewhat by pressure of the hands. Acute hydrocephalus is an indication for Apis and here it vies with Helleborus. The latter remedy exhibits a more stuporous picture, however. There may be a complaint of shooting pains in orbits, cheeks and chin.

Eyes
Acute swelling of the lids is apt to be accompanied by intense chemosis, much photophobia and scalding lachrymation. The lids smart and burn. Puffy swellings like 'bags of water' form below the eyes. Bathing the eyes in cold water affords some relief. The remedy has also been used in chronic eye troubles such as trachoma, ectropion, and kerato-iritis. Eye symptoms are aggravated when looking at a fire or at white surfaces, such as snow. The remedy might well be of service in snow-blindness with its picture of intense pain, lachrymation, photophobia and oedema of the lids. A similar condition, of course, may arise from exposure of the eyes to ultraviolet light in arc-welders and electricians.

Respiratory System
Violent sneezing is associated with acute blockage of air passages and only scanty discharge. The nose feels numb or stinging and the tip of the nose is cold. Throat symptoms are important. The pharynx acquires a mottled, glossy or varnished look and swallowing causes pain in the ears. Acute oedema of the throat may occur, the uvula looking like a bag of

jelly, and oedema may extend to the glottis; this produces a choking feeling, and makes swallowing even a sip of water almost impossible. The sufferer cannot stand anything tight around the neck. Ulceration may ensue, perhaps with a dirty grey or 'wash-leather' type of exudation on the fauces, such as may be present in diphtheria or scarlet fever. A chest symptom is a sense of oppression or constriction, as if 'would suffocate', and this is much worse in a warm room. Respiration may be panting in type, with a feeling as if every breath would be the last. The distress is made worse by leaning either forwards or backwards. Voice tends to be hoarse, rough, husky. Sputum is scanty and must be swallowed.

Alimentary System
There is a burning and stinging sensation in the mouth, which feels 'scalded'. Clusters of blisters may be formed on the back of the tongue. Acute glossitis may occur with sudden, rapid and alarming swelling of the tongue. A similar process may involve one or both lips. Acute inflammatory conditions in the abdomen may be present; the belly is tense, swollen, sensitive to touch and sore with burning pains; it hurts to sneeze. Diarrhoea accompanies low debilitated states, such as occur with fevers, and a stool is passed with every movement owing to a patulous anus, which becomes sore and raw. Watery, yellow or green stools which smell like carrion may be passed, worse in the morning. Painful prolapsed piles are relieved by bathing in cold water.

Cardiovascular System
Sudden pain is described below the heart, extending to the right. Palpitations occur with great irregularity of pulse and, possibly, dropped beats. The remedy may be called for in pericarditis with effusion, possibly associated also with hydrothorax. The sufferer cannot lie down, the chest feels constricted, there is a dry cough, suffocative dyspnoea and a feeling of imminent death.

Lymphatic and Glandular Systems
Thyroid dysfunction may occur associated with ovarian trouble. Acute mastitis presents a picture of erysipeloid inflammation with burning and stinging pains.

Genital System
Ovarian lesions occur, mostly on the right side, associated with much soreness in the right groin. The remedy has been found of service in relation to cystic ovarian disease accompanied by burning and stinging

pains, numbness down the thigh and over the right side of the trunk, and a feeling of constriction in the chest with a reflex type of cough, deriving from pelvic irritation.

Urinary System

Urination is scalding and urgent – can scarcely retain the urine for a single moment. This is very similar to the Cantharis picture, but in the latter the symptoms and burning are even more violent. Urinary incontinence in old men may also call for Apis. The remedy may be indicated in nephritis with scanty urine, albuminuria, tubular casts and, possibly, anasarca with puffy eyelids, general soreness, burning pains and probably marked absence of thirst. Oedema of scrotum is probably also present. The absence of thirst helps to distinguish the picture from that of Arsenicum Alb., another valuable remedy in nephritis.

Locomotor System

Stiffness and stitching pains affect the nape of the neck and are also felt deep to the shoulder-blades. The whole dorsum may feel tired and bruised, with a tendency to hot flushes alternating with shuddering. Acute synovitis may occur in joints, which become swollen with a wax-like appearance and feel as if 'stretched tight'. Pains occur in the limbs with much pricking and burning. Hands and feet feel swollen, numb, woolly and tremulous. Toes are red and burning, despite the fact that the feet are cold. Apis is indicated in paronychia when the pains are stinging and burning and relief is obtained from cold water.

Skin

Fulminating urticaria is associated with intolerable itching and burning and great sensitivity to touch. Even the hair is hypersensitive. Necrotic lesions may occur, boils, carbuncles, cellulitis, erysipelas with gangrene in spots. Erysipelas on the face is apt to start below the right eye and spread to the left, the affected part rapidly becoming oedematous. There are burning, stinging pains, high fever, and the initial pink colour changes to purple.

MODALITIES

Heat in any form, heat of fire, heat of hot stuffy room, hot bath, local application, causes severe aggravation. This is an important difference from Rhus Tox., with its definite amelioration from warmth. Aggravation is also caused by getting wet, by touch or pressure, when lying down.

Symptoms are worse about 5 p.m., during the night and after sleep.

Relief is obtained from contact with cool air, in the open air, by cool applications, and to some extent by uncovering, by change of position, by sitting up or walking about. Movement, of course, improves the circulation and aids the resorption of fluids.

CLINICAL NOTES

Apis is a remedy for acute exacerbations of chronic toxic conditions. It will clear up the acute outbreak but not prevent recurrences. For this the exhibition of a more deeply-acting remedy will be necessary, such as Natrum Mur., Pulsatilla or Tuberculinum. Incidentally, the preparation of Tuberculinum (Marmorek or Tuberculum Koch) should not be given too early after the acute episode and should usually be preceded by Natrum Mur. or Pulsatilla.

Experience has shown that Apis is contraindicated in direct sequence to Rhus Tox. It is said to follow well after Arsenicum Alb.

A special indication will be sickness resulting from the suppression, or delay in appearance, of the rash in one or other of the exanthemata.

Apis may be called for in severe adynamic conditions associated with such illnesses as scarlet fever, diphtheria and typhoid fever.

Warning is given that Apis in low potency or in frequent doses should be avoided in the early months of pregnancy, on account of a risk of abortion.

In acute conditions response to the drug may be expected within an hour or two. Otherwise Apis is somewhat slow in action, and a switch to another remedy must not be made too hurriedly. The favourable action of the remedy is first shown by a greatly increased flow of pale urine.

Argentum Nitricum

SOURCE

This remedy is prepared from silver nitrate, known in medieval times to the alchemists as Lunar Caustic. It forms flat transparent rhombic crystals which turn grey or greyish black on exposure to light. The crystals are odourless but have a bitter metallic taste. Organic matter, for instance the skin, is stained black by contact with the crystals.

The molten substance, when cooled to 71°C, suddenly solidifies with such violent expansile force as to burst a test tube.

PHARMACOLOGY

The salt is highly soluble in water. In strong solution it is astringent or actually caustic; it is described as a powerful disinfectant from its action in coagulating the proteins of bacteria.

In relation to the tissues of the body, it is an irritant poison with a special affinity for mucous membranes, causing violent inflammation; for red blood corpuscles, leading to haemolysis and ecchymosis; and for the nervous system, giving rise to cramps, convulsions, loss of peripheral sensation, and paralysis.

PROVING

Silver nitrate only obtained a few symptoms in Hahnemann's hands, the 15th potency being employed. But it has received an extensive proving from Dr J. O. Müller of Vienna, the record of which was published in the second volume of the *Oesterreichische Zeitschrift*, and may be read in Hempel's translation of Stapf's *Beiträge*.

APPEARANCE

The physical features associated with the remedy are less important than the mental and emotional factors.

A typical appearance is described as one of malnutrition, with sunken facies. There is a prematurely old, withered, weak and tremulous look, seen perhaps especially in children.

Blue lips, cold, blue hands, forearms, feet and legs may be seen in women during menstruation.

Discoloration of the skin of grey-blue, violet or bronze hue may occur. The discoloured skin is tense and hard in texture.

PSYCHOLOGY

The Argentum Nit. subject lives in a state of perpetual agitation, always feeling driven, never having enough time for what he wants to do or feels he ought to get done, wanting to have a job finished almost as soon as it is begun, darting off with unnecessary precipitation to carry out an assignment, and generating an atmosphere of turbulence, tiring and exasperating to his entourage whether at home or at work.

If any kind of ordeal is coming up, this agitation is intensified into a peculiar type of fear, namely apprehension ante. It is really an apprehension of what may happen – fear lest he miss the train; fear lest the guests do not arrive on time for the dinner party; fear lest he forget his lines on the stage; fear lest memory fails at a viva voce examination; fear of what the physician may reveal, or may conceal, if he goes to see the doctor; and other such possibilities of embarrassment.

This peculiar apprehensiveness finds expression in other ways. There is a fear of crowds, lest one be crushed or trampled on; a fear of certain places such as streets or high buildings, lest 'the corners of houses will bump into one' or 'the high building will topple over onto one'; a fear of heights both when looking up and when looking down, lest someone fall from a high window or a girder high up in space, or lest one be impelled by a sudden urge to jump over a cliff or off a bridge.

Water draws, and a bridge with low parapets, or a wharf side is avoided sedulously. The reaction to heights is often accompanied by giddiness and even by a loss of muscle tone, so that the knees give way and the subject finds himself on all fours.

Claustrophobia is also a prominent feature, with resulting feeling of panic if shut in a telephone booth or caught in a tube train which has stuck in between stations, and a general objection to being confined in close quarters.

The hurried, restless feeling often impels its victim to walk and walk and walk, until becoming quite tired out. Moreover there is a liability to irrational behaviour; does strange things or comes to odd conclusions, and is harassed by a constant flow of troublesome thoughts. All this is further evidence of the deep-seated agitation and apprehension.

PHYSIOLOGY

As to food and drink, there is a great desire for sweets, which tend to disagree (infants at the breast develop diarrhoea if the mother eats a lot of sweets). There is also a craving for salt, and a fondness for icecream and cold drinks. Considerable thirst may be associated with dryness of the mouth.

Nervous insomnia is frequent, and sleep is disturbed by horrible dreams, often of violence in some form or other. He feels chilly in bed when lightly covered, yet smothered when heavily covered. On waking up the limbs are apt to feel 'bruised'.

There is a liability to sudden profuse nervous sweats.

SYMPTOMATOLOGY

General

A peculiar symptom met with under this remedy is a distressing sensation of expansion, expressed in various ways – as if 'squeezed in a vice', as if 'constricted by an iron band round chest or waist', or as if the part affected is 'blown up', 'too big', 'going to burst'. A prominent feature is extreme fatigue ensuing on quite mild exertion, accompanied by a sensation of great weariness in the lower limbs. Emotional distress or over-exertion mentally is apt to result in widespread disorder affecting digestion, circulation and other functions, and possibly resulting in a state of chronic psychosomiasis as evidenced by palpitations, pulsations, paraesthesias, and tremor. Pains are sharp or splinter-like, come and go slowly, and are often left-sided. Discharges tend to be thick and muco-purulent. Ulcers tend to bleed. Haemorrhage may occur from various sites such as nose, lungs, uterus.

Head Region

Giddiness is a very prominent symptom, especially when looking up at or down from a height, or when over water. The vertigo tends to be accompanied both by trembling of the limbs and tinnitus in the ears. Headache may be hemilateral, of throbbing type and aggravated by warmth. Concomitants may be a feeling as if the head is 'expanded', or seems 'too large'. Contact with cool air and tight bandaging afford relief. Facial neuralgia occurs, affecting especially the areas supplied by the intra-orbital and mandibular nerves, and often accompanied by a sour taste in the mouth.

Eyes

Eye symptoms are various and tend to be severe – photophobia, purulent conjunctivitis, chemosis, adherent lids on waking in the morning, corneal ulceration, ophthalmia neonatorum. The eye symptoms are worse in a warm room or from the heat of a fire, but alleviated by cold bathing or in cool air.

Respiratory System

Rhinitis is associated with severe itching in the nose and an irresistible desire to rub the nose till the nostrils become raw and sore. It may proceed to ulceration with purulent, blood-streaked discharge. The throat is especially vulnerable, becoming sore and raw, even ulcerated. The fauces and uvula are injected and dark red. There is complaint of a sticking sensation in the throat, or of 'the presence of a splinter or a hair lodged there'; the larynx feels 'clogged'. Cold fluids are desired, a point of distinction from Hepar Sulph., with which remedy there is a preference for warm fluids. Burning and heaviness may be complained of in the chest, or painful cramp-like pains in the thoracic muscles. Nervous asthma may be brought on by being in a stuffy room or in a crowd.

Alimentary System

The tip of the tongue may be markedly red and also sore. Gums become tender and bleed easily but are not swollen. Nausea is relieved by taking a good meal. Belching is violent but ineffective. Food is vomited in mouthfuls. Haematemesis may occur, with 'coffee-grounds' vomit. Pain or distress felt in the epigastrium is apt to come on soon after meals and be accompanied by flatulence with excessive distension, not relieved either by belching or by passing flatus. Both procedures are violent and noisy. The remedy has proved useful in alcoholic gastritis. Diarrhoea occurs with noisy, spluttery stools, characteristically green in colour and very offensive. The stools may be dysenteric and contain membraneous casts or shreds. The condition is likely to be precipitated by eating sweets or drinking even small amounts of water. Nervous diarrhoea may occur before an ordeal of some sort or from emotional stress.

Cardiovascular System

Anginal pain may be felt around the heart, accompanied by intense dyspnoea. Violent palpitation may be brought on by quite slight mental exertion or by sudden muscular effort. This tends to be worse in the afternoon and better when walking out of doors. This is just the reverse of the anginal pain of Arsenicum, which is brought on by walking even on the level. There is inability to lie on the right side in bed, as this position induces fresh palpitations and pulsations, which drive the sufferer from bed.

Urinary System
Dysuria is quite severe, with pain and scalding both during and after urination. Urine tends to be scanty in association with gastro-intestinal affections and profuse in nervous disorders, with frequent passage of pale urine or even incontinence. The remedy may be called for in relation to urethral discharge or in the presence of haematuria.

Genital System
An indication here is very severe dysmenorrhoea, associated with copious yellow corroding vaginal discharge and bleeding from the cervix. Ovarian pain associated with feeling of being blown up on the affected side. Painful inflammatory conditions of external genitalia are accompanied by the sensation of 'sticks' or 'slivers' in the parts affected.

Locomotor System
Rending, shooting pains are described in the limbs, and a tendency to stagger in the dark or when the eyes are closed. Hands tremble and legs are weak, with a bruised feeling in the calves. Pain in the lumbar region is worse when sitting, and especially in the act of rising from the sitting position, but is relieved by standing or walking. Pains may be felt in and around the joints, particularly the smaller joints.

Skin
There is hypersensitivity of the skin, but at the same time a loss of acute discrimination of sensations, which produces a feeling of numbness. Dermatitis is specially liable to occur on the neck and at the hair margins, as is the case with Natrum Mur. There is erythema with burning, itching and a tendency to pustule formation.

MODALITIES

There is aggravation from warmth in any form, and a craving for cold air. The Argentum Nit. subject wants the doors and windows open, suffocates in a stuffy room, wants his head in a cool place, loves to be out in a wind and to be lightly clad. Further aggravating factors are sugar or cold food, the menstrual period, both before and at the time, any unusual mental effort or emotional stress and, chronologically, at night and on waking up in the morning.

Relief is experienced from cold, in the fresh air, and also from pressure on the affected part.

CLINICAL NOTES

The remedy is of special value to those who do a lot of active brainwork, to artistes, and nervous people of the type described above.

It is to be considered in connection with the luetic diathesis ('constitution fluorique' of Vannier). Thuja is a complementary remedy in affections of the genito-urinary tract and nervous system, and Lycopodium in digestive troubles.

Ill effects of the use of silver nitrate can be antidoted by Natrum Mur.

It is said to be of value in epilepsy when the attack is preceded for hours or days by dilatation of the pupils, and when the attack is followed by great restlessness and tremors of the hands; also if the attack is induced by a fright or associated with the onset of the menstrual period.

Arnica Montana

SOURCE

Arnica montana is a member of the vast Compositae family. It is known as Leopard's bane, fall herb, Panacea Lapsorum. Its value in relation to wounds was known to the Greeks and Romans. Mountain dwellers especially appreciated its value in this respect. It was reported of the dwellers in the Andes that it was customary in the event of an accident to gather the herb, which grows conveniently at high altitudes, pour on boiling water and give the resulting infusion to drink to the injured person.

Its bright yellow flowers make it conspicuous; the ligulate florets, notched at the tip, are in such untidy disarray as to give the impression that the head of the plant had been bashed, perhaps by the mountain gusts. The stem is a foot high or somewhat less, with twin ovate opposite leaves; it springs at the base from a rosette of dark green leaves, the reverse side of which are of lighter colour. The root is woody, with a number of small radicles; when macerated it has a peculiar odour like apples, and an astringent taste.

The mother tincture is prepared from root, flowers and leaves after removal of the larvae of the Arnica fly, which are commonly found on the plant.

Although recognized primarily as the remedy par excellence in wounds and injuries, Arnica has also been proved in the accepted manner and has its own materia medica picture.

PHARMACOLOGY

There is a marked affinity with blood vessels, leading to dilatation, then stasis and finally increased permeability. As a result of these changes purpura and various types of haemorrhage can ensue. Alterations in tone of the walls of blood vessels may produce either pallor or flushing.

Involvement of the alimentary system induces nausea, vomiting, diarrhoea or dysentery. Action on the central nervous system gives rise to agitation, prostration, visual disturbance, tremors or even convulsions.

Affinity with muscle tissue causes over-contraction and hypertrophy, e.g. enlarged heart. A further effect is to produce myalgia with a bruised sensation and tenderness, the result of localized hyperaemia. A local action on the skin is to cause severe irritation and eruptions which are erysipeloid, vesicular or pustular in type.

PROVING

Arnica was proved by Hahnemann, and is described in the first volume of *Materia Medica Pura*.

APPEARANCE

Both pallor and flushing are described. A peculiar feature is a hot head and face associated with a cold nose and body; or the upper part of the body is hot and the lower part cold.

Mottled areas like bruises may be observed in various sites.

Backward jerking of the head may be present. There is constant turning and twisting in bed; this is not due to restlessness, but to the odd and characteristic sensation that the bed is distressingly hard and full of lumps.

PSYCHOLOGY

The patient is morose, wants to be left alone and in peace, is unwilling even to be spoken to. Pain is intolerable and there is great fear of being touched or even approached.

There is inability to concentrate and aversion to any kind of effort, even talking. Normal self-confidence is lost.

Forgetfulness is frequent; he has to go back and see if he has turned off the gas. Is easily startled. May develop a horror of imminent death.

Characteristic is a curious mental attitude when seriously ill – says, 'I'm all right. Why bother to get the doctor?'

A French physician describes the Arnica subject thus: 'Over-excitable, laughs without cause, when told something disagreeable gets mad and shouts at the top of her voice. Capricious; wants a whole lot of things and then has no use for them. Quarrelsome, up against the whole world. He wants to know better than everybody; no one can take him up; is disdainful and imperious. Worried about the present and the future; in despair; becomes indifferent towards everything, lazy, averse to and incapable of all forms of work; extremely opinionated and obstinate. Foolishly gay, fickle, mischievous.'

Altogether quite a mixture, with ill-humour predominating. Agoraphobia is also mentioned.

PHYSIOLOGY

There is a general hypersensitivity to heat and cold, not to mention touch.

Appetite is variable. There may be a loathing of food, with definite distaste for meat, broth, milk.

Anorexia may be present, or easy repletion. Canine hunger is recorded. As also desire for vinegar, for alcohol.

Thirst again may be excessive, especially for cold water, or may be absent altogether.

Sleep may be delayed till 2 or 3 a.m., and then liable to being disturbed by anxious or horrific dreams. Drowsiness during the day is accompanied by much yawning.

SYMPTOMATOLOGY

General

Feels bruised all over, as if suffering from multiple blows or knocks. Moreover, the bruised sensation is accompanied by great exhaustion and weariness. There is widespread hypersensitivity and soreness, also throbbing and burning with muscular twitchings. The condition is aggravated by any sudden movement or jolt. Haemorrhages from various surfaces are of dark venous blood; spontaneous bruising and purpura are characteristic. Sepsis may be a feature, especially of the putrid variety. Stuporous states occur, with incontinence of urine.

Head

Whirling giddiness occurs chiefly on rising after sleep, on moving the head or when walking. It may be accompanied by nausea; there is a tendency to fall to the left; it is worse on closing the eyes. Headache can be severe, as if the head was being distended from within or as if a nail was being driven into the skull; it is often unilateral, worse in the morning, and accompanied by fibrillary twitching of facial muscles. A neuralgic type headache is aggravated by the least movement of the head.

Eyes
Eye symptoms relating to the remedy are subconjunctival or retinal haemorrhage; diplopia following injury; conjunctivitis with burning tears; eye strain from watching television or over-use in other ways.

Ears
Shooting pains occur in and around the ears. Deafness and buzzings after a blow.

Respiratory System
Much tingling inside the nose may precede nosebleed. Epistaxis may follow injury, or occur during whooping cough or in association with typhus fever. Stitches in the chest are felt, especially on the left side, and are aggravated by respiratory movements and by coughing. A dry tickly cough is accompanied by blood-stained sputum; it is worse in the morning. In whooping cough the child cries before the paroxysm.

Alimentary System
Lips may be chapped with a sensation of burning heat. There is a foul taste in the mouth and foetor oris. Tongue shows a slimy yellow coating. Eructations have the odour of rotten eggs. Salivation is excessive. Dysphagia is associated with nausea, possibly with empty retching and gagging. Epigastric pain and pressive discomfort extends to the back. Vomit may contain dark coagulated blood. Cutting or colicky pains occur in the abdomen. Flatulence with odour of rotten eggs. Diarrhoea is associated with tenesmus, offensive brown or blood-stained stools, possibly involuntary; has to lie down after every stool. Dysenteric symptoms are accompanied by ischuria; there is a considerable interval between stools. A 'typhoid state' may supervene with foul eructations, tympanites, tender belly, decubitus as if moribund, horribly offensive stools, often passed in sleep, melaena.

Cardiovascular System
Cardiac pain as if the heart was being squeezed. Heart action becomes irregular and feeble. Palpitation occurs at night.

Urinary System
Dysuria is caused by spasm of sphincter at base of bladder. There is frequency of urge and delay in starting the act. Nocturnal enuresis may occur during sleep. Actual retention of urine may occur after exertion. Haematuria may be present.

Genital System

Severe soreness in the uterine region may prevent the patient from walking in the erect position. During pregnancy foetal movements are especially painful at night and interfere with sleep. The menopause is associated with great fatigue and extreme asthenia, palpitations, heat of head, coldness of body and bruising on least contact.

Locomotor System

A curious symptom is a deathly coldness of the forearm. Pain in muscles is accompanied by a bruised feeling; it may result from over-use or unusual use, or from exposure to cold and wet; it is aggravated by any movement. The pains are sharp and shoot down the limb. Feet or hands may become swollen and feel sore and bruised. The wrist or the hip hurts as if dislocated. Limbs feel very heavy as if from fatigue. Spinal hyperaesthesia is accompanied by sudden spasms in the neck and the paraspinal muscles. Muscular weakness may affect grip and gait.

Skin

Various lesions may be met with: eczematous, pustular, papular, psoriatic, or ulcerative such as bedsores. These eruptions are apt to show a symmetrical distribution. Important are successive crops of small, extremely painful boils.

MODALITIES

Is worse in damp cold weather; from exposure to hot sun; from movement and any exertion; from least contact; from wine.

There is amelioration when lying down with the head low (although the bed still feels hard).

CLINICAL NOTES

The uses to which this remedy can be put are multiple. Paramount, of course, is its unique and outstanding value in relation to every variety of wound or injury. Not only does it aid in the arrest of bleeding and promotion of healing, but it is also of value in allaying shock and counteracting the emotional trauma associated with the injury.

It has a limited use as an external application in contusive types of injury where the skin is not broken. For this purpose a lotion is prepared of five or ten drops of the mother tincture, or preferably of the 1c potency, to a pint of water or weak alcohol. Contact with the skin should not be prolonged beyond twenty-four hours lest an erythematous eruption be caused.

The remedy should be given before and after dental or surgical operations. It is also of value for the effects of a remote injury.

It is of special value in cases of concussion with or without fracture of the skull, in muscle trauma resulting from sudden strain, in all cases of fractures to reduce swelling and allay pain.

It is a remedy for persistent tiredness, whether physical or psychological. It is called for in cerebral haemorrhage, gout with fear of being approached, and after childbirth.

Arsenicum Album

SOURCE

The background of this remedy is a remarkable one. It illustrates in a striking manner the homoeopathic contention that what a drug can cause in the way of symptoms it can also cure, when used as a therapeutic agent in suitable doses. Put succinctly in this particular instance it is a case of 'the killer cures'.

Arsenicum Alb., arsenious oxide, has a galaxy of cures to its credit, but this harmless-looking, tasteless, colourless, white powder possesses a most sinister background of lethality. For decade after decade white arsenic held the pre-eminent role as the first choice of the homicidal poisoner.

In the fifteenth and sixteenth centuries those 'Olympic' poisoners, the Borgia family, made full use of arsenic in their cantarella, acqua di Napoli and other subtle poisons that could kill quickly or by slow degrees, as seemed most expedient. There was no Marsh Test to detect the presence of arsenic, and the victims appeared, as far as symptoms went, to have died of natural causes. Such was at any rate claimed to be the case.

A famous vendor of poisons in the seventeenth century was La Tofania, who distributed her 'Acqua Tofa'na' to 'distressed, adulterous, neglected or jealous wives over wellnigh all Europe. Apparently her poison was merely crystallized arsenic compounded, for no apparent reason, with the herb cymbalaria.' She was executed at the age of 70. 'After La Tofania's death fewer husbands died suddenly in Italy.'

So common was death by poisoning in the glamorous era of Louis XIV, Le Roi Soleil, that the period was known as the Age of Arsenic.

The popularity of arsenic as a convenient and not too readily suspected poison extends into the present century. Sir Sydney Smith records that murder by poisoning was very common in Egypt, where he was Principal Medicolegal Expert to the Ministry of Justice from 1927 onwards. He states, 'I do not think there was a day during my eleven years in Cairo in which no case of arsenic poisoning was under examination in my laboratories.'

A twentieth-century epidemic of poisoning took place in a district in

Hungary enclosed in a loop of the river Tisza. An old witch-like woman, known as Auntie Fazekas, dispensed doses of what she called the 'water of inheritance' for a charge of 80 pengo. She did a steady trade in these fatal doses for about twenty years until in 1929 the authorities took belated action. A sample batch of fifty bodies were exhumed, of which no less than forty-six were found to contain arsenic. Her brew was made by stewing a few pennyworth of arsenical fly-papers.

In *Strong Poison* by Dorothy Sayers, that master of meticulous detail, there is an excellent description of acute arsenic poisoning in the opening chapters. The plot centres round the fact that a dose of arsenic which can be swallowed by an arsenic habitué with impunity will be lethal for an unprotected individual.

Arsenic does in fact provide a striking example of the phenomenon of acquired drug tolerance. Small doses of the substance administered to horses will encourage a sleek glossy coat. Small doses are given to turkeys as an aid to breeding and to combat turkey disease. The birds become immune to the poison but their flesh, if eaten inadvertently, might prove deadly.

The term poison is a relative one. The degree of toxicity will depend on several factors – the size of the dose, the form in which it is administered, the portal of entry into the body, and of special significance, the susceptibility or otherwise of the dosee.

Schenk, in his book on poisons, records – 'I have seen and spoken to many arsenic eaters in Styria, Lower Austria and Carinthia. Woodcutters, hunters and mountain guides in these districts believe that arsenic makes the breathing easier and the step more certain. I myself saw a porter in Deutsch-Landsberg at the foot of the Kor Alp consume a lump of arsenic the size of a pea. I estimated it at almost half a gramme – four times the fatal dose.'

It is obvious, therefore, that in Arsenicum Alb. we are dealing with a drug of no mean potentialities.

PHARMACOLOGY

Cases of both acute and chronic arsenic poisoning provide a wealth of information on the tissue affinities of the drug and the symptoms it is capable of causing. These are very varied and only too easily apt to be ascribed to 'natural causes'.

In acute poisoning the main symptoms are a burning sensation in the mouth, followed in about half an hour by nausea, faintness, burning in the throat, severe pain in the stomach, increased by pressure, shortly accompanied by frightful retching, vomiting, diarrhoea and tenesmus. Dehydration and cramps with collapse ensue and death occurs in some six to twelve hours. A picture of acute gastroenteritis, with involvement of the vasomotor system resulting in rapid exhaustion, anoxia, and collapse.

In chronic poisoning, which may be homicidal with sub-lethal doses, or accidental, even perhaps iatrogenic, the symptoms are multiple and reveal a variety of affinities with different tissues, notably mucosa, skin and appendages, peripheral nerves, and bone marrow.

The oral, nasal and pharyngeal mucosa becomes progressively dry and unusually red in colour. Constant thirst is an accompaniment.

The eyes become red and injected, smart and burn, and the eyelids show oedematous swelling. Dimness of vision is complained of.

Both acute and chronic gastro-intestinal symptoms occur, leading to confusion in diagnosis.

Neuralgias occur in various sites and tend to be persistent. Peripheral neuritis may result in the onset of paraesthesias or localized paresis.

Very occasionally the skin may be clear and transparent-looking. More usually it acquires a dry, dirty appearance with associated pigmentation and keratosis, the latter change especially affecting palms and soles.

There is a great liability to urticaria with long weals which itch and burn unbearably. Later actual eczema may supervene. Hair and nails become brittle and may be shed.

Progressive loss of weight, malnutrition and anaemia lead to cachexia and myocardial degeneration. Finally death ensues, being ascribed to progressive ill-health, probably accompanied by gastrointestinal disorder.

This sequence of pathological events may result from one large (but not at the time lethal) dose or, what is more likely, from oft-repeated smaller doses.

PROVING

Hahnemann published provings of Arsenic in the second volume of *Materia Medica Pura*, and in the second edition of *Chronic Diseases*.

APPEARANCE

Typically the Arsenicum individual is spare, stylish, neat and well-groomed, possibly of rather sallow complexion.

There is a general air of tension, unease and restlessness – the restlessness of the hard-pressed executive rather than the fidgetiness of the dilettante, suggesting Phosphorus.

The Arsenicum patient makes quick movements, walks across the floor rapidly and takes a quick look round the room; on sitting down seems fidgety, does not wait calmly to be questioned but starts straight in to relate his tale of symptoms.

The countenance appears lined and drawn. Skin and mucosa look shrivelled and dry. Face and hands look skinny. Expression is anxious, worried, perhaps even terrified. The physical restlessness is obvious, even in grave illness with marked prostration.

The picture may be one of collapse with pale, cold, clammy skin and a pervading cadaveric odour. Discharges are acrid with an offensive putrid smell.

Puffy oedema may be noticed affecting the lower eyelid or the limbs.

Speech is apt to be rapid and precipitate, with special emphasis on accuracy and detail.

PSYCHOLOGY

The Arsenicum subject is restless in mind as well as in body, unduly anxious and worried about many things, sure there is something definitely, even seriously, wrong.

May be rather hopeless and despairing about the situation. Doubtful if there is much point in relating the symptoms as it will not be possible for anything to be done.

Is excessively tidy to the point of tiresomeness, fastidious, fussy, addicted to fads.

Is extremely sensitive to circumstances and immediate surroundings, irritated beyond measure by slackness or idleness on the part of others, given to alternations between hilarity and despair. Oversensitive to pain, noise and odours, especially the smell of food. Severe pain may cause fainting.

Fear is a prominent and important feature. Apt to be full of apprehension and dread, gets all worked up if anything goes wrong or simply over fear that something will go wrong; especially liable to panic at night.

There may be a sudden wave of fear, especially when alone, fear of death, or fear of being alone, especially in the dark; may search the house for robbers. Fear too, possibly, of doing hurt to someone, especially if a knife or other weapon is lying handy.

Despair of recovery may result in actual fear of certainty of death, so that both medicine and food are refused – 'What's the use anyway?'

All this fear, horror and apprehension tends to get worse in the evening as darkness comes on.

Causeless fear of impending evil may be associated with utter weariness of life, accompanied by suicidal feelings.

Features mentioned by a French author are – critical of everything and discusses the faults of others; scruples of conscience, feels he has offended everyone; goes round asking everybody's pardon; subject to sharp regrets and bitter remorse; likes to cause suffering both to people and to animals.

May see ghosts both by day and at night. May complain of a feeling as if the bed was turning over and tipping him onto the floor. May have delusions of vermin.

PHYSIOLOGY

Inadequacy of the cutaneous circulation and irregular distribution of blood-flow produce an extremely chilly individual, sitting over the fire in the winter, wanting to be well wrapped up, subject to ice-cold waves which surge through the body and give place to sensations of burning heat from scalp to soles.

Appetite is often poor with desire for fat, vinegar and pickles, but aversion to fat is just as likely. May go off all food.

Thirst is characteristic, with a desire for frequent sips of water rather than a long drink. Keeps water by the bedside at night. Prefers warm or hot drinks. Children may not be thirsty at all. In fever may develop an unquenchable thirst for quite large quantities during the sweating stage, or in states of severe dehydration.

With regard to sleep, although drowsy by day is apt to be extremely restless at night, being driven from bed to get up and wander about, make a cup of tea and so on, perhaps several times during the night. Dreams are often terrifying.

Apt to wake about 1 a.m., thirsty, agitated, with fear of death, and possibly sweating. May sleep with hands raised above the head.

SYMPTOMATOLOGY

General

Certain general features should be noted. Pains are characteristically burning, whether in stomach, bladder, vagina, lungs – 'as if coals of fire were burning one's vitals'. Or the pains may be described as like 'hot needles or hot wires piercing the flesh'. Typical is the rapid onset of grave prostration, seemingly quite out of proportion to the rest of the symptoms, or even without any very apparent cause at all. Secretions and excretions tend to be excoriating, causing burning and redness, with an offensive odour of putrefaction and decomposition. There is a tendency to the development of gangrene in inflammatory conditions or erysipelas of severe type. Inflammations are of sudden onset, violent and prostrating in nature. Periodicity of symptoms is an important feature, with a tendency to recurrence at the same time each day, at intervals of one, two or more weeks, or at the same season of the year. There is a liability to haemorrhage with easy bleeding from any surface, but especially from mucous membranes. The blood tends to be black and offensive. Serous or synovial effusions may occur, or oedema may develop in various sites. Symptoms tend to be right-sided.

Head

There are two main types of headache associated with Arsenicum Alb. One is a periodic congestive headache of migraine type, accompanied by throbbing, burning, anxiety and restlessness, and also possibly by severe nausea, retching, and vomiting. It is aggravated by light, noise and movement, and there is a desire to lie quietly in a dark room, with the head raised on pillows, and for cool air and cool applications. The headache may be unilateral, or there may be a dreadful pain in the occipital region which makes the sufferer feel dazed or stunned. These headaches are apt to occur soon after midnight, or be triggered off by excitement, over-anxiety, over-exertion, or by becoming over-heated when walking. They may come on in the afternoon, get gradually worse and last all night. The pain is paroxysmal. Prostration is marked. Pallor is usual. The other type of headache is a neuralgia of the frontal or supra-orbital region. It is associated with extreme sensitivity of the scalp – a comb or hairbrush seems to penetrate to the surface of the brain – possibly a sensation as if 'the brain flaps against the inside of the skull when walking'. This type of headache is aggravated by cold and relieved by warmth.

Eyes

Symptoms for which Arsenicum may be needed are acute conjunctivitis with swelling of the lids, excoriating sanious discharge, and much redness of the canthi with burning sensation. There is bag-like swelling of the lids or below the eyes (in contrast to Kali Carb. with bag-like swelling above the eyes). Pain in the eyes on first opening the lids after sleep, aggravated by turning the eyes to one side or the other; severe photophobia; corneal ulcer; these also are mentioned under this remedy.

Respiratory System

There are a number of conditions in which this remedy may be curative. Acute coryza, as in hay fever, with paroxysms of violent sneezing and profuse watery discharge which is excoriating to nostrils and upper lip. Old chronic nasal catarrhs, with a tendency to constantly take fresh colds of acute type with rapid spread to throat and larynx, accompanied by hoarseness and burning pain, which is increased by drinking cold fluids and relieved by taking something warm. The catarrh may spread downwards and cause a dry cough, aggravated by either eating or drinking and worse out of doors. There may be a suffocative cough at night with wheezing respiration and much frothy white sputum. In asthmatic attacks Arsenicum may also be curative, especially when the attack occurs soon after midnight and causes the sufferer to sit bolt upright in bed or even get out of bed and walk about in search of relief. The asthma is liable to be of psychogenic type, attacks often being precipitated by some emotional stress, such as hearing bad news over the phone. Other chest indications are stabbing pain like hot needles in the upper third of the right lung, gangrenous pneumonitis with haemoptysis, and horribly offensive prune juice sputum containing clots.

Alimentary System

As would be expected there are many indications for the remedy. Ulcerative stomatitis with easily bleeding gums. Blue discoloration of gums. Acute gastritis, everything taken being vomited immediately, even water. A sip of hot water may be retained for a minute or two, but cold fluids are returned promptly. (By comparison with Phosphorus, when cold fluids are desired but are vomited as soon as warmed up in the stomach.) With the Arsenicum gastritis there is burning in the oesophagus, whether swallowing or regurgitating. The stomach is extremely sensitive and the least touch is resented. Local heat is comforting. Enteritis is associated with tympanites, great tenderness to touch, marked restlessness with endless tossing till too exhausted to move. Stools are dysenteric, blood-stained, watery, colour of prune juice, smelling like putrefying flesh. Every stool burns like fire in the rectum, and there is in fact burning throughout the whole length of the bowel. Despite the burnings the pain is ameliorated by warmth and the application of external heat. It is, however, aggravated by the least amount of food or drink, from taking a deep breath, and from least touch or pressure on the belly wall. A very similar state of affairs is recorded under Secale, but this is distinguished by a desire for ice-cold drinks, wanting to be uncovered, preferring a cool room and open windows, and relief from cold water sponging. Vomiting and diarrhoea may occur together, with the typical pallor, restlessness, prostration and cadaveric odour, fearful anxiety and expectancy of death. Other conditions to note are piles which protrude like grapes, burn like fire, are hot, dry and bleeding; anal fissure; pruritic eczema around the anus.

Cardiovascular System
The remedy may be called for in relation to heart failure associated with great weakness and prostration, a very irregular pulse, and relief by sitting bolt upright. Palpitation may occur on least exertion. The remedy is especially effective when agonizing precordial pain occurs while walking, even on the level. A curious symptom is a sensation as if 'waves of ice cold blood or of boiling water, were flowing through the vessels.

Urinary System
Acute nephritis with suppression of urine, possibly resulting from excessive loss of fluids by vomiting and purging, may respond to the remedy. It has also proved effective in chronic renal disease when orthodox remedies have failed.

Genital System
The remedy is called for in acute inflammation of the external genitalia associated with oedema, erythema of erysipeloid type, and much burning, smarting and stinging. It is also related to vaginitis with a whitish, thin, watery discharge which excoriates the skin and is so profuse as to run down the thighs. The remedy has been found palliative in connection with carcinoma of uterus and also of breast.

Nervous System
Neuritic symptoms are met with, burning neuralgic pains with numbness and tingling – fingers feel 'like sausages' – also localized pareses with resulting disability. The remedy may be considered in connection with chorea, also with epilepsy.

Locomotor System
There are a great many indications for this remedy. It may be of use when there is a complaint of severe drawing pain in the back between the shoulder-blades, relieved by lying down. Also when great unease in the lower limbs prevents sleep, impossible to lie still or get comfortable at night in bed.

Skin
Eruptions of various types may call for the remedy, especially if accompanied by much burning and itching with desire to scratch, but scratching only makes matters worse – psoriasis, urticaria, herpes, and other scaly dermatoses.

Ulcers that burn, become necrotic and tend to spread in all directions, and exude very offensive discharges.

Itching and burning of the skin; after rubbing the itching is relieved but the burning remains.

MODALITIES

Cold in any form aggravates, cold air, cold food, cold fluids, as do also alcohol, the least draught and wet weather. An important chronological aggravation occurs at or after midnight up to 2 or 3 a.m.

Relief is obtained by warmth, local heat, warm or hot drinks; by sitting bolt upright, standing erect; by movement; after sweating.

CLINICAL NOTES

This is a very widely used remedy. The characteristic physical and psychological features and the modalities are the chief guides to its selection.

It is said to be incompatible in sequence with Pulsatilla. Complementary remedies are Carbo Veg. and Phosphorus, notable respectively for states of collapse and prostration.

Arum Triphyllum

SOURCE

This plant, Indian turnip, is the American variety. It is similar in most respects to the plant found in Britain, *Arum maculatum*, a plant which by reason of its astonishing appearance is the proud possessor of no less than sixty local names.

It is a plant possessing remarkable characteristics. For the first four or five years of growth only leaves are produced, rising from the root, a thick white tuber which when fresh has a very acrid juice.

One year a larger bud arises in the axil of a leaf to form the flower spike. The leaves have long thick stalks and are pointed with a broad notched base suggestive of a barbed arrow head. The colour is dark green, often spotted with purple or black blotches.

The flowers are highly specialized. Some two months after the appearance of the leaves in February, a light green pointed tip is seen emerging from the centre of the plant. This forms a long narrow olive green cone rather like a dunce's cap. Later the upper part unfurls to form the spathe, and reveals a short central poker-like rod backed by the hood-like spathe. This erect rod is sometimes purple and sometimes yellow. The unusual appearance of the plant at this stage gives rise to such names as Lords and Ladies, Jack-in-the-Pulpit, Wake Robin and so on.

The flowers are arranged around the lower part of this stem or spadix, and enclosed at first in the unopened lower portion of the spathe. This forms a trap to enclose certain insects which are attracted by the scent emitted by the spadix and enter the trap to feed on the nectar of the flowers. Later the insects escape when the hairs at the entrance of the trap lose water, shrink and wither. In doing so they become loaded with pollen and carry this into their next port of call, thus effecting cross pollination.

This ingenious procedure works like clockwork and is completed in less than twenty-four hours. Later the spathe shrivels and withers, leaving the lower end of the spadix exposed bearing a cluster of shiny bright red berries.

The plant favours moist shady localities and soils rich in bases, slightly alkaline and containing plenty of calcium and phosphorus. The root or corm, the part used in the preparation of the mother tincture, contains calcium oxalate, starch, fat, mucilage and an acrid volatile substance.

PHARMACOLOGY

This is a definitely poisonous plant. Henslow records, 'All parts of the plant are poisonous; the leaves when bruised exhale an unpleasant odour; the fruit also contains needle-like crystals of calcium oxalate.'

Quelch says, 'The bright green leaves of this little plant are to be seen in most hedges in the spring. Those leaves are often spotted and are easily recognized by their strange, halberd-like shape. The berries, first green and later red, last long after the leaves have died. The berries are very poisonous.'

Cornevin (1893) says, 'The fruits which are berry-like and of a fine red colour have poisoned children who have eaten them, despite the unpleasant odour they give out on crushing. If the quantity is sufficient to cause death, there appear terrible stomach pains, cramps, severe diarrhoea, together with a burning sensation at the back of the mouth. Death follows in ten to twenty hours after eating the fruit.'

Quelch mentions three children who having eaten some of the berries 'were seized with horrible convulsions, their throats becoming so swollen that they were unable to swallow anything. Two of them quickly died, while the third was saved with great difficulty.'

Gerrard (1597) writes, 'The most pure and white starch is made from the roots of Cuckow-pint; but most hurtful to the hands of the Laundresses that hath the handling of it, for it choppeth, blistereth, and maketh hands rough and rugged and withal smarting.' This was obviously due to the presence of the fine needle-like crystals of calcium oxalate in the starch powder.

A case of poisoning from eating the root was reported from Italy in 1860. A child of three complained of burning pains in the mouth and lips immediately after eating. Three hours later it was in a state of profound torpor, to which a violent febrile reaction succeeded. Later the child became quite prostrate, unable to speak, raising its hands frequently to its mouth and throat, uttering at intervals a sharp cry, and starting up as if suffocated. The caustic action of the plant had extended to the lips, the palate, the tongue and the tonsils.

A case of 'accidental proving' occurred in 1913. Dr O. Schlegel of Stuttgart, walking in the woods with his father, came across a plant they could not identify. His father bade him pluck a leaf, bite off a portion, chew it well, and then spit it out. This he did.

Within a very short time he noticed an unusual burning and pricking on the tongue, which soon disappeared. A few days later he was overtaken by an unwelcome drowsiness and listlessness, and found his temperature was 38°C. He spent a day in bed, mouth being very dry and amount of urine passed very scanty.

After this the dryness in mouth and throat increased, was not relieved by a swallow of water, and was associated with much swelling of cervical lymph nodes. The gums and lining of mouth and throat looked red and inflamed and 'quite spotted', especially on the gums.

A red eruption then spread over arms and entire chest, giving a picture resembling scarlet fever. The painful dryness of mouth and throat caused much distress and finally broke out in painful sores. After eight days he began to feel better, and gradually the listlessness and tired feeling cleared up.

He had been back at work for several days when he woke one morning with an unusual sensation on the tongue, which felt like a piece of wood and seemed entirely too big to its very root. It was sensitive, tight, and practically immovable. The sublingual gland was swollen, and on raising the tip of the tongue expelled a double gush of milky fluid.

From the foregoing it is clear that the plant contains a powerful irritant poison capable of acting on a variety of tissues. It appears to possess an alkaloid similar to coniine but less potent, also a saponin (arin), traces of HCN, and crystals, as mentioned before, of calcium oxalate.

The main tissue affinity of the plant is, therefore, with mucous membrane, especially that of the mouth and upper respiratory tract, inducing a very violent reaction evidenced by pricking and burning, acute redness and swelling, and acrid discharges.

There is also a tendency for involvement of lymph nodes, resulting in acute swelling. Furthermore an irritant effect on the central nervous system finds expression in twitchings, cramps, convulsions and stupor.

PROVING

Arum Triphyllum was proved by Dr Lippe. His results were given in Allen's *Encyclopaedia*.

APPEARANCE

The picture may be one of grave illness. The lips are dry and cracked; there are scabs round the nostrils; there is constant picking at nose and lips until they bleed; a tendency to pluck aimlessly at the bed-clothes and to bore the head into the pillows.

'Strawberry tongue'; bright red mucosa which easily bleeds. Foetor oris; acrid discharges which excoriate the skin; possibly a scarlatiniform rash.

PSYCHOLOGY

The sufferer is restless, irritable, and may be delirious.

PHYSIOLOGY

A widespread sensation of heat and burning is usual, but the patient may complain of chills and much aching in the bones.

SYMPTOMATOLOGY

General

A grave toxaemic state may be present, associated with suppression of urine and stupor. The prostration is accompanied by incessant restless movements of head, limbs and fingers. Symptoms tend to be more severe on the left side.

Head

A headache is made worse by warmth, also by taking hot coffee and from too warm clothing. Relief after a meal.

Respiratory System

Ulceration is present inside the nose with much pinching and irritation, leading to constant rubbing and boring into the nose with a finger, especially on the left side. Removal of scabs leaves raw areas of increasing extent. Coryza and hay fever may occur, associated with similar concomitants. Nasal obstruction may be marked and discharges excoriate the skin of the upper lip.

The pharynx and larynx are especially liable to be involved, leading to sudden hoarseness with aphonia. This is made worse on any attempt to use the voice. If the vocal cords can be cleared of mucus the voice will improve. The laryngitis is accompanied by tearing pain on coughing. (This is to be compared with Causticum, under which remedy the coughing is painless. Furthermore with Arum the throat symptoms are usually associated with rhinitis; with Causticum the nose is not usually involved.)

Tickling and burning are felt in the throat; much mucus is secreted, and is raised in lumps and with considerable pain; rawness and soreness is experienced when swallowing; talking is painful; attempts to phonate are not only futile but painful. Burning and rawness may also be felt in the chest.

Alimentary System

The corners of the mouth are cracked and sore. The tongue becomes swollen, fissured, raw and bleeds easily. Salivation is profuse and acrid. There is much pricking, burning and stinging in lips, tongue and palate. Constricting burning pain may be felt in the stomach, or a sense of 'oppression' rising up from the belly to fill the whole chest. Diarrhoea occurs with brownish-yellow stools which redden and excoriate the perineum and intergluteal folds.

Lymphatic System

The lymph nodes are liable to be involved and acutely swollen, especially in the cervical region.

Skin

A widespread or patchy erythema may be present, or raw, haemorrhagic patches occur on the skin.

MODALITIES

Symptoms are aggravated by heat, by a wind in the north-west, and also when lying down.

CLINICAL NOTES

The main sphere of usefulness is in affections of throat and larynx. High potencies are said to give prompt relief. The remedy is also of service in malignant types of scarlet fever and diphtheria, and in typhoid states. Impetigo may be an indication for its employment. A complementary remedy is Nitric Acid.

Aurum Metallicum

SOURCE

Aurum, gold, is the sun metal, the sovereign of the world of metals. This metal is mainly found in a pure state, and nearly always very close to the surface of the earth, for instance in desert sand and in river beds. Gold miners are well aware that the deeper they tunnel the less gold they find.

Gold is extremely resistant to chemical action. It requires two strong acids in concentrated form, hydrochloric acid and nitric acid (Aqua Regia), to convert the metal gold into the water-soluble chloride.

The sun is at the heart of physical life and gold can be a central force in human history. In ancient Egypt and in more modern times in Tibet the private ownership of gold was forbidden – on pain of death. Gold was kept in the temple coffers or used in sacred buildings and debarred from common usage or possession.

Nevertheless, all down history wars have raged round the precious metal in the pursuit of what gold can buy in the shape of power and material possessions. The pure and beautiful metal which should have been the symbol of purity of heart and motive has been debased to become the overweening objective of human greed and pride.

Gold has been at the very heart of things in more senses than one; as a therapeutic agent in potency it is closely associated with affections and disorders of the heart in both the physical and the emotional spheres.

PHARMACOLOGY

Pure gold in bulk is medicinally inert. This is evidenced by its ineffectiveness when swallowed in the form of gold ornaments with suicidal intent. This is quite a common occurrence in the Orient. In subdivided or colloidal form the metal and its salts are extremely active. Affinity with connective tissue, mucous and synovial membranes, produces inflammatory changes and ulceration; with bone, induces caries and necrosis; with the heart, liver and kidneys, results in fatty degeneration; with skin, may cause an exfoliative dermatitis; with the central nervous system can bring about severe depression.

70

PROVING

The first proving of Aurum appears in the fourth volume of Hahnemann's *Materia Medica Pura*.

APPEARANCE

The Aurum subject in health is alert, glittering, erect in stance; in sickness is bowed and furtive with grief and gloom.

The face may be ruddy with a puffy, shiny appearance. The hair is dark and so are the eyes. Nose may be knobby and red. Foetor oris may be noticed. Ulcers, if present, are foul-smelling.

PSYCHOLOGY

The Aurum person craves sunshine, finds dull cloudy days unbearable. Is characteristically depressed, dejected, tired of life, discontented. Suffers from a profound inferiority complex, which results in self-condemnation or laying the blame on contrary fate. Is easily frightened, and the fear persists. Is restless, hurried, fidgety, quarrelsome, may indulge in wild outbursts of rage with subsequent remorse. Cannot bear to be contradicted. Is hypersensitive to all stimuli and especially to pain and cold.

Causal factors may be grief or severe emotional stress.

PHYSIOLOGY

The Aurum subject likes to be well wrapped up but also craves fresh air. Is usually ravenously hungry and tends to gobble his food, especially at the beginning of a meal. Is also intensely thirsty for cold fluids.

Sleep is restless, often disturbed by frightful dreams. The patient may thrash around in bed as if desiring to do himself an injury.

SYMPTOMATOLOGY

General
The Aurum pains are boring in character and tend to be quite unbearable. They are worse at night, especially when getting too warm in bed.

Head
Vertigo is worse on stooping and when attempting to walk; it is accompanied by a tendency to fall to the left. There may be complaint of

a maddening headache and the face becomes flushed, bloated and shiny. There may be a sensation as if air were blowing on the head, which has to be well wrapped up. The scalp and skull are sore and tender to the least touch. Alopecia is common.

Eyes

Catarrhal conjunctivitis is accompanied by scalding lachrymation. The eyes are very sensitive to touch, and vision is apt to be blurred or double. There may be a sensation of a black veil over the upper part of the visual field, so that only the lower part of objects can be seen. Tensive pain may be felt in the eyeball and severe pain in the bony orbit. Other eye conditions which may occur are trachoma, corneal ulcer, exophthalmos, inequality of pupils.

Ears

There may be complaint of cracking in the ears. Otitis media of chronic type is accompanied by discharge of foul foetid pus.

Respiratory System

Nasal obstruction may be accompanied by ulceration, which is very painful, especially when breathing through the nose. The nasal discharge is foetid. Necrosis of the nasal bones may occur. Ulcers also occur on the palate and in the fauces. A sensation of constriction is felt in the chest, resulting in a constant desire to take a deep breath. There may be a feeling of weight on the sternum, aggravated by going up stairs or ascending a slope. It is worse also in the first part of the night.

Alimentary System

Salivation is excessive, associated with foetor oris, having the smell of old cheese. Abdominal distension is accompanied by painful, indurated enlargement of the liver. Tabes mesenterica may be present. Meals are often followed by an urge to stool, and the stools are pale yellow or ashy white in colour.

Cardiovascular System

Aurum may be indicated when there is complaint of heat flushes followed by sweating and chilliness. Cardiac crises occur, characterized by violent palpitation, agonizing pain of anginal type, a sensation as if the heart stood still, throbbing carotids and acute dyspnoea. The sufferer is forced to sit up in bed and lean forward.

Lymphatic and Glandular Systems
Involvement of lymph nodes or glandular structures is characterized by hypertrophy accompanied by induration. The affected tissues are also painful.

Urinary System
Frequency and urgency of micturition are described, the urine being watery, or perhaps of the consistency of buttermilk with an ammoniacal odour and showing a copious thick deposit on standing.

Genital System
Orchitis occurs, especially affecting the right testicle. The swelling is painful and of stony hardness. Shooting pains in the uterus are aggravated by using the arms. Concomitant mental depression is probable. Uterine prolapse occurs as a result of chronic congestion and fibrosis.

Locomotor System
Prominent in the Aurum symptoms are severe bone pains; these wander from site to site and may build up to an acute cardiac seizure. The pains disturb sleep and may drive the sufferer from bed in search of relief despite the fact that the pains are aggravated by movement. The feet often feel bloated and heavy.

MODALITIES

The Aurum patient is worse in cold air, on cloudy days, in winter, from sunset to sunrise, when recumbent. In the case of women there is an aggravation at the time of the period.

Conversely, amelioration is felt in warm air, in sunny weather, and in summer, if the weather is summery.

CLINICAL NOTES

The remedy is often called for in syphilitic lesions. The mental factors are also of primary importance. Complementary remedies are Lueticum and Sulphur.

Baptisia Tinctoria

SOURCE

This remedy is prepared from the plant known as wild indigo, horse-fly weed, rattlebush, indigo-weed. It is indigenous to the eastern area of North America, and was formerly used as a dye – hence the name Baptisia, from the Greek word meaning 'I dip or immerse'.

The plant is found growing in dry woods or fields, often in a hilly region; it bears yellow flowers on a spike; the root is fleshy, brown to black in colour, and is the part used in the preparation of the mother tincture. It is non-odorous but has a nauseous acrid taste. The whole plant emits an unpleasant odour if bruised.

PHARMACOLOGY

There is evident affinity with mucous membranes, tending to necrotic, ulcerative, even gangrenous lesions; with the circulation, causing interference with normal flow of blood and consequent relative or absolute anoxia of tissues; with the nervous system, inducing rapid and grave prostration.

PROVING

Short provings of Baptisia, made by seven persons, may be found in the fifth and seventh volumes of the *North American Journal of Homoeopathy* (1857 and 1859).

APPEARANCE

The Baptisia subject is obviously a desperately sick individual. He is stupidly dull, and often delirious at night. He looks drugged, almost drunk, with dusky mottled visage, and the mucous surfaces are of a peculiarly dark red hue.

In the early stages of the rapidly developing illness there may be an anxious, frightened look with sweat on face and forehead.

Tremulousness is evident, both of tongue and limbs, and progressive weakness causing the sufferer to slide down in the bed. This is the case despite a tendency to toss from side to side in search of ease.

A notable feature is the pungent, penetrating, pestilential odour of all discharges and indeed of the whole body, a stench which is noticeable on first entering the house and almost unbearable in the sick-room.

The tongue is swollen, raw, stiff and protruded with difficulty. Sordes form on the teeth. Foetor oris is extreme.

The jaw drops and the mouth sags open with dribbling of saliva on to the pillow. Livid blotches may appear on trunk and limbs.

PSYCHOLOGY

A feature here is an extreme restlessness of both mind and body; the sufferer's thoughts are wild and wandering; it is difficult or impossible for him to follow a coherent train of thought. But the most characteristic feature is a curious disorder of body-sense; he feels as if there are two people in the bed, or as if his body is scattered about and he must try and get the pieces together again.

A further sensation may be that the bed feels too hard, is full of lumps or like a hard wooden board. There is also a feeling of being sore and bruised all over.

In addition there is often a fear of being poisoned by food or medicine offered.

PHYSIOLOGY

While chilly in the daytime the patient becomes hot and feverish at night. He is drowsy all the time, and if roused will drop off to sleep again while being questioned.

There is a tendency to wake between 2 and 3 a.m. and toss around, unable to get off to sleep again, while endeavouring to assemble those scattered limbs.

Thirst is marked. Sweat is offensive in odour.

SYMPTOMATOLOGY

General

The patient is taken suddenly and fearfully ill, and the condition deteriorates with alarming rapidity. There is early stupor, early appearance of sordes on teeth, early bloating of belly, early delirium, and the sufferer complains of aching and feeling bruised all over. The pulse rate tends to increase with any rise in temperature. Symptoms may be mainly right-sided. Grave illness presenting such a picture may occur in influenza, typhoid fever, typhus, diphtheria, scarlet fever, septicaemia or other forms of infection.

Head

The scalp may feel numb and tingling. The head may feel too big and so heavy that it cannot be lifted off the pillow. The skin across the forehead feels tight, or as if being pulled backwards towards the occiput.

Respiratory System

There is much mucous discharge from nose and throat which is sanious and very offensive. The throat is swollen, dark red in colour, ulcerated, but oddly enough not painful. The chest feels tight and compressed; breathing is difficult and there is air hunger.

Alimentary System

The mouth is ulcerated and in a foul state. The gums ooze blood and are dark red or purple in colour. The tongue is coated yellow or brown down the centre with red glistening edges; it is often studded with aphthous ulcers and may be swollen and stiff, feeling as if made of wood or dry burnt leather. Gangrenous stomatitis may develop. There is excessive secretion of thick ropy saliva, which dribbles all over the pillow. A notable feature is a complete inability to swallow solids as the result of spasm of the muscles of deglutition. Only liquids can be taken. The abdominal wall is tense and tender and tympanites is marked. There is definite soreness in the right iliac fossa. A foetid exhausting diarrhoea may be present, with dark sanious stools which excoriate the perianal region.

MODALITIES

These are not as important as the overall picture. Is generally worse after sleep, and worse from movement, despite the urge to toss about. A rise of temperature is likely about 11 a.m., accompanied by shivering.

CLINICAL NOTES

The range of usefulness of this remedy is more limited than that of many others, but when called for by the picture detailed above its use is of undoubted value, and may indeed prove life-saving.

It is especially indicated in the early stage of a fulminating infection. Complementary remedies which may follow well are Crotalus Horridus, Hamamelis, Nitric Acid and Terebinth.

Baryta Carbonica

SOURCE

Barium is described as the most poisonous of the alkaline earths. The carbonate is a soluble salt and quite toxic in its reactions; hence its unsuitability as an opaque medium for X-ray work.

PHARMACOLOGY

The salt has an affinity with various tissues. It increases the force and duration of muscle contractions and induces violent vomiting and purging. Effects on the central nervous system are to cause both clonic and tonic muscle spasms which pass on to paralysis. The action on the heart is at first to cause acceleration of the heart beat, but irregularity of cardiac action ensues and the heart stops in systole. Degenerative changes are produced in the walls of the arteries leading to hypertension. Lymph nodes and glands are involved, resulting in hypertrophy and induration. In cases of poisoning a condition of hypokalaemia has been noted.

PROVING

Baryta Carb. makes its first appearance in the first edition of Hahnemann's *Chronic Diseases*.

APPEARANCE

The Baryta Carb. patient is apt to look prematurely old with a withered, dried-up, sickly appearance. But the face may be bloated and of purplish hue.

The child is emaciated, with a hard bulging belly. Adults tend to obesity. The child is obviously shy, bashful, sits around idle and uninterested.

PSYCHOLOGY

The child is backward, retarded, late in learning both to talk and to walk, owing to poor muscular co-ordination; is inattentive, forgetful, just cannot remember things.

77

The adult finds it difficult to think clearly and consecutively; is irresolute, unable to come to a decision about anything; has a poor memory and forgets well-known names; dislikes meeting strangers; gets lost in familiar surroundings.

Trifles frighten; there are vague fears that 'something is going to happen'; develops imaginary cares and worries; thinks everyone is noticing and laughing at her; gets angry over trivialities.

May complain of a sensation of cobwebs on the face which cannot be brushed off.

PHYSIOLOGY

Is very chilly; wants to be well wrapped up, like the Psorinum person.

Has a poor appetite and is soon satisfied, despite quite enjoying the food. Dislikes cold things and fruit, especially plums. Is constantly thirsty.

Is sleepy in the daytime; sleep at night is uneasy, disturbed by frequent waking from anxious dreams. Cannot lie on the left side. Sleeps with the mouth open, dribbles saliva onto the pillow, wakes with a dry tongue like a nutmeg grater in consequence.

Foot sweats are offensive.

SYMPTOMATOLOGY

General
Physical weakness is apparent; there is a constant desire to lie down; is exhausted by the least effort. There is a curious tendency to the formation of lipomatous or fibrotic growths or nodules.

Head
Troublesome, pressive headaches occur, especially in old people, aggravated by heat and better out of doors. There may be a sensation as if the brain was flopping from side to side within the skull, or was moving up and down. Premature baldness may be present.

Eyes
Heaviness of the upper lids; agglutination of lid margins on waking; aching or burning pain in the eyes; muscae volitantes; dimness of vision; opacities in cornea; corneal ulcers. There may be a sensation as if the forehead was pressing down on the eyes.

Ears

Ears crack when swallowing or chewing; pulsation is felt in ears when lying on side at night. Ears may itch; tinkling and roaring tinnitus may be present; eruptions occur on or behind the pinna.

Respiratory System

Chronic nasal catarrh is accompanied by swelling and soreness of nose and upper lip with crust formation; the nasopharynx is often involved. There may be perversions of smell such as the odour of pine woods. The Baryta Carb. subject takes cold very easily and the cold goes to the throat. Tonsillitis ensues with great soreness of throat, especially on the right side, and progressive enlargement of tonsils; there is burning, sticking pain in the throat, worse on empty swallow; and a tendency to quinsy. Involvement of the larynx results in huskiness or aphonia; tracheobronchitis is accompanied by a great accumulation of mucus and rattling respiration, especially in old people. A sensation as if inhaling smoke or dust may be noticed. A very persistent type of cough is probably secondary to enlargement of hilar lymph nodes, and is only relieved by adopting the prone posture.

Alimentary System

Oesophageal spasm may cause an inability to swallow anything but fluids, and induces a strangled feeling. The digestion is 'weak'; there is discomfort in the stomach after eating. Inveterate constipation is associated with hard, knotty, inadequate stools. Piles protrude when passing urine. Urge to stool may be sudden and irresistible. Tabes mesenterica may be present, with passage of undigested matter in the stools.

Cardiovascular System

There is a complaint of frequent palpitation, aggravated by attempting to lie on the left side, and also by moving about. Definite hypertension may be present.

Lymphatic and Glandular Systems

Enlargement and induration of lymph nodes and of salivary glands is common; the enlargement is progressive without any tendency to suppurate.

Urinary System
There is a constant urge to urinate, associated with incontinence of greater or lesser degree.

Genital System
Atrophy of testicles; impotence; prostatic enlargement. In women there is a tendency to enlargement and induration of uterus.

Nervous System
The remedy has been employed in relation to multiple sclerosis associated with high systolic and low diastolic blood pressure. A further indication is the paralysis following a stroke.

Skin
Eruptions on the scalp in puny infants. Eruptions on or behind the ears. Ulcers with indurated edges. The skin is often sensitive and tense, giving a 'hide-bound' sensation. Soles and toes are tender. Intertrigo may be present.

MODALITIES

Aggravating factors are cold, especially damp cold, also great heat or exposure to hot sun; when standing or sitting still; by lying on left side; after eating; when thinking about symptoms.
   Relief is obtained from warmth, from movement and in the open air.

CLINICAL NOTES

The remedy is of special value in both childhood and 'second childhood'. It is complementary to Antimonium Tart. It should not be given in sequence to Calcarea Carb. or Calcarea Phos. It has proved of benefit in high blood pressure.

Belladonna

The source of this invaluable remedy is the plant *Atropa belladonna*. It is the common deadly nightshade, a member of the Solanaceae family, as also are its sinister sisters, the hairy henbane (*Hyoscyamus niger*) and the thorn-apple (*Datura stramonium*). Other, but less lethal, members of the family are the red pepper (*Capsicum*), bittersweet (*Solanum dulcamara*), black nightshade (*Solanum nigrum*), mandrake (*Mandragora*) and tobacco (*Nicotiana tabacum*).

The plant is widely distributed throughout most of Europe. It is striking in its appearance and remarkable in its manner of growth, revealing a nature that corresponds in a most interesting way with the character of the disturbance, both physical and psychological, which calls for its aid as a remedy.

It is found growing usually in chalky soil and prefers a shady site, beside a high hedge or in the lee of a wood. The tall stem, upright, somewhat hairy and of reddish purple tinge, may reach a height of six feet and do so in one season. It bears a plethora of dull darkish green leaves with entire margins; these are solitary below, but higher up the stem are found in pairs, though of unequal sizes, one of the pair being larger than the other. Some of the leaves may be as much as ten inches in length.

The flowers which appear in July and August are bell-shaped, quite large, up to one inch, and of a sinister cyanotic pinkish-purple hue. The plant has a long, thick, fleshy branching root of whitish colour, possessing a mawkish, slightly bitter taste and exuding a faint peculiar odour.

It is, however, the berries which arrest the eye and may prove all too alluring to the unwary. They are large, globose, shiny black in colour and seem to stare at the passer-by to challenge and entice. In size they resemble a small cherry, and indeed have been given such names as 'devil's cherries', 'naughty man's cherries' and 'boutons noirs'.

The plant presents a remarkable picture of violent growth, springing into intense activity in the early part of the year from its underground root, bearing leaves, flowers and both ripe and unripe berries all at the same time in a furore of growth, and attaining in one short season perhaps to the height of a man.

The fresh plant when crushed exhales a disagreeable odour which almost disappears on drying. The leaves have a bitter taste both when fresh and dried. One author describes the berries as tasting intensely sweet, thus tending to encourage their consumption, especially by children.

For preparation of the mother tincture the whole plant is used, gathered at the commencement of flowering.

The name 'bella donna', 'belle dame', 'beautiful lady', arose in Venice from the custom of the Italian women of the Renaissance to employ the juice of the berries to widen the pupils and render their eyes larger, darker and more brilliant. The juice is still used for a similar purpose by the veiled beauties of North Africa.

But the plant has other names, suggestive of the fact that its criminal significance far outweighs its cosmetic attractions. It was known as Dwale, from the Danish for delirium, and Manicon, from maniacum – madness. Indeed, so vehement were the poisonous effects when a number of the berries were eaten that death was almost inevitable. Hence the full name of the plant, *Atropa belladonna*, from Atropos, the third member of the three fates, who cuts the thread of life so carefully woven by Clotho and Lachesis.

There always was a sinister aura of lethality associated with the plant, as mentioned by Step: 'The herbalists regarded the plant less as a medicine than as a terrible poison, useful mainly for disposing of enemies and obnoxious relations.' Gerrard wrote: 'But if you will follow my counsell deale not with this plant in any case; banish it from your gardens and the use of it also, being a plant so furious and deadly, for it bringeth such as have eaten thereof into a dead sleep, where many have died, as hath been often seen and proved by experience.'

It is recorded that the plant was a favourite homicidal weapon among the Lithuanians of the 17th century, thus: 'They have also a plant which they call maulde, and when they owe money to someone they find means of introducing it into his drink. Whoever receives this plant into his body must die; the whole pharmacopoeia cannot help him.'

One berry is known to have caused severe illness in a child and three to have caused death.

PHARMACOLOGY

The poisonous proclivities of the plant have provided a wealth of information as to its symptom-inducing powers. Among other constituents are the alkaloids hyoscyamine, atropine, apo-atropine, belladonnine and hyoscine or scopolamine. Hyoscyamine is actually the principal constituent, but atropine which has the same chemical formula, is probably the most potent of the alkaloids.

It is stated that 'The action of atropine and belladonna go a long way together, and those of the alkaloid will prove to be a valuable guide. In atropine we have something highly characteristic of belladonna and its sister species.'

Accidental provings have occurred without number, both as the result of eating the berries and also in the employment or preparations of belladonna or of atropine in unwise dosage in therapy. Space forbids lengthy reference to these enlightening and enthralling happenings, but one quotation provides a fairly typical example. In an old book on flowers it is stated: 'For those who have unwisely eaten the berries the following consequences may be predicted – a complete loss of voice, continuous restless motion, an inability to swallow, but yet a great feeling of thirst, the vision impaired, a catching at imaginary objects, delirium passing presently into insensibility, and finally death.'

The plethora of provings, accidental as well as planned (there are fifty-three pages of Belladonna symptoms in the *Materia Medica Pura* of Hahnemann), show that the drug has a striking and profound action on the whole nervous system.

It acts on the autonomic system, causing stimulation of the sympathetic and inhibition of the parasympathetic nerves, with resultant paralysis of certain muscles and drying up of secretions. Thus there is relaxation of muscle tone in the bronchi and bowel wall, dilatation of the pupil, loss of power of accommodation for near objects, dry eye, dry skin and mucosa, dark red flush on face, neck, throat and trunk.

These effects are mainly due to the action of atropine, which interferes with the activity of acetylcholine and blocks all parasympathetic nerve impulses. In addition, sympathetic stimulation of sweat glands and vasoconstrictors is interfered with by blockage of impulse transmission at the terminal end organs.

There is also a direct action on the sphere of the psyche, producing such effects as restlessness, wakefulness, talkativeness, delirium, mania and finally stupor, coma and death.

Interference with the heat control centre induces fever. The respiratory centre is stimulated by small doses but depressed by a larger dose. Irritation of centres in the spinal cord gives rise to muscular twitching, jerkings or actual convulsions.

There is also direct action on the peripheral nerves, varying from irritation causing pain to inhibition of sensory impulses, with resulting dulling of pain and sensation of numbness. Hence the employment of Belladonna plaster to allay pain by local effect.

The effect on the circulation is most marked, with a tendency to sudden, intense hyperaemia, often in localized areas.

PROVING

Hahnemann devoted early attention to the pathogenetic effects of Belladonna, and published his results first in *Fragmenta de Viribus Medicamentorum Positivis*, and later in the last edition of the first volume of *Materia Medica Pura*.

APPEARANCE

The Belladonna patient presents a picture of ebullition. The face is fiery red, the pupils huge and black and staring, like the black shining berries of the plant. The initial bright red colour may change to a dusky tint and the countenance become mottled in appearance. The appearance is one of fury rather than fear, as would be the case if Aconite was indicated.

A bright red erythema suffuses the skin all over, and the surface feels burning hot to the touch.

The pulse is full and bounding and there is marked throbbing of the carotid vessels.

Local areas of inflammation show great heat, redness, swelling and extreme tenderness to the least touch.

Muscular twitching and jerking may be localized or widespread with resulting convulsions.

Incessant incomprehensible chatter may be a prominent feature.

In general, the Belladonna type of individual is said to be plethoric, vigorous, with a capacity for sudden violent reactions, and a proneness to acute illness of fulminating type.

PSYCHOLOGY

The Belladonna subject manifests acuteness of all the senses – starts at the least stimulus, noise, touch, bright light, jar or jolt. Easily becomes over-excited with rise of temperature as the result.

There may be furious bellicose delirium with a tendency to bite and scratch, tear things to pieces, or make attempts to escape. This phase may give place to one of mental dullness and semi-stupor.

Hallucinations are the rule, further confused by the loss of normal visual accommodation, with consequent distortion of the image of objects looked at.

Clutching sensations may be complained of, especially in the throat and in the region of the liver and the uterus.

The turmoil in the circulation may produce a feeling as if the bed were swaying up and down. (Arsenicum Alb. has the sensation of the bed turning over, Lachesis of the bed swaying from side to side, and Lac Caninum of the bed moving about.)

The person specially amenable to the influence of Belladonna is said to be quickly reacting, highly strung, sensitive, of sanguine temperament.

PHYSIOLOGY

Curiously enough the Belladonna subject, although seemingly in a state of boiling heat, feels worse in cold air, from cold applications, from the least draught. This is presumably due to the fact that the surface of the body is hypersensitive to any kind of stimulus. Uneven distribution of blood flow may give rise to cold extremities in association with a burning hot head.

Sometimes taking food will quieten the delirium.

Quite often there is a craving for lemons and lemon drinks.

Thirst is usually not marked, but there may be a desire to moisten the dry, even parched, mucous membranes of the mouth. A curious dread of running water may be a feature.

Sleep is very restless, often disturbed by screaming. Grinding the teeth during sleep, jerking awake when just dropping off to sleep, talking or moaning in sleep, even sleepwalking, may all suggest the desirability of considering the remedy.

Sweats occur on covered parts of the body, but without affording relief to symptoms.

SYMPTOMATOLOGY

General

Complaints presenting the Belladonna symptom picture may be induced by exposure to cold air. Symptoms characteristically manifest suddenness of onset and are violent in nature. Pain, headache, pulsations, inflammations, mental disturbance are all violent. Heat is also a noticeable feature. Sweats are hot. In haemorrhage the blood is hot. In fevers head and skin surface are burning hot to the touch. Inflamed areas are acutely hot. Belladonna pains are throbbing in nature and are typically aggravated by the least jar or movement. They both start and cease with abruptness. Swellings also come up rapidly and are associated with much stinging, burning and throbbing, great sensitivity to touch and a sensation as if the part affected 'is going to burst'. Symptoms tend to be right-sided.

Head Region
Headache of violent throbbing type is associated with great sensitivity of the scalp, so much so that the sufferer refuses to have the hair combed or brushed. Firm pressure, however, may be tolerated and bending the head backwards may give relief. It is often found that this type of headache is relieved by cold applications and in the open air, which is contrary to the usual modality of the remedy. The headache is aggravated by stooping, inclining the head forward, from the least jar, by lying down and in direct sunlight. It may be accompanied by a muzzy feeling in the head as if semi-intoxicated. The type of vertigo associated with Belladonna is noticed on movements of the head or on turning over in bed. Everything seems to be 'going round'. This too is relieved in the open air. The remedy may be indicated in early meningitis when the patient rolls the head from side to side on the pillow or manifests definite head retraction. It would be considered in heat stroke.

Eyes
Various disturbances of vision may occur, associated with enlargement of pupils, heat and redness in the eyes. Muscle spasm may cause diplopia or squinting or twitching of lids. Throbbing deep in eyeball may be present, or the eyes may feel swollen and protruding.

Ears
The remedy is of value in acute earache, especially on the right side, with a bright red and possibly bulging tympanic membrane. The sense of hearing is often extremely acute and the voice seems to reverberate in the ear.

Respiratory System
Epistaxis may occur with hot blood and red face. The nose may be swollen with a shiny red tip and very tender and sore. Frequent violent sneezing may occur. The sense of smell may be very acute or perverted, with an awareness of foul odour in the nose. Throat symptoms are

important. Great dryness of the throat, which burns like fire, and sudden hoarseness or even complete loss of voice. There may be an unpleasant clutching sensation in the throat with difficulty in swallowing, especially liquids. There is a constant desire to keep swallowing despite the pain and difficulty. The tonsils may be acutely inflamed, swollen and even ulcerated, especially on the right side. A dry, spasmodic, barking cough tends to be worse at night, on lying down, on taking a deep breath. It is also aggravated by talking or crying and in a dusty atmosphere. It may be relieved temporarily by the expulsion of a pellet of mucus. An acute tickle in the larynx may precipitate a bout of coughing lasting minutes.

Alimentary System
The remedy may be called for in sudden, acute swelling of the lip with redness and great pain. Mouth and tongue tend to be excessively dry, causing difficulty in deglutition. Typical 'strawberry tongue' may be present and a scarlet appearance of the pharynx. The sense of taste may be intensified. Toothache especially affects the upper teeth on the right side, and is accompanied by much throbbing and a very red face. Cramping pains occur in the stomach which extend through to the back and impel the sufferer to bend backwards for relief. On the other hand, biliary or intestinal colic may be eased by bending forward. Griping or clutching sensations may centre round the umbilicus or predominate in the hypogastrium. In acute peritonitis the abdomen is burning hot to the touch and also extremely sensitive to touch or pressure of bed covers. This sensitivity is present also with severe pain in the ileo-caecal region. Stools may be dysenteric with much ineffectual urging. Acutely inflamed piles may be so painful and sensitive that the sufferer is forced to lie with the legs widely apart.

Lymphatic and Glandular Systems
Acute enlargement of the cervical lymph nodes usually accompanies sore throat, with local heat and redness. Lymphadenitis elsewhere or acute parotitis may call for the remedy. Acute mastitis is associated with much heat, extreme sensitivity to touch and red streaks running from the nipple.

Cardiovascular System
As Kent observes, 'Belladonna especially affects the whole vascular system'. Violent palpitations may occur, especially on going up a hill or ascending the stairs. The palpitations are apt to reverberate in the head and throbbing pulsations may be felt all over the body.

Urinary System
The bladder symptoms are severe – violent distress with clutching sensations, burnings and constant urge to urinate. There is liable to be retention from spasm of the sphincter urinae, or else paralysis of the sphincter with resultant loss of bladder control. Tenesmus is felt in the bladder after passage of urine. Involuntary dribbling occurs while standing or walking. The urine may be dark and turbid with presence of blood.

Genital System
Violent bleeding from the uterus may occur in association with abortion or labour, in the latter case accompanied by hour-glass contraction of the uterus. The blood is hot, the flow profuse, the colour bright and clots are present. A violent bearing-down sensation may be complained of, with a feeling as if the genital organs would prolapse in entirety. Right-sided ovarian pain may occur. Also spasmodic dysmenorrhoea in plethoric subjects. The menstrual period is liable to be too early, with profuse loss of bright red, hot blood.

Nervous System
Belladonna subjects manifest marked hyperaesthesia with extreme irritability of tissues. This results in an extensive array of peculiar nervous reactions – twitching, jerkings, trembling, subsultus tendinum, cramps, spasms, convulsions, all of which are apt to supervene with unexpected suddenness. The convulsions are usually associated with head symptoms and are relieved by warmth. Dentition or worms may be precipitating factors.

Locomotor System
The remedy may be indicated for stiff neck, especially when this has resulted from impact of cold air, possibly following a haircut. Tearing pains are described from hips down thighs, keeping the sufferer restlessly walking to and fro in search of ease, the pains being worse at rest. Acute rheumatism may call for the remedy when accompanied by tearing pains and associated with red, sensitive, swollen joints; impact of cold air is resented. There is a desire to lie perfectly still and local heat affords relief.

Skin
The chief sign is erythema, either in patches or widespread, associated with heat and hyperaesthesia. A cutting sensation may be felt as if the

skin were 'sliced with a sharp knife'. A morbilliform eruption may occur, or blister formation associated with intense pain. The remedy may be indicated in relation to boils, erysipelas, acne rosacea, acute cellulitis.

MODALITIES

There is definite aggravation from bright light, any form of noise, and the least jolt or jar. As would be expected, symptoms are aggravated by lying on the affected part. Chronologically there is an aggravation about 3 p.m. and fever peaks are at 9 p.m. and 8 a.m.

There is amelioration in a warm room, by warm wraps, by rest and avoidance of movement, also by bending the head backwards.

CLINICAL NOTES

This remedy is effective in a wide range of potencies and over an extensive range of illnesses. Dr Edward Hamilton wrote in 1852, 'The chief affections in which Belladonna is indicated are the following: Phlegmonous and erysipelatous inflammations, the more delicate the inflamed organ or tissue the more suitable is Belladonna. Catarrhal affections. Affections consequent upon fear, fright and chagrin. Nervous affections. Spasms of every kind.'

A special sphere of usefulness is in the treatment of scarlet fever; pioneer work in relation to the use of Belladonna as a prophylactic in relation to this exanthem was carried out by Hahnemann. Opinion varies as to the efficacy of Belladonna in this respect, but either Belladonna 30c or the nosode Scarlatinum 30c could be employed in contacts, three doses spread over twenty-four hours and a further single dose a week later.

Belladonna is a quickly-acting remedy of undoubted value in acute states of sudden onset. It will often abort inflammatory processes if given early.

Complementary remedies are Calcarea Carb. and Sulphur. The plant has a neutral affinity with calcareous soils, growing best on dry limestone.

Berberis Vulgaris

SOURCE

Berberis vulgaris, barberry, pipperidge bush, is a spiny shrub of wide distribution in Europe, Asia and North America. It grows to a height of 3 to 6 feet. The branches are strongly grooved, yellowish to start with but turning grey in the second year. The leaves arise in bunches, are dull green in colour, obovate with sharp fine teeth along the edges and very veiny; they reach a length of 1½ inches. At the base of the bunch of short-stalked leaves there are three wicked-looking, very sharp thorns.

A drooping flower raceme arises from the centre of the leaf bunch in a cluster of small pale yellow blossoms; it is some 3 inches in length and the flowers give rise to red egg-shaped berries, half-an-inch in length, which are very acid in taste due to the presence of oxalic acid.

The flowers appear in May and June; each blossom possesses six stamens which show a peculiar irritability. Should the base of the stamen be touched on its inner aspect, e.g. by a nectar-seeking insect, it immediately rises up and strikes its pollen-bearing head against the stigma. Stamens stimulated in this manner subsequently return to their original position under cover of the petals.

The plant is found in woods and hedges and also on bushy chalk hills. The parts used in preparation of the mother tincture are the small branches of the roots, or the bark of the branches of the roots of moderate size.

PHARMACOLOGY

There is an affinity with the body as a whole. One grain given to a healthy girl three times a day for four days gave rise to a feverish condition, shivering along the back, heat in the face towards evening, inflammation of the conjunctiva, great thirst, anorexia, some griping in the belly and pains before urination.

Affinity with the throat results in redness and swelling of tonsils, pharynx and uvula; with liver and alimentary tract leading to increased flow of bile, intestinal inflammation and dysentery; with uterus causing congestion; with kidneys and bladder giving rise to nephritis and haematuria; with venous system causing pelvic congestion and haemorrhoids.

PROVING

A proving of Berberis was published by Dr Hesse in the first volume of the *Journal für Arzneimittellehre*.

APPEARANCE

There is a sickly appearance with poor colour, sunken cheeks and bluish discoloration around the eyes. The inner aspect of the lower lip shows a reddish livid hue, and bluish red spots appear in the vicinity of the corners of the mouth. The patient is apt to sit with both hands clasping the head.

PSYCHOLOGY

The individual is inert, listless, lethargic, with a particularly poor memory; finds it difficult to recall incidents of preceding years; is incapable of sustained mental effort. Becomes very nervous at dusk with a tendency to see visions of animals or monsters.

PHYSIOLOGY

Appetite is variable; hunger alternates with anorexia; thirst alternates with thirstlessness.

SYMPTOMATOLOGY

General
The pains are radiating in type, constantly shift from one site to another, often emanate from the small of the back, seem deeply placed. The pains are sharp, sticking (like thorns), burning, tearing, pinching; not made worse by pressure but aggravated by certain postures, especially standing upright and also by active exercise. Symptoms are apt to alternate rapidly, e.g. a thirsty feverish condition can change quickly into a thirstless prostration, a voracious appetite can suddenly give way to complete anorexia, acute polyuria can alternate with oliguria. Symptoms tend to be mainly left-sided.

Head
Vertigo with attacks of fainting may be troublesome. A peculiar feature is a feeling as if the head was encased in a helmet or as if growing puffy

and too large; this gives rise to what are described as 'tight hat' headaches.

Eyes
There is extreme dryness of the eyes, associated with burning and a sensation of sand beneath the eyelids.

Ears
There may be lacerating pain in the auricle, with the presence of gouty concretions.

Respiratory System
The nose is unduly dry or there may be an obstinate catarrh affecting the left nostril. A crawling sensation may be noticed inside the nose. Laryngitis may occur with hoarseness, or possibly a laryngeal polypus. Tearing stitches may be felt in the chest.

Alimentary System
The mouth feels dry, with sticky, frothy saliva, like filaments of cotton. The tongue feels scalded and may show the presence of vesicles. Nausea may be present first thing in the morning. Stitches occur in the region of the liver, acute pains coming on suddenly and with instant intensity, aggravated both by movement and by pressure. The left lobe may be especially affected. Catarrh of the gall-bladder is associated with constipation and a degree of jaundice. There is a constant urge to stool, which when passed is white. Colourless diarrhoea is accompanied by sharp pricking pain in the region of the anus before, during and after stool. Haemorrhoids are associated with burning pain after going to stool, and the pain radiates to the surrounding area. Anal fistula may be present. Perianal eczema may prove troublesome. A sticking pain is described, felt first anterior to the kidneys and spreading to liver, spleen, stomach, groins and the inguinal ligament.

Urinary System
Renal colic is accompanied by sensations of burning and boiling; it is aggravated by the movement involved in travel by car or by train. It is often left-sided. There is urgency of urination accompanied by pain and burning, especially during the act; the pain passes down into hips and thighs. There is a sensation of incomplete emptying of the bladder after the act. The urine varies; may be turbid containing thick mucus and a bright red sediment on standing, or may be yellow with a chalky whitish

deposit or, perhaps, a sediment that is reddish and contains blood. There is frequency of urination and burning in the urethra, even when not passing water.

Genital System
Pains shoot down the spermatic cords into the testicles, sometimes on one side and sometimes on the other. Smarting, burning, stitching pains may involve testicles, prepuce and scrotum. In women, pinching sensations may be felt in the mons veneris; vaginismus may occur with tenderness of the vagina. There may be actual burning and soreness in the vagina. Libido is diminished, and cutting pain may be experienced during intercourse. Menses are scanty with grey mucus and accompanying pain in kidneys and down the thighs. Leucorrhoea occurs with much greyish mucus and painful urinary symptoms.

Locomotor System
Stitching pains occur in neck and back, aggravated by respiratory movement. Lumbago type pain is accompanied by pains shooting down the lower limbs and by red sand in the urine. Burning, stinging, tearing, stitching pains occur in joints indicating early signs of multiple arthritis. Neuralgic pains are felt deep to the finger-nails, associated with swelling of the digital joints. Paralytic pain of rheumatic type occurs in shoulders, arms, hands, fingers, legs and feet. Heels may be painful as if ulcerated. Stitching pain may occur in metatarsus as if standing on a nail. Walking only a short distance may induce intense weariness and lameness in legs.

Skin
Flat warts occur. Itching eruptions burn and smart, made worse by scratching; cold applications afford relief. Eczema especially afflicts arms and hands; affected areas show circumscribed pigmentation when inflammation has subsided.

MODALITIES

Symptoms are aggravated by movement, by walking or driving in a vehicle; by any kind of jar or jolt; by the effort of maintaining the erect posture.

Rest affords a measure of relief.

CLINICAL NOTES

The lower potencies are often effective. Complementary remedies are Lycopodium and Sulphur.

Bromium

SOURCE

Bromine is the liquid member of the non-metallic halogen group. It is a brown, fuming liquid, which when vaporized forms an evil-smelling, powerfully pungent brown gas, from which its name derives, viz. *bromos*, Greek for 'stench'.

It is found in combination with iodine in seaweed ash, in sea-water and in the effluent of certain salt springs. It also occurs in compound form as the purple dye obtained from the sea-snail *Murex brandaris*, formerly used to colour the togas of Romans of Imperial rank.

Salts of the element are used in medicine, in the dye industry and in photography.

PHARMACOLOGY

Bromine, like chlorine, is a general protoplasmic poison. On the mucosa of the respiratory tract it has a violently irritating action leading to laryngeal spasm, formation of pseudo-membranous exudates, and possibly acute pulmonary oedema. Affinity with lymph nodes and glandular structures produces enlargement and induration. The mouth, throat and stomach are similarly inflamed and irritated; likewise the skin, which becomes red and blistered.

The local reactions are due to the formation in situ of hydrobromic acid and, later, bromides formed in the process of absorption.

APPEARANCE

The physical appearance in Bromium subjects varies. In general the type is lean, pale with delicate skin, very light hair and eyebrows, and blue eyes. But the appearance may be plethoric with red face, easy flushing and a tendency to become easily over-heated.

In types manifesting a chronic broken-down state, possibly suffering from goitre, lymphadenitis or malignant disease, the patient looks old with a sickly, grey, ash-coloured visage.

Fan-like movements of the alae nasi may be noticed, as is the case with Lycopodium. Pimples may be present on nose, tongue, fingers and around the anus. Emaciation may be marked, in association with tremulous limbs.

PROVING

Dr Hering published a proving of Bromium in the second volume of the *Neues Archiv*.

PSYCHOLOGY

Here too the picture is variable. At times there is cheerfulness with a desire for mental activity, or the subject is depressed, fatigued and unable to tackle a job. The general weakness induces a state of indifference, sadness, boredom and lack of any interest in household affairs.

Fear of ghosts may obtrude in the dark. Peculiar sensations occur, such as a feeling as if 'there was somebody behind or beside her', or a sensation as if 'there were cobwebs on the face, which cannot be brushed off'.

PHYSIOLOGY

The reactions to heat and cold are curious. Icy cold limbs are present with a hot head. If chilled when over-heated, the least draught seems to 'freeze him to the bone'. At the same time any over-heating, especially indoors, induces great discomfort.

Yawning is very frequent, and drowsiness may be quite irresistible when reading. Vivid dreams are common at night.

SYMPTOMATOLOGY

General
Predominant features are weakness, lassitude, shivering, yawning, desire to stretch and tremulousness. There is progressive prostration. Symptoms tend to be left-sided.

Head
Vertigo is curiously aggravated by proximity to running water, and is liable to be accompanied by the sensation mentioned above of someone or something unusual nearby. A good nose-bleed gives relief. A severe left-sided migraine may occur, made worse by stooping and also aggravated by drinking milk.

Ears
Affections of the ears are associated with enlargement and induration of the parotid lymph nodes.

Respiratory System
Acute coryza is accompanied by much sneezing with profuse, watery, excoriating nasal discharge. The nostrils become blocked, first on one side, then on the other. There is considerable soreness both inside the nose and at the nostrils, and the alae nasi become swollen. Pressive pain is felt at the root of the nose. An attack often coincides with the onset of hot weather and is frequently accompanied by headache. The throat is a special sphere in which this remedy can prove of value. Trouble tends to start in the larynx and spread upward. Tonsillitis is accompanied by swelling, injection and deep red colour; the throat feels raw and swallowing is painful. Chronic hoarseness occurs, the throat feeling raw as if 'scraped'. A rough dry cough gives trouble in the evening with much rattling of mucus but no expectoration. Spasm of the glottis may occur, leading to wheezing, rattling, rasping respiration and spasmodic croup. The remedy may be called for in malignant diphtheria with very rapid membrane formation; the process often starts on the left side. Asthma may occur. The sufferer jumps up gasping for breath, the larynx feels as if 'covered with down'; air passages seem 'full of smoke'; the air breathed feels cold as if 'coming off ice'. Warm drinks afford some relief. Sailors get asthma on coming ashore, especially on entering heated rooms. Respiratory symptoms are aggravated by exposure to dust and in a hot, stuffy atmosphere. There is a sensation as if enough air could not be drawn into the lungs.

Alimentary System
The remedy may be called for in chronic peptic ulcer which is accompanied by considerable vomiting or by diarrhoea, worse after taking food; the gastric symptoms are aggravated by acids, hot food or drink, oysters and tobacco smoke. There tends to be urge to stool soon after a meal; melaena may be present. Painful piles which constantly prolapse may give trouble. Mucus may be seen in the stools.

Cardiovascular System
Palpitation accompanies many symptoms. Cardiac hypertrophy may be present, associated with palpitation on rising from sitting, or on exertion.

Lymphatic System
Enlargement and induration are the prominent features of lesions in this sphere, but suppuration is unusual. The inflammatory process is slow and infiltrating, whether affecting lymph nodes, salivary glands, breasts or thyroid.

Genital System
Orchitis is accompanied by smooth, hard, hot, painful swelling, the pain being aggravated by the least jar. In women dull pain occurs in the region of the left ovary which becomes tender and hard, especially before the menstrual period. Membranous dysmenorrhoea may be present. A curious symptom, shared by Lycopodium, is a loud emission of air from the vagina.

Locomotor System
The limbs are apt to become progressively weak, wasted and tremulous.

Skin
Erosive ulcers have an indurated base. Pimples, pustules and boils may occur.

MODALITIES

There is aggravation from both heat and cold, from hot weather, a stuffy atmosphere, or too much clothing on the one hand and, on the other, from cold air, cold food and drink. An important aggravation is an adverse reaction to dust, especially in relation to respiratory troubles. Chronologically, symptoms tend to be worse from evening till midnight.

The Bromium subject feels better at the seaside, when riding on horseback and after shaving.

Actual illness may be brought on by over-heating in any way.

CLINICAL NOTES

The larynx and bronchial tubes are the main sphere of usefulness for this remedy, the great sensitivity to dust being one of the chief indications.

Bryonia Alba

SOURCE

There are some twenty-two varieties of *Bryonia* found in different parts of the world, but only two of these find a niche, albeit a very prominent one, in the homoeopathic materia medica. These are *Bryonia dioica,* found in Britain and also on the continent, and *Bryonia alba,* found only on the continent of Europe. Both are known as white bryony; it was the latter that Hahnemann used to make his provings.

However, careful and extensive provings were made by the Austrian school using both species and 'no difference in their actions could be established'. It therefore appears justifiable to use the root-stock of either species for preparation of the mother tincture.

Bryonia belongs to the Cucurbitaceae, the gourd family, of which *Colocynthis* is also a member.

Bryonia dioica is a climbing hedgerow plant, creeping quietly and slowly and somewhat unobtrusively on its way, often hidden by the foliage of the hedge shrubs. In this respect it is very different from the furiously growing *Belladonna,* and is suggestive of the Bryonia type of illness which is slow and insidious in onset, and the Bryonia patient who manifests inertia and desires to be left in peace and quiet.

The stems are annual and grow to a great length. The whole plant is covered with minute hairs. It contains an acrid milky juice which has an unpleasant odour. It is particularly nauseous when dried, and also irritant if coming in contact with the skin.

The leaves have a short curved stalk, shorter than the blade, which is divided into five finger-like lobes, all rather angular in shape, the middle one being by far the longest.

The flowers, which bloom in May, are small, greenish-yellow in colour and not at all showy. Those of *Bryonia alba* are paler. Stamens and pistils are never found in the same flower, the pollen flowers and ovary flowers being in separate sets. In the *dioica* variety they are on separate stems – hence *dioica* (two dwellings).

A unique feature of the plant is its method of climbing, which depends on the possession of long tendrils or feelers. These extend from the stem in search of some support and, having become attached to it contract into a coiled spring, one half of which is curled in a clockwise direction and the other half anti-clockwise. This provides fixation and stability for the parent plant.

The berries, often found hanging about the bushes after the stems and leaves have withered, are about the size of a garden pea. They occur in little clusters, changing from green to a striking yellow and finally crimson; they are covered with a dry delicate bloom. The berries of the *alba* variety are black when ripe.

The berries, when ripe, are filled with a juice of a foetid unpleasant odour; they contain three to six large seeds, greyish-yellow in colour and mottled with black. The berries are described as emetic and unwhole-some to eat. It has been estimated that forty berries would cause the death of an adult and fifteen prove fatal for a child.

It is important to distinguish the plant from another with a similar name, black bryony. This latter is *Tamus communis*, also a hedgerow climber but not using tendrils for its excursions. The plant climbs by twining its stem round any available support as it reaches higher and higher. Its leaves are very distinctive, being large, long, glossy and smooth; they are broad at the base and taper to a point at the tip. They turn to bronze or almost black before withering. The berries are bright red when ripe, much larger than those of white bryony and distinctly shiny, lacking any bloom on the surface. The root is black.

To return to white bryony, the root is white and large, possessing an unpleasant odour and a nauseous taste. It is thick and fleshy and may attain an enormous size, growing to a length of two feet and becoming 'as thick as a man's arm', weighing perhaps several pounds. Gerrard wrote, 'The Queen's chief surgeon, Mr William Godorus, a very curious and learned gentleman, shewed me a root hereof that waied half an hundredweight, and of the bigness of a child of a year old.'

The milky juice of the root possesses violent purgative and cathartic properties, shared in some measure by all parts of the plant. Many fatal cases of poisoning have been recorded. In France especially many accidents occurred among women at the time of weaning their infants, because of popular belief that a decoction of the plant would diminish milk secretion. The French name for the plant is 'Navet du diable' – Devil's turnip – which is suggestive.

The old herbalists recognized that the use of the plant was not unattended by danger. Culpeper speaks of it as 'a furious martial herb which purges the belly with great violence, troubling the stomach, burning the liver, and therefore not rashly to be taken.'

Nevertheless, it was used extensively by many notable physicians of former times. Dioscorides employed it in epilepsy, vertigo and melancholia. Galen in gout, hysteria and hypochondriasis. Caelius Aurelianus in jaundice. Sydenham in disorders of the mind, delirium, mania, insanity and imbecility. Alexander Trallian in deafness, diarrhoea, dropsy, pleuritis, stitches in the side, sciatica, white tumour of the knee. Hartman in diseases of the womb and tardy delivery. Loniger in asthma, pain in the neck, haemorrhage and spitting of blood.

This remarkable list of ailments is of interest in that the various conditions for which the drug was prescribed are all simulated by the type of symptoms Bryonia is capable of producing in healthy provers. In other words, these uses of the drug were in effect examples of inadvertent homoeopathy.

PHARMACOLOGY

The active principle of the plant is a glycoside, bryonin, which is a drastic purgative. Present also are an amorphous alkaloid and a resin, both of which are purgative, a volatile oil and an alcohol.

The chief affinity of the drug is with epithelial tissues, mucous, serous and synovial, tending to inflammatory change with the production of either fibrinous or serous exudation.

This tends to extreme dryness of mucous surfaces in air passages and alimentary tract, and in other locations to the formation of adhesions, which incidentally will limit or prevent movement of the affected part. Effusions in joints or serous cavities will also tend to limit movement by exerting fluid pressure.

The drying-up tendency is further manifested by interference with the free secretion and free flow of fluids, resulting for example in biliary stasis and damage to the tissues of the liver.

There is also affinity with fibrous tissues in muscles and ligaments around joints, inducing inflammatory reactions which provoke spasm, with resulting limitation of movement and avoidance of pain.

PROVING

Bryonia was one of the early remedies to be proved by Hahnemann; its pathogenesis occurs in the second volume of *Materia Medica Pura*.

APPEARANCE

The Bryonia patient will usually be found lying perfectly still, afraid to move a muscle because movement increases pain.

In fevers the face is swollen, puffy, purplish and drunken-looking. Pupils are dilated but lack the glint and stare of Belladonna.

Lips are dry, cracked and bleeding. The child constantly picks at his lips. Although scared to move there may be some fidgeting of the arms and legs. Constant side-to-side chewing movements of the lower jaw may be observed.

The gait is staggering, especially when going up or down stairs.

PSYCHOLOGY

The Bryonia type of individual has been described as 'persistent, pigheaded, choleric, bursting with plans and activity but afraid of poverty and fearful about the future'.

Gutman gives a most apt description: 'The typical Bryonia personality is not the artist or scientist or philosopher, the explorer of beauty or the unknown. He is the businessman, the insurance man, the stockbroker, the man without much imagination but with much 'calculation'; a dry fellow, sober, reliable, methodical, tenacious, weighing his steps, concerned in everything he does with safety, stability, security. Lacking a safe basis for his economic existence he becomes irritable, angry, anxious, depressed, always on the lookout for something which promises a hold to provide stability and security . . . Worried about his security, he holds on to his back, he holds on to his belly, he holds on to his pocket-book.'

In illness the individual characteristics are often exaggerated, so it is not surprising that the Bryonia patient is anxious both about his condition and about current affairs. He becomes irritable, morose, angry if crossed, his poise and sense of stability being upset.

There is aversion to making any effort, even that of conversation – inertia of mind as well as immobility of body.

There is a desire to lie still in a quiet room and not be disturbed or interfered with. But at the same time he is ill at ease, discontented – doesn't really know just what he does want. Often expresses a wish to 'go home' when he is actually in his own bed at home.

PHYSIOLOGY

Although the symptoms may be brought on by exposure to dry cold, especially cold east winds, the Bryonia patient prefers to be in a cool atmosphere and dislikes a warm room or being over-warmly wrapped up.

There is a tendency to overeat but sometimes this is replaced by an aversion to all food or, perhaps, a craving for something that is unobtainable.

Thirst tends to be excessive, for large drinks at fairly long intervals, not constant sips, as for instance with Arsenicum Alb.

Sweats are profuse, especially during the night at about 2 a.m., and the sweat has a sour smell.

Drowsiness is marked during the day, but sleep is often delayed at night and unrefreshing. There is a tendency to start awake in fright when dropping off to sleep, or during sleep. Somnambulism may occur, also nightmare.

SYMPTOMATOLOGY

General

Illness calling for Bryonia may be induced not only by exposure to cold east winds but also by weather changes from cold to warm; causal factors such as fright, anger or resentment may also be responsible. The onset of symptoms is gradual and insidious rather than sudden and abrupt, and may be delayed till a day or two after exposure. Moreover the illness progresses slowly rather than with violence and rapidity. Pains are plentiful and typically sticking or stitching in character; twinges of pain may cause actual wincing. The pains are notably aggravated by the slightest movement, and are accompanied by soreness of the affected part and sensitivity to touch. Firm pressure, however, is tolerated and gives relief. Acute effusions occur into serous or synovial cavities. Symptoms tend to be right-sided.

Head Region

The Bryonia vertigo is noticed, particularly on rising from sitting; it is worse in a warm room and better when lying flat. Headache is noticed on first opening the eyes in the morning and is of bursting or dull throbbing type, frontal or occipital in site, with a tendency to spread to the nape. Again, the ache may start above the right eye, spread backwards to the occiput and further involve the whole body in discomfort. The headache tends to be aggravated by stooping, after meals, from any exertion and on going to stool. It is better in cool air, by cool applications, by firm pressure and when lying down. On occasion more relief is obtained by local warmth than by cold. The scalp is also sore and sensitive.

Eyes

Pain and soreness in the eyeballs is greatly aggravated by moving the eyes. Letters tend to run together when attempting to read. The eyes feel hot and full of dust.

Respiratory System

A dry coryza may cause nasal blockage, or a fluent coryza may occur, associated with shooting pains in the forehead. The nose is apt to become swollen and sore. Epistaxis may be frequent and is especially likely to occur just before the menstrual period, or during pregnancy at the time when the period would normally be due. It may also occur in association with amenorrhoea from other causes. Dryness of the air-passages may result in laryngitis or tracheitis, with a tiresome tickle felt low down behind the sternum. There is tenacious mucus only shifted with difficulty. Downward spread may lead to a dry cough with much gagging and vomiting, and the cough is aggravated on entering a warm room. Involvement of lungs or pleura may lead to pneumonia or pleurisy, with or without effusion. When coughing the sufferer is apt to hold on to the chest with one hand and on to the head with the other. Eating, drinking, laughing, talking, smoking are all apt to aggravate the cough. With involvement of lung or pleura the patient prefers to lie on the affected side. There may be a sensation of pressure on the chest, with difficulty in breathing and a frequent desire to take a deep breath in search of relief. Stitches are felt in the chest when breathing in or when coughing.

Alimentary System

Lips, tongue and pharynx are excessively dry. Soapy, frothy saliva accumulates in the mouth. The tongue is loaded with a white or yellow coating. There is an unpleasant bitter taste in the mouth. Burning blisters may occur on the edge of the tongue. The Bryonia toothache tends to shoot from one tooth to another, or extend to head and cheeks. It is worse at 3 a.m. and aggravated by smoking. Firm pressure on the affected side affords some relief. With indigestion there is a distressing sensation as if the food taken lies like a stone in the stomach – gastric secretion is in abeyance and this is the result. The patient often has a craving for ice-cold water but it is a drink of something warm which gives relief. Eating makes things worse. With liver involvement there is much biliousness, nausea and vomiting, associated with yawning and a feeling of faintness. Recumbency affords relief, but on lifting the head from the pillow the dreadful sickness returns and the attempt to sit up has to be abandoned. Jaundice may be evident and tenderness noticed on palpating the liver. A feature may be hiccough associated with much belching; the eructations taste of food. They afford some relief for a time. The epigastrium is often sore and tender to touch. Burning, shooting, sticking pains may be felt in the belly, associated with extreme tenderness, aggravated by both touch and pressure, compelling the sufferer to lie motionless with the legs drawn up – the picture of acute peritonitis.

The Bryonia diarrhoea drives the patient from bed in the morning or comes on soon after rising. There is profuse purging accompanied by great exhaustion. The stools may be dysenteric in type, associated with griping pains in the belly and severe rectal tenesmus. The exhaustion compels the sufferer to lie down; but if while lying he makes the least movement he must hurry to stool again. An attack of diarrhoea may be brought on by eating sour fruit or drinking cold water when over-heated. Stools are apt to smell like old cheese and may have a yellow mushy appearance. The Bryonia constipation is characterized by large, bulky, dry, hard crumbly stools, brown to black in colour as if burnt. The stool is passed only with great difficulty.

Cardiovascular System
The remedy may be called for in pericarditis with effusion.

Lymphatic and Glandular Systems
With mastitis the breast is heavy, pale, hot, painful, stony hard. Local heat gives relief, as does also firm bandaging. The remedy is useful when the breasts become painful before and during menstruation. It is also of value in the lying-in period in relation to milk fever – breasts tense, headache, tearing pains in limbs, great fatigue and desire to lie still.

Urinary System
Urgent micturition is described with cutting pains, and the urine feels hot as passed. It may be dark brown in colour.

Genital System
Pain is felt in the groins before the onset of the menstrual periods. When the period starts, this involves the hypogastrium, and burning pain is felt in the uterus. Suppression of menses is apt to result from overexertion either shortly before or at the time of the period.

Locomotor System
Sticking, stitching, tearing pains occur in the muscles of nape, back and limbs. The pains are so violent that the sufferer cannot keep still, yet when he makes the least movement he cries out with worse pain. Heat gives relief. Arthritis or periarthritis is accompanied by swelling, possibly effusion, and severe pain. The joint affected is pale red and tense. The

least movement causes intense pain. Walking may be interfered with by severe weakness of the muscles of the thighs, also possibly by soreness in soles and heels.

MODALITIES

Aggravation from heat and relief when cold and from cool drinks or cold applications. Any muscular effort causes aggravation, even that required for standing or sitting erect, so much so that the legs seem hardly able to support the body. This is especially noticeable on first rising from sitting, or after a period of rest. Aggravation occurs at 3 a.m. and 9 p.m. A profuse urination may occur at 6 to 7 p.m.

Relief is obtained by lying motionless, also by firm pressure. The sufferer lies on the affected side, as this helps to restrain movement and diminish pain. Free perspiration also affords relief.

CLINICAL NOTES

In acute pulmonary affections Bryonia will follow Aconite with advantage, and in turn may give way to Kali Carb., Pulsatilla or Phosphorus as the symptoms develop.

In fibrositic or arthritic conditions the remedy will often be followed by Rhus Tox. as the symptoms change to the picture of that remedy – that is, pains worse on first movement but relieved by continued movement.

Bryonia is the acute remedy in relation to Natrum Mur. Its complementary remedies in chronic conditions are Alumina and Lycopodium, and in acute illness Sulphur and Sulphur Iod.

Cactus Grandiflorus

SOURCE

The source of this extremely valuable remedy is that somewhat amazing plant *Selenicus grandiflorus,* the night-blooming Cereus. The plant grows wild in Jamaica as a creeper or as a climber. Its succulent cylindrical stems of bluish-green colour are armed with clusters of sharp spines. The curiously short-lived flowers burst forth from the tip of the stem at sundown. Blooming through the night they are withered by the next morning. These flowers are large, up to ten inches in diameter; the petals are white, the lance-shaped sepals are brown on the outer surface and yellow on the inner side; the flowers exhale a quite strong odour redolent of vanilla.

The fleshy fruit is egg-shaped, of vivid orange-red hue, and covered with scaly tubercles. The extremely small seeds have an acid taste. The plant contains a milky acrid juice. The mother tincture is prepared from the more tender stems and the flowers, collected in summer. Tartaric acid is one of the constituents of the plant.

PHARMACOLOGY

Toxic symptoms are described as gastric irritation, mild delirium, hallucinations, mental confusion, diuresis. There is an affinity with the plain muscle of the arteries and with heart muscle, tending to induce spasm.

PROVING

Dr Rubini, of Italy, after observation of the physiological and therapeutic effects of Cactus for twelve years, published a pamphlet relating his experiences, which was translated by Dr Dudgeon for the twenty-second volume of the *British Homoeopathic Journal.*

APPEARANCE

The patient may be found pale, pulseless, panting and prostrate. Or at times, owing to instability of circulatory control, the face may become red and bloated.

PSYCHOLOGY

The subject is usually sad, taciturn, hypochondriacal, desiring solitude and made worse by consolation. At times the suddeness and intensity of the pain may induce a fear of death and despair of recovery. Tears may be profuse.

PHYSIOLOGY

As a result of the extremely labile circulation there may be swirls of blood in one or other direction, producing perhaps a hot head with cold extremities, or sudden localized flushes of heat.

Anorexia may occur associated with nausea. Excessive thirst may accompany fever.

Sleep may be disturbed by violent dreams, perhaps of falling; is apt to wake startled and frightened. Pulsations may interfere with sleep.

Profuse sweats occur in feverish states.

SYMPTOMATOLOGY

General

The most characteristic feature is a sensation of constriction, generalized or local, as if the parts were bound by wires squeezing tighter and tighter. Accompanying pains are shooting, darting or squeezing in character, and so violent as to elicit cries or screams. This sense of constriction may be induced by the slightest contact. There is a tendency to congestive haemorrhage of dark blood which coagulates readily, from nose, lungs, stomach, rectum, bladder or uterus.

Head

Periodic congestive headaches of throbbing nature affect especially the right side or the vertex; they are aggravated by noise, by strong light, by taking food. Firm pressure affords relief. There may be complaint of a feeling of weight pressing on the vertex. Vertigo may be severe, increased by exertion, by stooping, by rising from recumbent posture, by taking a deep breath.

Eyes

Vision may be dim, distant objects appearing blurred.

Respiratory System

The throat feels constricted, with full throbbing carotid vessels; this may amount to globus hystericus, a sensation of a ball or lump in the throat which cannot be shifted either up or down. The whole chest may feel oppressed as by a great weight, or tightly bound as by an iron band. This may cause a frequent desire to take, or attempt to take, a deep breath. Actual suffocating attacks may occur, accompanied by fainting, cold sweat on face and thready or impalpable pulse. Diaphragmatic pleurisy is accompanied by sharp shooting pains and a sensation of a wire or cord bound tightly round the waist. Haemoptysis may occur, associated with throbbing palpitations. There may be acute congestion of the lungs with inability to lie down.

Alimentary System
Spasm of the oesophagus causes dysphagia, or perhaps constant desire to swallow. Pyrosis, vomiting, haematemesis may occur. Pulsations are felt in the stomach. Neuralgic type pains may be felt if an accustomed meal is missed. Sometimes the sufferer complains of a sensation as if being disembowelled. There is often a feeling of painful pressure in the hypogastrium. Constipation occurs with stools which are hard and black. A feeling of constriction in the rectum is accompanied by much ineffectual urging to stool. Piles tend to bleed.

Cardiovascular System
This is the sphere in which the remedy is especially valuable. The heart feels as if constricted by an iron band with accompanying pricking, sticking or anginal pain, perhaps spreading to the left hand. The whole left upper extremity may be numb and tingling. The heart feels as if it had no room to beat. Palpitation is present both day and night and is worse if lying on the left side. The heart action is apt to be very irregular with an intermitting pulse. Pulsations are felt all over the body. Cardiac hypertrophy and failing compensation may be accompanied by oedema, especially of the left hand, foot and leg.

Urinary System
Retention may occur from spasm of the sphincter. Constriction at the neck of the bladder may result in a constant urge, with drop by drop urination. Frequent haematuria may occur, with the formation of clots.

Genital System
Dysmenorrhoea may occur, with violent clutching cramps causing the sufferer to scream with the pain. Cardiac symptoms are aggravated before menstruation starts. The menstrual flow ceases when recumbent.

Locomotor System

Polyarthritic rheumatism occurs, starting usually in the upper extremities. The rheumatic pains are not relieved by rest, by motion or by change of posture. There is much restless unease of the legs.

MODALITIES

Aggravation results from heat, from exposure to direct sun, from damp; is worse often after a meal; also when walking, going upstairs, lying on the left side; peak aggravations occur at 11 a.m. and 11 p.m.

Feels better in the open.

CLINICAL NOTES

The association of the illness with heart symptoms provides the chief indication for the use of the remedy.

Calcarea Carbonica

SOURCE

This extremely important remedy can be classified as of animal source, in association with Sepia and Murex, its aquatic confreres. Just as Sepia is prepared from the dark fluid secreted by the cuttlefish, and Murex from the dried secretion of the purple gland of *Murex*, the purple fish, so this remedy, also known as Calcarea Ostrearum, is prepared from the secretion of *Ostrea edulis*, the oyster.

The source of the remedy, the soft, snowy-white calcareous substance in the middle layer of the oyster's shell, is excreted by the mantle of the mollusc and is in fact a deposit of finely crystalline calcium carbonate.

This mollusc, placed between the snail and the cuttlefish, squats on the ocean bed with the two halves of its shell widely gaping in seemingly indolent inertia. It is, however, capable of one form of movement – if there is the slightest disturbance of the water in its vicinity it closes its shell with vice-like firmness, obviously manifesting a capacity for strong muscular spasm.

It is noteworthy that the Calc. Carb. subject is unduly sessile, exhibits an air of toneless inertia, and covers with a mask of clam-like unresponsiveness the turmoil of fears and anxieties that are seething within. The tightly-shut shell of the oyster conceals the agitation within, which gives rise to the spasmodic closure as a shield for its defencelessness.

As well as manifesting lack of tone and muscular weakness, the Calc. Carb. subject may also present conditions of muscle spasm affecting both skeletal and plain muscle.

PHARMACOLOGY

The predominant mineral form of calcium in nature is the carbonate. As such, next to aluminium and iron, it is the most abundant metal in the earth. Calcium is also the most important inorganic element in the body and occurs in the highest amount. The cyclic fate and behaviour of calcium in the earth and in the body are, on broad lines, analogous. The calcium processes in the body swing either to precipitation, calcium becoming bound in the tissues, or to diffusion, free calcium ions being available for cell-action. Calcium is stored in the skeleton mostly as phosphate and carbonate; the active ions combine as required with bicarbonate, acid phosphates and, to a lesser extent, with chlorides.

Sufficient supplies of calcium, for instance in the form of food additives, lime-water or calcium tablets, do not necessarily guard against disorders of calcium metabolism. Many factors enter into the processes of calcium absorption, assimilation and utilization. It is essential for the calcium to be present in the right proportion to the other members of the metabolic quartet – sodium, potassium and magnesium; these four must be maintained in active equilibrium and, for this, calcium assimilation and excretion must be kept adequately balanced.

Calcium antagonizes sodium and potassium ions, which induce cell colloids to imbibe water. In this way calcium acts as a bar and decreases the permeability of the cell membranes, thus upholding the tone of the cells and preventing them from becoming waterlogged.

Preponderance of calcium, however, makes the exchanges between cells and fluids over-difficult, and thus slows down metabolism. The membranes are altered as it were from filter paper to parchment, and excretion of water and solutes is cut down. Combustion is reduced and the picture of a person with a tissue-blocked calcium imbalance is produced – a sluggish, cold, flabby, pale, pasty, obese, phlegmatic, 'oyster-like' individual.

The retarding depressant action of calcium is also evident in the neuro-muscular sphere. Without the brake imposed by calcium the un-restrained influence of sodium and potassium ions would keep the skeletal muscles in a constant state of hypertonus, resulting in tetany and leading finally to paralysis through exhaustion. Too little circulating calcium is, therefore, as productive of disturbed metabolism as too much. Homoeostasis – electrolyte balance – is the aim, and when this is out of order, Calc. Carb. in potency may be able to restore essential equilibrium.

An understanding of the multiple functions of calcium in the body, or rather of the multiplicity of functions (for they are none too well understood) is a help in appreciating the varied symptomatology presented by this remedy.

Calcium is a main constituent of bone, where it is present in the form of apatite, a crystal lattice composed of calcium carbonate and calcium phosphate, which gives bone its hardness.

Calcium is essential for clotting reactions whether in blood or in milk. In optimal concentration, calcium accelerates the action of several enzymes, but if present in excess it inhibits enzyme activity.

Calcium is also considered to play a leading role in the development of bio-electric potentials, due to the existence of a calcium electrode in the calcium proteinate of the cell cortex. In fact it is likely that the abililty of calcium to combine with proteins to form compounds which occur almost everywhere in the body is the most significant biological property of the element. This accounts for its vital participation in so many physiological activities.

A wide range of disorders may stem from imperfect calcium absorption, distribution or utilization. These include such conditions as inadequate nutrition, inhibited growth and development, imperfect formation of bone, decreased coagulability of blood, increased excitability of nerves and liability to tetany.

The balance of calcium equilibrium in the body may thus swing in either of two directions, towards calcium repletion or towards calcium depletion. Not only do these disorders help to explain the varied symptoms manifested by Calc. Carb. patients, but experience has shown that the remedy administered aptly and in potency can effectively correct the disordered balance and restore health.

PROVING

The first pathogenesis of Calc. Carb. appears in the first edition of Hahnemann's *Chronic Diseases*.

APPEARANCE

The Calc. Carb. subject is often an obese blonde with blue eyes, a pale waxy complexion, pale lips, pale ears and pale fingers, though the face may at times have a red tinge. Sometimes the Calc. Carb. patient may be a thin scrawny brunette with a sallow skin.

Babies appear soft, flabby, pasty-faced and are constantly sweaty about the head.

The Calc. Carb. child appears lethargic, is sessile, stays put wherever dumped by its parent, picks at its fingers, fiddles with small objects. It displays delayed dentition, late closure of fontanelles, hot breath, cud-chewing movements of the lower jaw, possibly signs of rickets. Walking is late and wobbly owing to weakness of muscles.

In general there is an appearance of fatness without fitness. Adolescents show obesity. But some children will be emaciated about the neck and limbs, with a protuberant taut belly.

Poor circulation is evidenced by a hand like a dead fish, cold, clammy, lifeless, lacking grip, and by damp cold feet. The hand may in some cases be soft, warm, moist and feel boneless.

Wide pupils manifest low parasympathetic tone.

Speech may be non-stop, a constant chatter about trivialities of a personal nature, or the subject may relapse into obdurate silence and become almost catatonic.

A noticeable feature is a peculiar sour odour of body, of vomit, of stools.

PSYCHOLOGY

The emotional attributes principally mirror the general retardation deriving from disordered calcium metabolism. The Calc. Carb subject is slow, dull, uninterested and timid, and shuns any form of mental effort. This is not due to inherent laziness but to the inability for effort, which is the affliction rather than the fault of the sufferer.

Children do not like to be laughed at, and if frustrated just give up. They are slow at school, slow at games, get scared in the dark, may see faces in the dark, and are given to night terrors. They may become low-spirited and weepy.

The Calc. Carb subject is apt to be fretful, obstinate, unable to think consecutively or remember things, and becomes quite incapable of arriving at a decision. Mental or any kind of effort causes distress, and this may reach the point where he feels he cannot continue, and quits.

Fear is a marked feature. The Calc. Carb. subject is full of fear — fear of people, fear of the dark, fear of being looked at, fear of solitude, a vague fear of 'scarcely knows what', a growing fear of impending insanity. In this latter condition the sufferer cannot stop thinking about his apprehension, cannot stop talking about it and thinks everybody is looking at him with suspicion.

Another feature is an unresponsiveness, the individual shutting up like a clam and assuming an air of indifference, which is in fact an attempt to camouflage the anxiety and agitation within. He may become discouraged, despairing and disgusted with life.

A state of over-sensitivity may supervene – jumpiness, easily startled at the least noise, exceedingly distressed on hearing of cruelty, scared at the sight of wounds, impulse to scream or indulge in causeless tears.

There may be a tendency to grouse and complain over ancient wrongs, to become peevish, take everything amiss, and develop an unreasoning antipathy towards certain individuals.

Calcarea Carbonica

PHYSIOLOGY

Calcium stagnation impairs heat production in the body. It is not surprising, therefore, that the Calc. Carb. subject is excessively chilly and quite miserable when cold. There is a desire to be well and warmly wrapped up, and an aversion to open air and the least draught. Direct sunlight also is disliked.

Irregular distribution of blood-flow may produce internal heat combined with external chilliness; cold is often felt in patches; feet, normally cold, may, however, burn at night and be pushed around in search of a cool spot or shoved out from under the bed covers – a symptom shared with Chamomilla, Medorrhinum, Pulsatilla and Sulphur. The hands may 'burn' on the dorsal aspect. The Calc. Carb. individual easily becomes over-heated and distressed, and then, on ceasing from activity, quickly feels over-cold.

Hunger is the norm, with a tendency to experience a faint, empty sensation at any hour, perhaps immediately after a meal. There is a fondness for sweet things and often a real craving for eggs, even in children. There is often an aversion to hot food, meat, coffee and tobacco, and to milk, which may disagree.

A peculiar feature in the sphere of appetite is a tendency to odd perversions – the child may eat dirt, coal, chalk, possibly manifesting in this way an impaired calcium assimilation.

Thirst may be marked, but drinking water can cause nausea. Iced water is, however, tolerated better, and preferred.

Sleep is liable to be disturbed by terrifying dreams; children wake from sleep screaming and can scarcely be pacified. The child may sleep-walk, grunt, or grind the teeth in his sleep, and may lie with his hands under his head.

There is often difficulty in getting off to sleep; a flow of anxious thoughts prevent sleep until 2, 3 or 4 a.m.; or sleep may be broken about 3 a.m. and give place to restless tossing.

Sweating is a prominent feature, often excessive and especially marked on the head and feet. This is most evident at night, when the child's pillow will be found quite soaked with perspiration during sleep. Sudden sweats also are liable to occur from exertion or from excitement or fright.

Calcarea Carbonica

SYMPTOMATOLOGY

General

The symptoms associated with this remedy exhibit one or other aspect of disturbed calcium metabolism, the effects of slowed-down functional activity and deficient oxidation of tissues on the one hand, or of hypertonus and hyper-sensitivity on the other. The picture, is one of lack of stamina, very easy fatigue associated with actual muscular weakness and poor development. As the result of this inherent weakness any exertion tends to produce distress in the form of dyspnoea, flushing, headache and general malaise.

Noticeable also is a great liability to catch cold and develop catarrhal troubles. Involvement of mucosal surfaces leads to the formation of polypoid or papillomatous growths, which are liable to bleed.

Head Region

While it is usual for the scalp to feel cold with a desire to have the head warmly wrapped, there may at times be a swirl of blood to the head accompanied by a sensation of burning heat, especially on the vertex. Vertigo is readily induced by extra physical effort or even by mental exertion, owing to the inability of the circulation to cope with increased demand. Headache is common, a tearing or splitting headache above the right eye extending downwards in a wedge towards the nose, or a periodic headache, recurring every seven or fourteen days and accompanied by biliousness. The headache is aggravated by daylight, and relieved by warmth or hot applications and by lying down in a darkened room. A unilateral headache is also described, aggravated by noise and by the effort of talking, and tending to be better by evening. Alopecia occurs, the hair coming out in patches rather than all over the scalp.

Eyes

Eye symptoms may be severe with involvement of the cornea, possibly going on to ulceration and extreme photophobia. Dimness of vision may precede these severe changes, a sensation as if there was a veil or a film before the eyes. The symptoms are much aggravated by any exertion or prolonged use of the eyes for reading or other occupation.

Ears

Catarrhal involvement of the middle ear may lead to perforation of the drum, with chronic discharge, thick, yellow and mucopurulent in type and liable to exacerbation from every exposure to cold. Regional lymph nodes are often involved, and eruptions may break out on the pinna or behind the ear.

Respiratory System

As already mentioned there is an undue liability to colds. These tend to be accompanied by sore throat of an obstinate type with enlarged tonsils and involvement of cervical lymph nodes. Colds tend also to extend downwards and cause hoarseness of voice, which is painless, and worse in the morning. There may be complaint of a feeling as if a lump was lodged in the left side of the throat. Nasal catarrh may become very chronic with soreness of the nose, swollen ulcerated mucosa and thick yellow discharge with presence of crusts. Nasal polyps may develop. A persistent tickling cough is likely to be especially tiresome at night, or cough may be productive with copious, thick, yellow, sweetish-tasting sputum, possibly stained with blood. Respiration may be rattling from excess of mucus, and the chest is apt to feel as if it were too full of blood.

Alimentary System

An unpleasant sour taste in the mouth is accompanied by foetor oris. Burning pain may be felt at the tip of the tongue. The digestion seems sluggish with a tendency to frequent sour eructations or even sour vomiting. There is a curious repugnance to hot food, a good deal of heartburn, and possibly a cutting pain deep to the right scapula, with spread to the right hypochondrium and epigastrium. The latter area is often quite tender to touch. Stubborn constipation may be present with pasty, clay-coloured stools, and associated sensations of crawling, burning and weight in the rectum. Recurrent diarrhoea is common, worse in the afternoon with whitish, watery, frequent stools, having a sour pungent odour and liable to cause excoriation of the perianal skin. The stool often contains curds and undigested food particles. The remedy has value in relation to tabes mesenterica, as well as in helminthiasis.

Lymphatic and Glandular Systems

Lymph nodes in various sites become enlarged, indurated, with burning and stinging pains. Masses of matted nodes can be palpated, especially in the cervical regions and in the mesentery. The lymphadenitis is often tuberculous in nature.

Cardiovascular System

In association with the general state of asthenia, cardiac response to effort is poor, and exertion such as going up stairs is accompanied by dyspnoea and palpitation. There is a liability to attacks of faintness while walking out of doors. Veins show varicosity, and varicose lesions are associated with much burning discomfort.

Urinary System
Cystitis is associated with dark, brownish-coloured urine which has a peculiarly unpleasant sour pungent odour.

Genital System
Menstrual periods tend to be previous, profuse, prolonged – too long and too strong. A period may be precipitated prematurely either by emotional stress or physical exertion. The breasts are apt to swell and be painful before the period and while it is continuing; dysmenorrhoea is characterized by cramping uterine pains and also general stomach pains. Pain in the region of the right ovary is apt to extend into the thigh, and is worse when reading or writing. Leucorrhoea is profuse, the thick discharge being accompanied by itching, burning and smarting. There is a tendency to develop uterine or vaginal polyps which bleed easily.

Nervous System
Calc. Carb. is mentioned in connection with convulsions which occur during the night, also with attacks of epilepsy preceded by a peculiar aura, as if a mouse was running up the arm or leg. Paraesthesia may be complained of – pricking, darting sensations, quivering of muscles, a feeling of 'cold, damp stockings on the feet', feeling as if 'the part would burst'.

Locomotor System
The muscular weakness militates against any prolonged effort. Lifting has to be avoided for fear of spraining a muscle. The ankles are weak and readily turn over. Spinal muscles are weak, leading to faulty position when sitting and encouraging spinal curvature. Cramp is liable to occur at night, especially in the calf muscles. Rheumatic pains in the limbs are associated with much stiffness. Joints may become hot and swollen. Gouty affections of small joints with nodule formation are met with. Post-rachitic deformities may be present. Disorders of bone metabolism may occur, especially formation of exostoses.

Skin
Chronic urticaria is mentioned in connection with Calc. Carb., also warts and papillomatous growths. The skin cracks easily, forming 'chaps'. Warning is given against the use of ointments and bandaging in skin complaints of Calc. Carb. children. The excess calcium is seeking a way out of the body through the skin and must not be dammed back.

MODALITIES

Aggravation is caused by any contact with cold air, by draughts, by a change from warm to cold weather, in wet weather and by contact with cold water. There is also aggravation before and during the menstrual period, from the standing posture and when a limb is allowed to hang down, all of which cause embarrassment of the circulation. Chronologically symptoms tend to be worse after midnight, and also at full moon.

There is amelioration in warm, dry weather, when lying on the same side as the lesion and, curiously enough, when constipated.

CLINICAL NOTES

This remedy affords a good example of the importance of treating the patient and not prescribing by disease label. It is the patient-picture of Calc. Carb., especially the constitutional and mental manifestations, that is the chief guide to its use.

Bryonia should not directly precede or follow Calc. Carb. Belladonna is its complementary remedy in acute exacerbations. Rhus Tox. or Pulsatilla may be indicated in sequence to the remedy, but it should not be followed by Nitric Acid or Sulphur. A satisfactory sequence is Calc. Carb.→Lycopodium→Sulphur.

In association with pyaemic abscesses in the deep tissues it is said to be able to induce resorption of pus.

Too frequent repetition in old people is unwise, but the remedy can be repeated quite frequently in children if called for.

Calcarea Fluorica

SOURCE

This remedy is prepared from calcium fluoride, fluorspar. In the body, crystals of this very insoluble salt are found in masses in the Haversian canals. These increase the hardness and brittleness of bone. It also occurs in the enamel of teeth, in elastic tissues and in the epidermis.

PHARMACOLOGY

The affinity with the above-mentioned tissues carries a liability to the formation of exostoses, enlargement of glands and lymph nodes with stony hard induration, and the development of varicosities and distended veins.

PROVING

Calcarea Fluorica was proved on three persons in the 15th potency by Dr J.H. Bell.

APPEARANCE

There are no special appearances, apart from the presence of an obvious swelling in the jaws or other site.

PSYCHOLOGY

The patient is likely to be obsessed with the fear of financial ruin and consequent poverty. Indecision is characteristic, with inability to come to a decision about anything, more so in relation to insignificant matters than to important issues.

PHYSIOLOGY

The only matter referred to in this category is sleep, which is frequently disturbed by nightmares; the subject wakes suddenly with a feeling as if threatened by immediate danger.

SYMPTOMATOLOGY

General

Pains are described as shooting or stabbing, aggravated by cold or by humidity and relieved by warmth. There may be a history of syphilis, congenital or acquired.

Head

Headache is associated with nausea and a tendency to fainting in the afternoon. A sensation as of a creaking or straining sound in the head may be noticed, especially at night.

Eyes

Spots or sparks may be seen before the eyes after writing. The eyeballs may be painful; relief is obtained by closing the eyes and pressing firmly.

Ears

Otosclerosis.

Respiratory System

Nasal discharge, which is copious, thick, offensive and greenish yellow in colour, may be associated with bony lesions. Post-nasal discharge may also be present. The throat is excessively dry with much burning and feeling of suffocation; this is made worse by cold drinks and is also worse in the evening. Warm drinks afford relief. Laughing or reading aloud is apt to cause hoarseness. A hacking cough may result from a tiresome tickle in the larynx as if a foreign body were impacted there; coughing gives no relief. Stabbing pain occurs in paroxysms at the level of the right hypochondrium, under the seventh rib; this tends to wake the subject about midnight; the pain is aggravated by lying on the affected side.

Alimentary System

Teeth are deficient in enamel. The mouth is very dry. Food may be vomited undigested. Flatulence is excessive, associated with urgent call to stool. Stabbing pain in the region of the liver is worse when sitting, but relieved when lying down at night; it may come on at about 8 a.m. Diarrhoea occurs in gouty subjects. Constipation is asssociated with vertigo and dull headache. Severe itching at the anus may wake from sleep; this is apt to alternate with the tickling laryngeal cough.

Lymphatic and Glandular Systems
Cervical lymph nodes may be enlarged and stony hard. Indurated lumps occur in the breasts.

Cardiovascular System
Varicosities may occur. Varicose ulcer may be present.

Urinary System
Passage of urine down the urethra causes smarting, especially at the external meatus.

Genital System
Hydrocele may be present. Indurated nodules occur in the testes. Menses are excessive, and associated with shooting pains in the hypogastrium and down the thighs. Bearing-down or dragging pains affect the uterus and thighs. Prolapsus uteri may be present.

Locomotor System
There is a liability for recurrence of low back pain from the least strain; the pain is worse for rest, but eased by movement and warmth. Joints may crack or develop a chronic hydrarthrosis. There is a tendency to easy dislocation.

Skin
The skin is harsh and dry; liable to chaps and fissures, especially in the palms of the hands. Scars become unhealthy and may break down.

MODALITIES

There is aggravation of symptoms when at rest; as the result of a change in the weather; in damp humid conditions; from cold; in a draught.

Is better from heat; from warm applications; taking warm drinks; when moving about; by being massaged.

CLINICAL NOTES

The special sphere of the remedy is in relation to bone lesions, especially exostoses. Induration of stony hardness in any type of lesion suggests the use of the remedy.

A complementary remedy is Syphilinum.

Calcarea Phosphorica

SOURCE

The remedy is prepared from a mixture of tribasic and other phosphates of lime, obtained by the addition of dilute phosphoric acid to lime water; the result is a relatively insoluble tasteless white powder. It is of note that apatite crystals, which form about one-third of the mass of bones, are composed mainly of calcium carbonate and calcium phosphate.

PHARMACOLOGY

There is affinity with tissues concerned with growth and cell repair, inducing a tendency to deficient assimilation, impaired nutrition, delayed development, poor memory and brittle bones.

PROVING

Calc. Phos. was proved by Hering.

APPEARANCE

A pale, sickly child, rather tall for its age; skin is waxy and dirty-looking. Adenoid facies. Large, unclosed fontanelles.

The child may be thin, even emaciated; scarcely able to stand; slow in learning to walk; head inclined to wobble; belly scaphoid; legs tottery; spine scoliotic.

Much involuntary sighing; child may scream and grasp head with hands.

Old people stagger about on rising from sitting.

There is a sour body odour.

PSYCHOLOGY

The child is nervy, sensitive, timid. Is a slow starter, but may have spurts of brilliance; has a bad temper; wants to be left alone; shows contrariness – when out-of-doors wants to return home, when at home wants to go out.

Has a desire for change of scene; requires constant watching – may show an almost insane desire to go off alone.

Memory is poor; there is difficulty in making sustained mental effort; consequently dreads mental exertion. Is apt to use wrong words in speaking and writing.

Mental or emotional strain or stress may precipitate an illness. Child may become sick as the result of disappointment or vexation.

PHYSIOLOGY

The subject is chilly and feels the cold.

There is a craving for bacon, ham, especially the rind, also for salted and smoked meats, and savouries. Appetite may be ravenous round about 4 p.m. Appetite may be lost just before and during menstruation.

There is a desire for cold drinks but these disagree, as do also ice-cream and fruit.

Is drowsy by day, but sleepless at night up to about midnight; dreams are very vivid; may start from sleep in fear; is heavy with sleep at time for rising.

Copious sweats occur at night, possibly on single parts.

SYMPTOMATOLOGY

General

There is general weakness, deriving from imperfect nutrition, associated with evidence of delayed development. Pains of rheumatic type are widespread; often located in small areas. Children complain of growing pains in muscles. Symptoms are often left-sided.

Head

Vertigo is worse on rising from sitting, when walking in cold air, from mental or physical exertion. School-children complain of a dull head-ache, aggravated by the least jar or jolt, even by the pressure of hat; it is worse when out of doors and from physical exertion. It is better when quiet and alone; washing the face and head in cold water also gives relief. Children develop headache from watching television. A rheumatic type of headache involves the whole head; it is worse in cold air, from a cold wind, when walking, from exertion and at night. A headache on the vertex is associated with a sensation as if a cake of ice were melting on the top of the head.

Eyes
There is a sensation of a foreign body in the eye, accompanied by a desire to rub the eye constantly. Finds it difficult to read; light hurts; lachrymation is aggravated by yawning.

Ears
Tearing pain in ears is worse when the weather turns cold. Sudden swelling of external ear with associated eczema. Discharge from ear excoriates the skin. Tinnitus.

Respiratory System
Clear fluid runs from the nose in a cold room, but stops in warm air or out of doors. The nasal discharge may be blood-stained, as with Phosphorus. Blowing the nose may cause epistaxis. The nose may be swollen with sore nostrils. Large pedunculated nasal polypi may be present. Every cold settles in the tonsils, which become enlarged, perhaps chronically so; the throat is sore and relaxed; swallowing is painful; throat feels constricted. Accumulation of mucus in throat causes hawking and hoarseness. A dry hacking cough comes on in fits and starts both by day and at night. It starts with hoarseness, is aggravated in cold weather and tends to be better when lying down. A feeling of suffocation comes on from even slight exertion, as when going up stairs. Stitching pains occur in the chest, especially at the level of the 5th and 6th ribs and in the cardiac area. There may be much rattling in the chest with difficulty in raising sputum, which is yellow. Chest symptoms may alternate with anal fistula.

Alimentary System
Delayed dentition is associated with teething complaints. Teeth are very soft; easy caries. Upper lip becomes swollen, painful, indurated and burning. Tongue is swollen, stiff, covered with little pimples or tiny blisters which burn. There is a disgusting taste in the mouth. The child vomits milk persistently, whether breast milk or artificially prepared milk. It suffers from colic after every feed. The stools are green, slimy, undigested, accompanied by the passage of much foetid flatus. Cholera infantum may supervene. Every attempt to eat is followed by belly-ache, which is worse if cold food is taken; there is relief by belching and by the passage of flatus. The belly wall is soft and flaccid. Heartburn comes on about one hour after a meal; nausea can be induced by taking coffee or by smoking. Epigastric pain may spread to the spine. Vexation may bring on an attack of diarrhoea with hot watery stools or spluttery green stools,

possibly containing offensive pus. Diarrhoea can be brought on by cold drinks or accompany dentition. Constipation may occur with very hard stools. Piles are present in the elderly patient. Anal fissure or fistula may occur; this may alternate with chest symptoms.

Lymphatic and Glandular Systems
Involvement of lymph nodes is common in children; it may become chronic.

Nervous System
Numbness may be a feature, either localized numb areas or a more general numb feeling all over. The tongue may feel numb. This sensation of numbness is likely to be accompanied by a feeling of paresis.

Urinary System
Enuresis is associated with debility. Urine passed may be copious and pale. Cutting sensation is felt in the urethra before and after urination.

Genital System
There is premenstrual pain with uterine cramps. Menses are early, copious, with bright red blood. Leucorrhoea occurs both day and night; the discharge resembles egg-white; is worse in the morning after rising; has a sweetish odour. Libido is increased in both sexes.

Locomotor System
Pains in neck and back are worse in cold, stormy weather, worse in the morning, from getting in a draught, from lifting or other strain. Rheumatic pains in limbs are worse from wet weather and are aggravated by movement. They occur especially in spring and autumn and are accompanied by a cold or numb sensation in the joints. The pains shoot along the muscles into the joints. Warmth and rest afford relief. Sacro-iliac pain as if 'broken' spreads to the lower limbs, accompanied by sensations of cold and numbness; it is worse at any change in weather, and when snow is melting. Mention is also made of pain at the root of the fingernails; fingers feel paralysed; hands tremble.

Skin
Acne is common in adolescents, especially young girls. Eczema may occur on scalp and external ear.

MODALITIES

Aggravating factors are cold wet; change of weather; east winds; melting snow; movement and exertion; dwelling upon symptoms.

There is amelioration in warm dry weather; when resting; from a really hot bath.

CLINICAL NOTES

The remedy is of special value in complaints of children and adolescents. It has been used for tonic effect and vies with Symphytum in relation to non-union of fractures.

Complementary remedies are Carbo Animalis, China, Natrum Mur., Ruta, Sulphur, Sulphur Iodatum.

Cannabis Indica

SOURCE

This remedy is prepared from Indian hemp, *Cannabis sativa*, a hallucinogenic plant widely distributed in use as indicated by its numerous names – Hashish, Bhang, Kif, Ganja, Dagga, Marijuana – to mention but a sample.

The Ismaili sect contacted by the Crusaders in the eleventh and twelfth centuries were a contemporary Murder Inc. society, known as the Hashishin or Hashish-eaters, the Assassins. The drug was employed to key their young bloods up to their nefarious job of political assassinations, carried out with fanatical ruthlessness and a reckless disregard of death. Later the drug was used by the Zulus to 'inspire' the Impi hordes in their terrible marauding raids, when whole communities were massacred at the point of the spear. In Basutoland* dagga was a known companion of witchcraft, responsible for ritual murder carried out with unmentionable savagery.

Down the ages, therefore, the drug has been eaten, drunk and smoked as a means of attaining a state of narcosis with colourful and fantastic visions. It is widely indulged in today in the form of cigarettes or reefers. Although not such a binding drug of addiction as opium and its derivatives it is nevertheless a drug of menace, owing to the unpredictability of its effects and the fact that its use may lead to more serious types of drug addiction.

The plant is well known in Persia, Bokhara, and the East Indies. It will grow, however, in almost any garden. The most powerful plants are found at heights of 6,000 to 10,000 feet in the Himalayas. A tough, rather untidy-looking plant, its angular stem may reach a height of twelve feet. The large palmate leaves have five long lance-shaped deeply serrated leaflets; the greenish, rather small flowers are peculiar in that pollen and seed flowers are found on separate plants. The fruit is a small seed.

For preparation of the mother tincture, the dried flowering or fruiting tops of the female plant are used; they contain a resin, a phenoaldehyde (cannabinol) which is presumably the constituent responsible for the effects of the drug.

*Now Lesotho, Eds.

127

PHARMACOLOGY

The drug has, of course, a strong affinity with the central nervous system, especially the higher psychic centres. It is characteristically pleomorphic in its effects, which may vary in type from abysmal gloom to celestial bliss, and which may switch with alarming suddenness from a state of peaceful contemplation to one of uncontrollable agitation.

It is interesting that the experiences induced by the drug are largely determined by the mental calibre of the recipient. In intellectuals it can produce a state of double consciousness, with the ability to abandon themselves to their illusions and at the same time observe their experience objectively. But after larger doses this control may be lost, with the result that senseless and even violent behaviour may ensue.

With regard to these illusions, they may differ from one person to another. The room may expand, the floor tilt. Atmospheric phenomena, such as vapour and opacity, arise. Colours become brighter, objects more beautiful. Everything appears to be bathed in radiant light. The affected person suddenly forgets what he has been talking about. He is incapable of clothing his thoughts in words. The situation may become so compellingly hilarious that the hashish eater becomes incapable for minutes at a time of doing anything but laugh. His usual way of expressing himself, his facial expression, his gestures, his whole motor activity is changed. Thus the record of two experimental observers.

Prolonged usage has indubitably deleterious effects. The chronic dagga smoker is described as a tired, listless person with sunken eyes, which are always shining. He is usually morose, but will often react violently when suddenly aroused. In course of time the addict loses all power of thought or concentration, and he may end in becoming a psychotic.

PROVING

Some provings of Indian hemp, made with the tincture and lower attenuations, were published by the American Provers Union in 1839.

APPEARANCE

The patient looks weary and exhausted, or perhaps drowsy and stupid. The pupils are dilated and the eyes have a fixed look. The face is hot and flushed or else pale and moist. Eyes are red and injected.

There may be frequent involuntary shaking of the head. Speech is incoherent; he is apt to lose the thread and be unable to finish the sentence. There is a tendency to pointless uncontrollable laughter.

PSYCHOLOGY

A great variety of disturbances may be encountered in this sphere.

These include absent-mindedness, fixed ideas, horror of darkness, fear of death, fear of going mad, intense anguish of mind.

Euphoric ecstasy may alternate rapidly with deep depression. All perceptions, sensations and emotions are exaggerated to the utmost degree. Distances seem infinite and time endless; surroundings are distorted; colours have increased brilliance.

Hallucinations abound, both visual and auditory. There is a sense of duality – the soul seems separated from the body – the voice is not one's own. Body-sense is altered – limbs or parts seem inordinately large; the whole body seems light with a sensation of levitation.

Dream states alternate with rationality. All mental symptoms are relieved when walking out of doors.

PHYSIOLOGY

The subject cannot stand heat in any form and is apt to feel faint in a hot stuffy atmosphere, but is also liable to sensations of heat or cold in various sites, possibly with actual shuddering.

Appetite is often ravenous and there is excessive thirst for cold water. There may, however, be a fear of drinking.

Drowsiness is prominent, and sleep tends to be noisy and accompanied by grinding of the teeth. The sleeper is apt to be woken by a sudden jerking of the limbs or by a sensation as if something exploded inside the head.

Perspiration is profuse and of sticky consistency.

SYMPTOMATOLOGY

General
A prominent feature is excessive lassitude; there is an overwhelming desire to lie down in the daytime and a complete disinclination for any kind of effort. The subject becomes fatigued after even a short walk.

Head
Vertigo is common, associated with a stunning pain in the occiput and a tendency to fall over on rising from sitting or lying down. The head feels heavy and confused; there may be a deep throbbing type of headache. A variety of odd sensations may be experienced – the skin of the face feels

tightly drawn over the bones; blood is boiling and streaming up into the head; the head is held in an iron cap; the skin of the scalp is taut and compressing the skull; the skull is alternately opening and shutting.

Eyes
Vision is disturbed; it is impossible to read print as the letters all run together. Pressure may be felt in the orbit.

Ears
An unpleasant feeling of fullness is associated with bangings and buzzings.

Respiratory System
The nose is very dry. Discomforts of different types have been recorded in the chest, together with dyspnoea of greater or lesser degree.

Alimentary System
Much white, thick, viscid saliva is present in the mouth; mouth and throat are so dry that there is a constant desire for cold drinks. Pain in the epigastrium is eased by pressure. Pinching and cutting pains occur in the belly, associated with much distension. The belly feels 'full of water'. Painless yellow diarrhoea may be present. A curious sensation noticed at the anus is as if sitting on a hard ball that fills the whole perineum and presses on the posterior urethra.

Cardiovascular System
There are variable disturbances of cardiac rhythm. The pulse may be full and bounding with rate increased up to 120-160 beats per minute, or it may be quite slow at 40 to 50 beats per minute.

Urinary System
Burning and smarting occur before, during and after passage of urine, and the act is accompanied by much straining. Dribbling may occur after completion of the act. Much slimy mucus may be present in the urine or it may be copious in amount and almost colourless. Pain may be felt in the region of the right kidney, and laughing may cause pain in the loins.

Genital System
Libido is increased. Dysmenorrhoea occurs with profuse flow of dark blood but without clots.

Locomotor System

Cramp-like pains are felt in the limbs. Pain across the shoulders causes the sufferer to bend forward and walk with a stoop. Limbs feel almost too heavy to lift up, weak also, and knees are inclined to give way. Movements become tremulous and co-ordination poor, so that it is difficult to hold objects firmly. Agreeable thrillings are felt in the limbs.

Skin

Paraesthesias occur – numbness, even anaesthesia – sensation as if being bitten by insects or as if birds' feet were clawing onto the knees.

MODALITIES

Aggravation in the dark; from noise; from taking liqueur or coffee; by contact with tobacco smoke; when lying on the right side; when urinating; in the morning.

The subject feels better when lying down in the quiet; also in the open air or when using cold water.

CLINICAL NOTES

The remedy obviously has a field of usefulness in certain psychotic states. It also has genito-urinary application. It has proved of value in delirium tremens.

Cantharis

SOURCE

This remedy is prepared from the Spanish fly, or blister beetle, used formerly as a vesicant and also employed, sometimes with dire results, as an aphrodisiac. The insect is a small beetle, 1–2cm in length, of an iridescent brilliant green or bluish-green lustre. It is found in large quantities on trees and shrubs of the olive and honeysuckle families growing in southern and central Europe and western Asia. It has a strong odour and the taste is pungent and acrid. Workers who collect the beetles in June and July wear masks for protection.

The mother tincture is prepared from the dried powdered insect. The main active principle is cantharidin; uric, formic and acetic acids are also present.

PHARMACOLOGY

The drug is a violent irritant with a special affinity for the urinary tract, the lower bowel and the skin. It causes severe inflammation accompanied by a marked tendency to the formation of blisters.

PROVING

Cantharis was proved by Hahnemann, and published in his *Lesser Writings*.

APPEARANCE

The sufferer requiring the remedy may present a red, flaming hot visage with staring eyes or, at a later stage, pallor with a sunken, collapsed appearance – facies Hippocratica.

A restless unease causes a constant change of position. The patient may be continually moaning or crying.

PSYCHOLOGY

The mental state may be one of confusion; has strange ideas; thoughts run riot. Or the state may be one of frenzy, delirium, wild excitement, furious rage, and especially sexual frenzy.

There may be sudden loss of consciousness with ensuing stupor.

The mental condition is aggravated by looking at dazzling light or bright objects, also from slight touch on the larynx or any attempt to swallow liquids.

PHYSIOLOGY

The subject feels 'on fire' and the surface is hypersensitive. In the stage of prostration, internal burning is associated with external coldness and shuddering.

The appetite may be affected with extreme aversion to food and tobacco. Great thirst is present from the burning in the throat, but there is aversion to drinking, owing to spasm of the muscles of deglutition which occurs with any attempt to swallow fluids.

Drowsiness is likely during the daytime, but at night sleep may be prevented by the intensity of the symptoms.

Cold sweat may be present on hands, feet and genitals; the sweat has a uriniferous odour.

SYMPTOMATOLOGY

General

The onset of symptoms is sudden, and progress rapid. The most characteristic feature is the burning nature of the pains in whatever site is affected. The picture is one of great violence and severity associated with prostration; urinary symptoms accompany any illness present as a prominent feature. Discharges from mucous surfaces are stringy and tenacious, and haemorrhage is a frequent complication. A seven-day periodicity in the recurrence of symptoms may be observed.

Head

Headache is violent, lancinating, burning, throbbing or stabbing in nature. It may seem to originate in the nape of the neck; it is relieved somewhat when walking about.

Eyes

An acute burning conjunctivitis is associated with yellow vision.

Respiratory System

The throat is inflamed with much burning, rawness and a sensation of constriction, this latter is felt especially on attempts to swallow fluids. Membrane formation may indicate the use of the remedy in diphtheria.

Involvement of the air passages is accompanied by profuse, tenacious, ropy sputum. Pleurisy with effusion may be present. Gangrenous pneumonitis is accompanied by much burning in the chest with putrid, thin, sanious sputum.

Alimentary System

The tongue may be covered with vesicles, deeply furred and red at the edges. Violent burnings are felt in the stomach, possibly accompanied by blood-streaked vomit. Cutting, burning pains in the belly cause the sufferer to bend double in search of relief. The abdomen is distended and tender, and peritonitis may be present. Diarrhoea or frank dysentery is associated with blood-stained, watery, excoriating stools and severe rectal tenesmus. An urge to stool may accompany urination.

Cardiovascular System

Palpitation occurs, associated with a feeble, irregular pulse. There is a liability to syncope. Pericarditis may be present with effusion.

Urinary System

This is the most noteworthy sphere of action of the remedy. Urinary distress is acute with frequency, urgency, and strangury. Burning and cutting pains are felt in bladder and urethra before, during and after the passage of urine. Similar pains may be felt in the kidney region, accompanied by tenderness, and along the course of the ureter. Such symptoms as described above may accompany acute nephritis or acute cystitis.

Genital System

Intense sexual excitement may occur in either sex. In men this may be associated with violent priapism, and cutting pains along the spermatic cords and down the penis. In women burning pain may be felt in the region of the ovaries.

Locomotor System

Stiffness and rigidity are felt in the nape of the neck. Pains in the limbs are associated with weakness and, possibly, oedematous swelling.

Skin

Vesicular or erysipeloid eruptions occur; blisters may be large and extensive with much burning.

MODALITIES

The condition is aggravated by movement, touch and drinking fluids, especially coffee.

There is some amelioration by warmth, as the result of belching or the passage of flatus, and at night.

CLINICAL NOTES

Involvement of the urinary system is a strong indication for the use of the remedy, especially if accompanied by burning.

The remedy taken internally relieves pain in scalds and burns, also in gnat bites and in sunburn.

Carbo Vegetabilis

SOURCE

This remedy is prepared from black charcoal – 'The charcoal obtained from any kind of wood which has been heated to a red heat to drive off the gases'. Hahnemann is reported to have used charcoal made from birch wood. More recently carefully-selected beech wood has been used, duly carbonized in a closed mortar.

Charcoal in the crude state is medicinally inert, though it has uses as a deodorant, a preservative and an absorbent of intestinal gas. It is not pure carbon, containing traces of mineral salts, notably potassium carbonate.

The first three centesimal potencies are prepared by trituration, one hour being expended over each procedure.

PHARMACOLOGY

Widely distributed through nature, carbon is also widely distributed throughout the body in a great variety of organic and inorganic combinations. When activated by trituration and subsequent succussion, with accompanying sub division, Carbo Veg. shows a number of affinities with various tissues of the body. Predominantly the circulation is affected, with loss of tone in the blood vessel walls, resulting stasis and consequent lack of oxygen and excess of carbon dioxide in the blood and tissues. One result of this is an impaired resistance to infection. A further result is a tendency to haemorrhages of dark coloured blood which does not readily coagulate.

Mucous membranes become catarrhal with a liability to bleeding and ulcer formation. Hypotonus in the plain muscle of the wall of the gut induces an extreme degree of flatulence. Glands and lymph nodes become enlarged and indurated.

PROVING

A pathogenesis of Carbo Veg. appears in the sixth volume of Hahnemann's *Materia Medica Pura*.

APPEARANCE

The impairment and hypoxia of the circulation is manifested by a purple, dusky discoloration of the face, or by pallor associated with blueness of the lips.

Circulatory instabililty is evidenced by a tendency to easy flushing, especially as the result of taking even a small quantity of wine or eating spicy food.

The eyes have a lacklustre appearance; the veins are prominent and sagging; there is a general puffiness; movements are awkward and clumsy owing to the state of general debility.

The picture may be one of frank collapse – face pinched, lips livid, surface covered with cold sweat, tongue and breath cold, marked air hunger, loss of voice, corpse-like appearance.

The skin around ulcers has a mottled look, and all discharges are foul-smelling.

PSYCHOLOGY

The asthenia associated with the remedy is manifested mentally and emotionally in various ways. The subject is listless, lazy, torpid, indifferent, too inert to take interest in anything, or on the other hand may be irritable and excitable with quick changes of humour. This latter phase is most likely to be noticed at night or after dinner.

There is aversion to the dark. Anxiety in the dark may be so acute that the sufferer does not dare to lie down and close his eyes. Fear of ghosts is a prominent feature.

There is difficulty with thought. The head feels confused, ideas flow slowly, memory is poor, tends to forget things almost immediately. Little wonder, therefore, that one author mentions lack of poise and lack of aptitude for speaking in public. He also refers to faint-heartedness, despair to the point of tears, sadness to such a degree as not wanting to live, even the urge to suicide.

PHYSIOLOGY

The Carbo Veg. subject is essentially chilly, a veritable block of ice – cold hands, cold feet, cold nose, cold ears, cold tongue, cold breath, and especially cold knees. But with this surface coldness there may be complaints of internal heat, notably in the chest.

Whereas the coldness related to Calc. Carb. is due to retarded combustion and defective nutrition, in the case of this remedy it derives from retarded circulation and defective oxygenation.

In relation to food there may be a desire for acids, coffee, sweets, salt and rich things, associated with a dislike of digestible food, meat and milk. Digestion is impaired and even plain food may disagree. Fat is especially liable to cause hepatic embarrassment.

Thirst tends to be absent in fever during hot spells, but during chills there is a desire for cold water.

Profuse cold sweats occur, especially on face and limb, but afford no relief.

Sleep is haunted by anxieties and horrors, and accompanied by twitching and jerking. Apt to wake feeling worried and bathed in cold perspiration; is afraid to go to sleep again and, if he does, wakes unrefreshed.

SYMPTOMATOLOGY

General

This remedy manifests an extreme degree of debility, both somatic and psychic. A lack of vital reactivity is very evident, associated with a general lack of tone and poor circulation. Burning pains are common and there is a great desire for air, especially air in motion. Haemorrhages of dark, fluid blood may occur, in frequent small amounts or in a very persistent oozing from inflamed or ulcerated surfaces in nose, lungs, stomach, rectum, uterus or the skin. There is a marked tendency to degenerative processes associated with tissue destruction and putridity. The exhaustion and debility, most marked in the morning or on the least exertion, and associated with much stretching, yawning and cold extremities, present a picture of hypoxia.

Head

A whirling, confused feeling is common in the head. Headache is often frontal extending to the eyes, or occipital. It is distensive in type with sensations as if 'the scalp was too tight', or 'the head could not be lifted from the pillow', or 'head was heavy as lead', or even 'head feels like the morning after'. Also described is a throbbing headache in the temples, associated with a 'tight band' sensation and relieved to some extent by firm pressure. There may be tearing pains in the jaws and ears. Headache tends to be aggravated by the pressure of a hat, from any exertion, or even by moving the head. There is a desire to have the head warmly wrapped up. The remedy may be indicated for headache in children who are sluggish, slow at lessons, scared to sleep alone, and afraid to go into a dark room. The scalp is apt to be sore and to itch. Alopecia may be marked. ⁻

Eyes

Burning pains may be felt in the eyes, which as already mentioned have a lacklustre look. The pupils are sluggish and non-reactive to light. Lids feel heavy and margins of lids often itch.

Ears

The remedy may be called for in chronic otitis media associated with a watery, excoriating, very smelly discharge. It may have dated from an attack of scarlet fever or malaria. The ears may feel stuffed up, and tinnitus is common.

Respiratory System

There is a liability to coryza with much sneezing and a watery discharge, both during the day and at night. This is often associated with bouts of epistaxis of thin, dark, almost black blood which shows little tendency to clot. The bleeding may be induced by blowing the nose, by a sudden jar or even by straining at stool. Crawling and tickling sensations may occur in the nose, accompanied by ineffectual attempts at sneezing. Nasal catarrh is usually associated with general malaise; a warm room causes distress and sweating, a cold room produces shivering and a feeling of severe unease. The nose feels cold and tends to be red at the tip. Colds often spread to the throat with rawness, burning sensation and hoarseness. The condition is aggravated by talking, by coughing and by attempts to clear the throat. It is also worse in damp, humid air and in the evening. There may be associated sensations of crawling and tickling in the throat, or a feeling as if the throat was full of sulphur fumes.

A further spread downwards will result in a teasing cough, and foul-tasting sputum which is at first thin, but later becomes thick and yellowish-green in colour. The cough may become paroxsymal with much gagging and vomiting, associated with redness of the face, and relieved by contact with cold air. Dyspnoea of suffocating type may occur with inability to lie down. There is a distressing feeling of weakness in the chest and a desire for air or to be fanned. As with Antimonium Tart., the cough may be rattling with tough, mucopurulent sputum which is difficult to raise, and Carbo Veg. may be called for when the former remedy has failed to give relief, especially if the sputum is foetid in type. Another indication is actual oedema of lungs with cyanosis. It may be needed in the presence of bronchitis or asthma, or both combined, especially in old people. With asthma, the sufferer has to sit by an open window and complains of great distress and a feeling of extreme exhaustion, or even collapse. The asthma is worse in warm, damp weather and at night; it is associated with much bloating in the belly and some relief from bringing up wind. Actual haemoptysis is accompanied by an anxious appearance but no restless tossing. It is likely to be associated with a burning sensation in the chest as from 'a glowing coal'.

Alimentary System

Asthenia may be evidenced by quivering of the upper lip, which is apt to become swollen. Other signs of tissue-degeneration are rapid caries of teeth, spongy, bleeding gums, separation of gums from teeth, associated with increased salivation and foetor oris. Teeth may feel 'too long' and be sore; the pain is aggravated by both heat and cold. Multiple small ulcers may occur in the mouth and throat, which cause much pain when attempting to swallow. The remedy may be called for in relation to the ill-effects of over-indulgence in food and drink. There is queasy nausea in the morning, waterbrash, burning in the stomach, constant belching, marked flatulence with the passage of offensive flatus. The condition is aggravated by lying down and about half an hour after meals; belching gives some relief; the eructations taste rancid.

Flatus may become incarcerated, especially below the left costal margin, at the splenic flexure of the colon. There are colicky cramping pains accompanied by dyspnoea and rumblings, and the pains radiate upwards into the thorax. Morning diarrhoea may occur with watery stools and much straining. Cholera Infantum may provide occasion for the use of the remedy, especially if exhaustion is marked and there is excoriation of the perianal skin. Piles tend to prolapse, burn and have a blue colour. Portal congestion may occur leading to enlargement of the liver.

Cardiovascular System

In this sphere the remedy is associated with right-sided heart failure and venous engorgement. Throbbings occur with flushes, which mount upwards and end in profuse sweats. Palpitations often accompany 'wind', owing to pressure of distended guts forcing the diaphragm upwards.

A special feature is circulatory collapse with cold breath, cold knees and air hunger. In this connection it may be of value to compare the somewhat similar state of collapse as met with under certain other remedies.

Aconite collapse occurs as the result of a sudden fright or other shattering experience. It is characterized by terror and tossing; the subject is prostrate with panic, frantic with fear, speechless from shock, dyspnoeic from dither, and manifests a rapid pulse, restless tossing to and fro and is liable to be soaked in sweat.

Arnica collapse occurs as the result of trauma. The sufferer is pale, panting, pulseless (or has a weak pulse, rising in rate). There is a curious fear of being approached, and a tendency to either belittle the situation and say, 'I'm all right. What's all the fuss about?', or to be convinced that death is imminent. It is well to look for signs of haemorrhage, obvious or occult.

Arsenicum Alb. collapse is associated with sudden illness. The prostration is out of proportion to the obvious symptoms, and is extreme. It is, however, accompanied by great restlessness of body and anxiety of mind; the surface of the skin is cold and clammy; the expression is worried, perhaps terrified; there is despair of recovery; the pulse is weak and possibly irregular; the lower eyelids appear puffy; and there is a corpse-like odour of the body.

Camphor collapse presents a picture of icy coldness; eyes are upturned or closed; lips are drawn back, displaying the teeth; skin is blue and shrivelled; the tongue is cold; the voice is high-pitched or husky, and questions remain unanswered; despite the icy coldness there may be a desire to throw off the covers; there is fear of impending death. The picture is that typically met with in cholera.

China collapse typically results from serious loss of body fluids, especially haemorrhage. The picture presented is one of pallor, sunken eyes, blue rings round the eyes, coldness and shivering, profuse prostrating sweats, puffy oedema, feeble pulse. A cold feeling is experienced in the belly with each inspiration.

Muriatic Acid collapse is liable to be met with in the course of a debilitating illness such as typhoid fever. The sufferer has a vacant staring look, cold extremities, slithers down in the bed with legs drawn up, displays a moaning or muttering delirium, a pulse which is rapid, weak and intermits at every third beat, a tongue which is dry, shrunken, pointed, paralytic and rattles in the parched mouth, and rapid, feeble rattling respiration.

Strontium Carb. collapse is typically the form of shock experienced in association with surgical operations, in the treatment of which it has proved of great value.

Veratrum Alb. collapse presents a very typical picture. The skin is cold like marble; the face is pale, drawn, sunken; beads of cold sweat are seen on the forehead; there is marked pallor associated with blue lips; the skin looks livid; hands and nails are blue; the pulse is thready or impalpable;

watery saliva dribbles from the mouth. The sufferer is so dehydrated that he can scarcely speak. Death seems imminent.

When Carbo Veg. is called for in its typical form of collapse it may prove a veritable corpse-reviver and avert almost inevitable death, at any rate for the time being.

The remedy also has a sphere of usefulness in relation to varicose veins, and varicose ulcers.

Lymphatic and Glandular Systems

Mastitis is accompanied by burning pain and marked induration. Lymphadenitis may proceed to abscess formation, when the pus will be thin and sanious.

Genital System

The menstrual periods are liable to be premature, profuse, painful, having a pungent odour, are associated with pruritus, and accompanied by generalized aches and pains. Metrorrhagia occurs as the result of uterine atony and congestion; there is continuous oozing of dark blood, accompanied by burning pain in the lumbo-sacral region and great craving for air. The remedy may be of service in relation to debility and prostration in nursing mothers with suppressed lactation.

Locomotor System

Drawing pains may occur in nape, back, deep to the coccyx, in forearms, wrists and fingers, giving rise to restless unease. The coccygeal pain is worse when sitting down. The limbs may feel 'bruised' and sore, and the part lain on, or pressed on, very easily 'goes to sleep'. This tendency to easy numbness and tingling is presumably due to further embarrassment by pressure of an already inefficient circulation in the part concerned.

Skin

Fine, moist eruptions may occur, associated with patches of burning sensation elsewhere on the suface of the body. Indolent ulcers burn, especially at night; the discharge is serous and smelly; the ulcers are shallow and tend to spread; the surrounding skin shows a brownish discoloration. Other conditions in which the remedy may be called for are intertrigo, carbuncle with bluish or livid discoloration, spontaneous bruising and petechiae formation, trophic ulcers and senile gangrene.

MODALITIES

These are related obviously to the circulatory asthenia. There is aggravation from cold, especially cold, frosty weather, but also in a hot, stuffy atmosphere and in humid weather, both of which intensify the lack of oxygen. Is worse by movement, when walking out of doors, after meals, from taking alcohol, quinine or mercury. The worst time of day is the evening.

Some relief is obtained by being fanned vigorously, by belching (for a short spell), and also after sleep.

CLINICAL NOTES

The remedy is of special service in patients who are desperately ill from typhoid fever, diphtheria, bronchopneumonia etc. Diabetic coma is also mentioned. In grave collapse it is recommended that the 30c or 200c be prescribed. It is of value in states of low vitality after a debilitating illness, in persistent ill-health stemming from an illness, stress or injury, perhaps of remote date.

The 3x potency has a good reputation in relation to flatulence.

Carcinosin

SOURCE

Carcinosin, the nosode of cancer, was used by homoeopathic physicians of the nineteenth century, but a comprehensive drug picture of the remedy does not appear in the early literature. Although Clarke, in *A Dictionary of Practical Materia Medica*, states that he used it more frequently than any other diathesic remedy, he only gives twelve lines on the indications for its use in the appendix to the main work. The remedy employed at that time was known as Carcinosinum, and although its source is uncertain, it is thought to have been prepared from a breast epithelioma. This substance was the subject of a proving by Dr W. L. Templeton in 1954, but it must be said that the drug picture now so frequently used consists mainly of a collection of clinical symptoms – viz. those symptoms often seen in patients whose conditions have improved after taking the remedy.

Dr D. M. Foubister, when paediatrician at the Royal London Homoeopathic Hospital, noticed a similar appearance in two children suffering from insomnia, both of whom had been born of mothers who during their pregnancy were suffering from carcinoma of the breast. These children had cafe-au-lait complexions, blue sclerotics, and many moles. For some years Foubister and his associates gave Carcinosin to children with a family history of cancer, and observed certain characteristics common to these patients. Later it was realised that children with the Carcinosin appearance did not always have a family history of cancer, but that a family background of tuberculosis, diabetes, pernicious anaemia, as well as malignant disease, is more common in such children than in the average population. Gradually the 'Carcinosin drug picture' evolved, and Foubister published two papers on the remedy in 1954 and 1958. They included symptoms observed in adults as well as children.

The family history of the subject is considered important; a background of cancer, tuberculosis, pernicious anaemia, diabetes or any combination of these, is an indication for the use of the remedy. The patient's past medical history may include glandular fever, whooping cough, any exanthem occurring more than once, or pneumonia at an early age. A severe reaction to vaccination is also significant.

APPEARANCE

The subject may have a bluish tinge to the sclera, a brownish café-au-lait complexion, many pigmented moles, and there may be blinking eyes or bizarre tics.

PSYCHOLOGY

Clarke mentions the use of Carcinosin in 'many mental cases, especially where the heredity points that way' and in cancer patients who have a suicidal tendency.

The provings produced dullness of mind, disinterest, difficulty in thinking, and aversion to conversation. Dr Foubister's observations include prolonged fear and unhappiness, worry in anticipation and obstinacy. The subject may be fastidiously tidy (Arsenicum Alb., Nux Vomica, Anacardium, Graphites,) or the opposite (Sulphur). He may enjoy storms, be sensitive to music, and sympathetic to others. Children are sensitive to reprimand (Medorrhinum) and sometimes aggravated by consolation. Foubister also mentions this remedy as useful for children with Down's Syndrome.

PHYSIOLOGY

Insomnia is common. The patient may be awakened by shudders, have excited dreams, or be kept awake by over-active ideas (Cuprum). Mental fatigue is better for a short nap. Children may sleep in the genupectoral position (Medorrhinum), or in the dorsal position with the arms raised above the head.

There may be a strong craving or aversion to one or more of the following foods: salt, milk, eggs, fat meat, fruit. Alternatively, a child may be averse to any of these at one time, only to desire it at another.

Secretions in general may be acrid and thick.

SYMPTOMATOLOGY

Head
The provings elicited a sensation of thumping, mostly on the right side. There were general feelings of tightness and constriction in the brain, with a throbbing pain deep inside the head.

Nose and Throat
Chronic sinusitis and tonsillitis ('where indicated', Foubister).

Eyes
General twitching of the eyes, as well as twitching in other muscle groups. Blue sclerotics.

Digestive System
Constipation with or without desire to pass stool. A feeling of tightness in the abdomen, with pain relieved by pressure, bending and hot drinks, worse between 4-6 p.m.

Cardiovascular System
General throbbing and a feeling of tightness and constriction in the region of the heart.

Respiratory System
Dr D. J. Cooper mentions its use in acute respiratory infections where an initial response to the indicated remedy had not been maintained. It may be useful in acute glandular fever (Ailanthus Gland.), or in the syndrome 'never well since glandular fever'.

Skin
The aforementioned brownish cafe-au-lait complexion is typical as well as an abundance of pigmented naevi. Eczema is common, especially in the sternal area and between the shoulder-blades. It has been claimed that Carcinosin reduces keloid formation if used pre-operatively in patients undergoing plastic surgery.

MODALITIES

Temperature: There is either aggravation or amelioration from heat or cold, or the subject may be sensitive to both.

Time: Symptoms are generally worse in the afternoon from 1-6 p.m. (Lycopodium, Arsenicum Alb.).

Geographical: The influence of sea air is said to be important – it may aggravate or relieve, or the subject may feel better on the east coast and worse on the west coast, or vice versa.

Laterality: Alternation of symptoms from one side of the body to the other may occur (Lac Caninum).

Carcinosin

CLINICAL NOTES

Related remedies are: Tuberculinum (*all preparations*), Medorrhinum, Syphilinum, Sepia, Natrum Mur., Calc. Phos., Dys. Co, Lycopodium, Phosphorus, Psorinum, Arsenicum Alb., Arsenicum Iod., Pulsatilla, Sulphur, Opium, Alumina, Staphisagria.

Foubister considers Carcinosin when one of the above remedies, although strongly indicated, does not work, or has only a limited action, or when a series of these remedies does not produce a satisfactory result. He also considers it useful where there are partial indications for two or more of these remedies, but where no single one covers the case.

PREPARATIONS OF CARCINOSIN

The original preparation previously known as Carcinosinum and used by Kent, Burnett and Clarke is thought to have been prepared from a breast epithelioma. It is this preparation which will be dispensed if the prescriber simply writes 'Carcinosin'. It is available in potencies from 30c upwards, and only a few doses are usually given.

However a number of new varieties of Carcinosin have been prepared from specimens obtained from the operating theatre of the Royal London Homoeopathic Hospital. They are as follows :

Preparation	*Origin*	*Potencies*
Carcinosin Adeno.Stom.	Epithelioma of Stomach	6c-lM
Carc. Adeno. Vesica	Epithelioma of Bladder	6c-30c
Carc. Intest. Co.	Epithelioma of Intestine and Bladder	6c-30c
Carc. Scirr. Mam.	Scirrhus of Breast	6c-200c
Carc. Squam. Pulm.	Epithelioma of Lung	6c-30c

Their drug pictures have not been differentiated, and it would seem that a strong family history of one of the above may be a pointer to its use.

REFERENCES

1. Templeton, W.L., 'Report on a Proving of Carcinosin.' BHJ *44*,108.
2. Foubister, D.M., 'Clinical Impressions of Carcinosin.' BHJ 44, 202.
3. Foubister D.M. 'The Carcinosin Drug Picture.' BHJ 47.
4. Cooper, D.J. 'The Nosode Carcinosin.' BHJ, *7l*, 175. (Possibly the most comprehensive review of the literature of Carcinosin, Eds.)
5. Cooper D.J., Ibid. 169.

Causticum

SOURCE

This remedy is prepared after the method of Hahnemann by the distillation of an intimate mixture of equal parts of slaked lime (calcium hydroxide) and potassium bisulphate. The resultant solution is stored in hard glass containers.

PHARMACOLOGY

The affinities of this product, as would be expected from its potassium content, are mainly with the neuromuscular system, inducing weakness and paresis of both voluntary and plain muscles. There is also an irritant action on the central nervous system leading to muscular twitchings, cramps, even convulsions, and neuralgic pains. Fibrous and ligamentous tissues are affected, with resulting stiffness and actual contractures.

PROVING

A pathogenesis of Causticum appears in the second volume of the second edition of Hahnemann's *Materia Medica Pura*.

APPEARANCE

The Causticum subject is liable to have dark hair, dark eyes, a sallow or dirty, pale skin, and to be of spare build. Children are often emaciated, especially about the face, with a large belly.

The child is late in walking and stumbles on making the attempt; it is also late in talking.

There is marked restlessness and inability to lie still; no ease can be found in any position. This is especially so at night. Moreover no relief is obtained by movement.

The sufferer looks weary, weak and wasted.

In speech there is a tendency to stammer or make Spoonerisms, and to repeat the question before answering.

Eruptions may be present on the scalp and the eyes may look red and inflamed.

PSYCHOLOGY

The Causticum patient is described as unhappy, weepy, hopeless, timid, nervous, anxious. Is easily upset emotionally and may become hysterical. Is hypersensitive to noise, to touch, to anything exciting or unusual.

Is full of foreboding and apprehension; jumps at the least noise; has fearful fancies in the dusk. The child is afraid to go to bed in the dark.

There is a tendency to become peevish, irritable, censorious, or suspicious and distrustful. A feature may be intense sympathy with the sufferings of other people.

Failure of memory is common; so is absent-mindedness.

It is worthy of note that a Causticum picture may derive from sudden emotional stress or, on the other hand, from long-lasting grief or worry.

PHYSIOLOGY

The Causticum person is chilly, but also averse to either extreme of temperature.

Appetite is capricious; sits down to a meal quite hungry, but the thought, smell, even sight of food, takes away all desire. There is an aversion to sweet things, and a desire rather for pungent delicacies. A similar revulsion from sight or smell of food is met with under Arsenicum Alb., Cocculus, Colchicum and Sepia.

Despite a burning thirst for cold drinks, especially beer, the subject may shrink from the act of drinking.

There is intense drowsiness accompanied by much yawning and desire to stretch the limbs during the daytime, but insomnia at night – cannot get comfortable in any position – legs constantly 'on the go'. May start suddenly awake during sleep; sees frightening images on closing the eyes.

Sweats are common and the perspiration has a sour odour.

SYMPTOMATOLOGY

General
The Causticum condition is apt to be brought on by exposure to cold dry winds, from the strain of night-watching and loss of sleep, from the exhausting effects of chronic illness or as the result of a previous illness from which the patient has not fully recovered.

Symptoms develop slowly and progressively, with an accompanying general deterioration and increasing weakness – must lie down.

Pains are severe, tearing or drawing, with much soreness and rawness, and accompanied by tenderness of parts touched or lain on. The pains are worse in cold windy weather, also when thinking about them. They are better when it is raining and on warm damp days.

There is a tendency to muscular weakness with tremors, also to actual paralysis of single parts, for instance Bell's Palsy.

Periodicity of symptoms may be a feature. The laterality of the remedy is right-sided.

Head

Vertigo may be present, with a tendency to fall forward or to one side. Headache may be so severe as to cause nausea, and is worse in a warm room. The scalp may feel tight and contracted, or there is a sensation as if 'there was an empty space between the brain and the skull'. This is relieved by warmth.

Eyes

Various visual disturbances have been recorded. There may be great heaviness of the upper lids, with involuntary closing of the eyes. Also mentioned are sensations of grit in eye, corneal ulcer, incipient cataract.

Ears

Earache occurs, tending to persist. Deafness is associated with tinnitus, and words spoken or steps taken seem to reverberate in the ear. Ears feel 'blocked'.

Respiratory System

Dry coryza is associated with nasal obstruction and accumulation of crusts. Itching may be prominent at the tip of the nose, at the nostrils and also intra-nasally. Postnasal discharge is thick, copious and yellow or yellowish-green in colour. Epistaxis may be a feature. Burning pain is felt in the throat with much rawness and soreness, which is worse in the morning. Tough mucus is hawked up from the larynx. Hoarseness is present and at times there is complete loss of voice. An annoying, dry, hollow cough occurs from a paroxysmal tickling in the throat. This is worse in the morning and when warm in bed. Urine may escape with each cough. Taking a sip of cold water may ease the cough. The cough may cause pain in the region of the hip. The chest feels unpleasantly tight with a constant urge to take a deep breath for relief. Sputum slips back when attempting to expectorate, and is swallowed.

Alimentary System

Stiffness and pain occur in the temporomandibular joints with resultant difficulty in opening the mouth. There may be dysphagia from paresis of the muscles of deglutition, or an inclination to keep swallowing because the throat feels 'too narrow'. Toothache is aggravated by drawing cold air into the mouth. There is a tendency to bite the tongue or the cheek while masticating. Cracks develop on the lips.

Nausea occurs with or without vomiting. There is burning in the stomach with waterbrash. Abdominal bloating may be extreme, made much worse after food. Griping, cutting colic is made better by bending double and is relieved entirely at night, when recumbent. Paralytic weakness may affect the rectum, which fills up with hard faeces coated with shiny mucus. The stool is apt to slip out unawares. Passage of stool is rendered easier by standing to defaecate. Piles occur with sticking, burning pain, aggravated by walking, by contact, when thinking about it, and when straining the voice. Anal fissure is apt to be accompanied by pruritus. A painful pustular eruption may be present around the anus.

Urinary System

Leakage of urine occurs when coughing or sneezing, owing to partial paresis of the sphincter urinae. Sudden enuresis may occur when laughing or from excitement. Enuresis is liable to occur at night during the first sleep, worse in winter and better in summer. There may be frequency of urination, with passage of large quantities but little awareness of the flow. Paralytic retention may occur. This may yield to a drink of cold water or be relieved by standing up to urinate. Itching at the urethral orifice may be prominent.

Genital System

Menstrual periods may be delayed and followed by severe exhaustion. The flow ceases on lying down.

Nervous System

Convulsions recur at full moon. Paralysis is preceded by twitchings and jerkings, or by cramps. Choreic movements tend to persist during sleep. Convulsions may follow a fright. Epileptic attacks are aggravated by emotional stress, from getting chilled, from bathing in cold water or being exposed to a cold wind.

Locomotor System

Drawing and tearing pains occur in the limbs, especially in the popliteal region; these tend to be better in moist weather and for warmth. Joints become enlarged and soft, with stiffness especially noticeable on attempting to rise from a chair. Joints creak on movement, especially knees. Actual contractures of muscles and tendons may develop, causing deformity such as wryneck. Pseudoparesis may ensue after over-use of muscles. Kent states that 'Causticum has also rheumatic complaints aggravated in warm damp days and in wet weather, but this is not so striking', i.e. in contrast to the usual, opposite, modality. This is probably worth noting.

Skin

There are several skin conditions associated with Causticum. Acne rosacea on cheeks and forehead. Eruptions occurring behind the ears. Thick crusty eruptions in the occipital region. Warts, especially on hands, face and margins of eyelids. Large, jagged warts, often pedunculated and apt to be moist and bleed readily. Old scars become sore again after healing.

MODALITIES

Causticum complaints are worse in dry weather and especially from contact with dry cold winds. Other causes of aggravation are going from cold atmosphere into a hot room, from exposure to draughts, from getting wet, after a bath, and from movement, or car travel. The symptoms are worse at night, in the early morning on waking, also from 6 to 8 p.m.; worse from taking coffee, and also after a stool.

The Causticum patient feels better in warm, moist weather, and when warm in bed.

CLINICAL NOTES

The remedy is seldom called for in acute conditions. It should not be given in direct sequence to Coffea, Phosphorus or Acids. Carbo Veg. and Guaiacum are complementary.

Chamomilla

SOURCE

The source of this remedy is the German Chamomile or Wild Chamomile (*Matricaria chamomilla*). It is a member of the daisy family, the Compositae. Growing in the wild state it is described as 'a modest little weed which flourishes about September in rickyards'. The plant loves the light and is often found at the edge of paths and in open fields. It prefers sandy or clay soil and shrinks from damp and shady places. It is also found growing on chalky ground, and thrives well on salt-impregnated soil.

The flower heads are about 20mm in diameter, with some fifteen or so white strap-shaped florets. These tend to straggle horizontally in a rather untidy manner or are coyly reflexed downwards to wrap round the flower stalk. In addition there are numerous tubular yellow perfect florets, forming a conical golden centre dome, which is hollow.

The plant is often found in cornfields and must be distinguished from the Corn Chamomile (*Anthemis arvensis*), which shows little chaffy scales or bracts among its florets and has a solid centre. Moreover, this plant is odourless whereas *Matricaria chamomilla* possesses a strong scent, somewhat like that of the Common Chamomile (*Anthemis nobilis*), but less aromatic. The scent of the latter plant is sweetish, and reminiscent of the smell of an apple room.

The flowers, despite their somewhat aromatic odour, possess a very bitter taste. They contain a volatile oil, a bitter extractive and a trace of tannic acid. The etheric oil distilled from the flowers is of a deep blue colour, unlike most etheric oils, which are pale yellow. The oil is said to be 'very effective in controlling inflammation'. Certainly the remedy is of signal value in controlling inflamed tempers.

The growth of the plant is interesting. From the first germination of the seed there is a very rapid growth, an energetic upgrowth of leaf, shoot and flower. After a very few months, with the formation of new seed, the cycle is completed. In cultivation the plant will bloom in two months from sowing and thus provide two crops in one season. This manner of growth is suggestive of energetic, even exaggerated, response to stimulus and lack of patience.

153

The foliage has a characteristic bushy, curly, feathery appearance. The leaf, although threadlike in length, when looked at transversely, is seen to be thick and succulent with a margin which is rolled inwards.

Sensitivity is the chief characteristic of the plant, as evidenced by its texture, its manner of growth and its habitat.

PHARMACOLOGY

The chief tissue affinity of the plant is with the nervous system, inducing an extreme degree of over-excitability and hypersensitivity.

PROVING

A pathogenesis of Chamomilla appeared in Hahnemann's *Fragmenta de Viribus*, and in the second edition of the third volume of *Materia Medica Pura*.

APPEARANCE

The Chamomilla subject often has light brown hair and a fair complexion.

The child is in a petulant, snapping, snarling mood, throwing things about; cries when approached or interfered with, but becomes quiet when carried in arms.

One cheek is apt to be red and hot while the opposite cheek is pale and cold.

The head is often warm and moist with sweat.

There may be a crack in the centre of the lower lip, a sign shared with Graphites, Natrum Mur. and Sepia.

When in pain the sufferer tosses to and fro in agony and is quite unable to stay still.

Muscular hypersensitivity may result in much jerking and twitching from mortification, chagrin or excitement; if punished the child may throw a fit of convulsions.

PSYCHOLOGY

The Chamomilla subject, whether child or adult, is morbidly sensitive. Temper becomes a turmoil, and restlessness is extreme.

Is intolerably irritable and impatient; everything is unbearable; pain is intolerable. The child cannot bear being looked at, spoken to or approached – flies into a rage at once.

Emotion may be so intense as to cause fainting.

Nothing pleases; every trifle annoys; child howls for a toy and, when it is brought, throws it away and demands something else.

Very easily chagrined or offended. Becomes melancholy, sits and broods and refuses to reply when spoken to – appears absorbed in thought, as the result of pent-up rage or resentment.

Symptoms of illness may arise from anger, either suppressed or vented, or from contradiction or interference.

PHYSIOLOGY

The circulation takes part in the turmoil, and heat and shivering may become intermingled. May feel 'on fire' although to the palpating hand the skin feels cold. This is unlike Belladonna, which shows a characteristically hot skin, burning to the touch.

Appetite is usually lacking. There may be a craving for coffee or for narcotics. Kent, however, speaks of aversion to coffee, warm drinks, soup and fluid foods.

There is a marked thirst for cold water, which is liable to be held in the mouth for quite a while before being swallowed. There may be a desire for acid drinks.

Sleep is disturbed by much moaning, starting and tossing; or may be unable to stay in bed, gets up to walk up and down in vain search for easement. May be sleepy but still unable to get to sleep. May dream with eyes wide open, and nightmares are common.

As with Pulsatilla and Sulphur, the soles of the feet tend to burn at night, and the feet are moved around in search of a cold spot or pushed out from under the bed-covers to cool off.

Profuse sweats occur on covered parts; the head perspires during sleep; the face sweats after eating or drinking. The perspiration is hot and sticky.

SYMPTOMATOLOGY

General
The Chamomilla pains are quite unbearable and seem out of all proportion to any obvious pathological lesion; the pains are drawing or tearing in character, and are often accompanied by a feeling of numbness or burning heat. Pains in head and belly tend to be eased by warmth. Pains are worse at night, especially from 9 p.m. to midnight, but usually ease off after midnight.

Head Region

A throbbing unilateral headache is brought on or made worse by anger, and gets worse in the evening. Heat and warm wraps afford some relief. A facial neuralgia, associated with pain inside the mouth, however, is relieved by cold. But if the pain is located in the side of the face or the ears it is better for heat.

Eyes

The eyes tend to be swollen in the morning with adherent lids. Blepharospasm occurs. There may be a sensation as if the eyeball was lightly compressed from all angles. The sclerotics may show a yellow tinge.

Ears

Earache is pressive in type, worse on stooping, with tearing pains which extort cries; the ears feel stuffed up. Tinnitus occurs, with tinkling or buzzing noises.

Respiratory System

Although the nose feels blocked, hot watery discharge drops from the nostrils. There is much dry sneezing, and the nose is extremely sensitive to any kind of odour. A constant tickle behind the upper part of the sternum causes a teasing dry cough. Suffocative tightness of the chest may be complained of, with paroxysms of coughing. At times there is a hard, hacking cough, worse when talking, on expiration and at night. Asthma brought on by anger or tantrums may call for the remedy. It may be indicated also when the child coughs in its sleep and wakes 'crabby'.

Alimentary System

Toothache is induced by taking anything warm into the mouth, is aggravated by talking and worse in bed; holding cold water in the mouth gives relief. Teeth feel 'too long'. An indication for the remedy is teething in children, accompanied by green watery stools which smell like rotten eggs. The tongue shows a yellow coating; foetor oris is noticeable. Attacks occur of severe vomiting associated with violent retching, as if the stomach would be torn to shreds; the sufferer is covered with cold sweat and becomes exhausted. A similar type of vomiting is caused by morphine in sensitive subjects. There may be complaint of pressure in the stomach as 'of a stone', accompanied by fruitless attempts to vomit; this type of distress is also met with in connection with Nux Vomica. Biliousness may be brought on by anger. Bloating may occur after meals, with painful belching. Colic is accompanied by tympanites; flatus is passed in small quantities and without affording any relief; local heat to the abdomen may give relief. The child doubles up, kicks and screams with pain. Colic is felt while urinating. Slimy diarrhoea occurs with grass-green stools containing particles of undigested food, mucus and blood. The stools are foul-smelling. The anus becomes sore and prolapsed.

Lymphatic and Glandular Systems
Breasts become tender and nipples sore and inflamed. Tenderness of breasts in infants.

Genital System
Uterine haemorrhage of dark blood with clots accompanied by labour-like pains. Early menstrual periods are accompanied by dysmenorrhoea; the flow is heavy, dark with many large clots; the patient feels hot, thirsty, cross. In labour, severe pains extend from the back to the medial aspect of thighs. The remedy may be called for in threatened abortion.

Locomotor System
The arms are apt to 'go to sleep' when grasping objects. Rheumatic pains drive the sufferer from bed to walk the floor; he is thirsty, hot, and almost beside himself with anguish. Cramps occur in legs. Ankles seem weak and easily turn over. Joints crack on movement and feel 'bruised'.

MODALITIES

There is aggravation from exposure to heat and also from draughts; from wind and from wet. Symptoms also tend to be worse from taking coffee, both before and during menstruation, at 9 a.m. or 9 p.m., and in the first part of the night.

Feels better in warm, moist, humid weather, a modality shared with Causticum, Hepar Sulph., Kali Carb. and Nux Vomica. Being carried or being driven in a car also affords relief.

CLINICAL NOTES

The chief indication for Chamomilla is provided by the psychological picture. The remedy is not called for in those who bear pain patiently and with resignation.

The remedy is often of great service in complaints of the newly-born and during dentition. (If Chamomilla fails, prescribe Belladonna.) Chamomilla will often give relief in nausea and vomiting or other ill effects of morphine. Also of use in irritable states resulting from abuse of narcotics or coffee.

157

Chelidonium Majus

SOURCE

Chelidonium majus is the greater celandine, a flower belonging to the poppy family. It grows in waste places. It has large bluish-green compound leaves. The four-petalled yellow flowers are found at the tips of hairy, slender, branching stems; they are a half to one inch across. The stems are brittle, and when broken exude a thick yellow juice which is acrid and irritating and has a disagreeable odour. The juice is reputed to cure warts when applied externally. The fruit is cylindrical and up to two inches long; the seeds have a large crest on one aspect.

The plant is said to be a drastic purgative and the flesh of an animal poisoned by the plant should not be eaten. It must not be confused with the lesser celandine, which belongs to the Ranunculaceae.

On analysis the plant is found to contain alkaloids similar to those found in the opium poppy; the juice also contains protein-digesting enzymes and mitotic poisons. The latter are capable of inhibiting cell growth.

The small black seeds gain a relationship to the ant world, and are carried along the ant routes to take root on walls, towers, castle ruins, willow stumps and other unexpected sites. The whole fresh plant is used in preparing the mother tincture.

PHARMACOLOGY

There is affinity with the liver, the base of the right lung and the kidney, causing irritation and inflammation; also with the nervous system, acting as a depressant.

PROVING

Chelidonium was first proved by Hahnemann, and published in the fourth volume of *Materia Medica Pura*.

APPEARANCE

A thin, spare individual with a light complexion, though the skin may be tinted yellow from the presence of jaundice.

A feature is a thickly-coated yellow tongue, having red edges indented by the teeth.

PSYCHOLOGY

Is sad and anxious, perhaps in agony of conscience as if 'had committed a great crime and must escape'.

Is sluggish in thought, in gait, in speech. Has a horror of movement.

Is quarrelsome, irritable, peevish, liable to uncalled-for outbreaks of temper.

There is forgetfulness, inability to think consecutively, fear of going mad.

Is weary, indolent, averse to any mental exertion or even the effort of carrying on a conversation.

PHYSIOLOGY

Is chilly internally, shivering; the right foot may be icy cold.

There is a bitter taste in the mouth, and a preference for hot food and hot drinks.

Seems to be dogged by a nauseating odour, as if everything in the environment were fouled by excrement.

Is drowsy in the daytime with great lassitude; sleeps badly, especially in the first half of the night.

Perspires during sleep, especially after midnight.

SYMPTOMATOLOGY
General

The general lethargy and unwillingness for effort of any kind are prominent features. Jaundice of skin and conjunctiva may be obvious. There is a liability to serous effusions, e.g. hydrocele. Symptoms tend to affect the right side of the body. Pains are pressive or stabbing, brought on or aggravated by change of weather.

Head

Vertigo is accompanied by a tendency to fall forwards and is often associated with bilious vomiting, and also by pain in the region of the liver. A right-sided sick headache is aggravated in the open air; the skull seems too small. Head feels too heavy. Icy coldness is felt in the occiput and there is a sensation as if the 'occiput was being drawn down into the nape of the neck'. Facial neuralgia is made worse by change in the weather. The pain is located especially over the right eye, in the right cheekbone and right ear, and is accompanied by excessive lachrymation.

Eyes

Neuralgic pain occurs in and above the eyes; there may be quivering of the right eyelid. Sclerotics may be tinged yellow. With lachrymation tears just gush forth. Eyeballs are painful when looking upwards. The neuralgic pain with nausea and vomiting occurs as soon as the head is turned. Eyes tire easily in artificial light and water profusely. Corneal opacities may be present.

Ears

Tinnitus can be quite troublesome, described as the sound of distant cannon, sensation of wind rushing out of both ears, or as if ears were stopped up.

Respiratory System

Flapping of the wings of the nose may occur. A paroxysmal cough is especially troublesome at about 4 p.m. A choking sensation may be felt in the throat, as if too large a morsel had been swallowed; this is accompanied by a constant urge to swallow. There may be hoarseness with a sensation of dust in the trachea resulting in a paroxysmal cough, hollow in type, dry or associated with lumpy sputum which is raised with difficulty. The cough is associated with pain in the right chest, especially near the angle of the scapula, worse on inspiration. Pneumonia, usually at right base with involvement of pleura; must sit up in bed, bending forward, and keep perfectly motionless; fever high; cough racking; sputum profuse but only raised with difficulty.

Alimentary System

Characteristic of stomach or liver complaints is a pain at the lower angle of the right scapula, aggravated by movement and better by heat. Complaint of pyrosis. Grinding, gnawing pain in stomach is relieved temporarily by taking food; it is accompanied by great sensitivity to touch and pressure in the epigastrium and both hypochondria. Acute pain in the epigastric notch shoots through to the angle of the right scapula. Drinking hot milk affords relief. There is congestion and enlargement of the liver associated with sticking pains and jaundice. Gallstones may be present, and biliary colic. The upper abdomen feels as if constricted by a cord and the pressure of clothing is resented. The belly is distended and girdle pain is felt at the level of the umbilicus. Flatulent rumblings occur with spasmodic pains in groins. Diarrhoea alternates with constipation. Stools are pasty and light-coloured, or golden yellow.

There are burning, crawling, itching sensations in rectum with constant urge to stool; faeces may be like sheep's dung, or loose and slimy and coloured as mentioned. They tend to float in water.

Cardiovascular System
Violent palpitations accompany other symptoms.

Urinary System
A dull, deep-seated ache is present in the loins, or pains which shoot along the length of the ureters. The first type of pain is relieved by lying in the prone positon. There is frequency of urination and spasmodic pain above the pubes; urine is dark yellow or beer-coloured.

Genital System
Labour-like pains occur with profuse discharge of clotted dark blood; the pains are spasmodic and pressing upward. There is intolerance of pain. The nipples may be inflamed and tender to touch. Bilious complications accompany gestation. Hydrocele may be present in the male.

Locomotor System
A tearing backache affects the lumbar region, worse bending either backward or forward. Neck muscles feel stiff. Rheumatic pains occur in extremities. Limbs feel heavy, stiff, bruised and are sore to the touch.

MODALITIES

Is worse from heat, open air, wind, movement, change of weather, anger, being touched, and at 4 a.m. and 4 p.m.

Is better in warm, wet weather, from being carried, by taking food, from hot drinks, especially hot milk, and by rest.

CLINICAL NOTES

Chelidonium is often indicated in disorders of the liver and gallbladder, particularly where there is jaundice, and in right-sided pneumonia. Complementary remedies are Bryonia and Lycopodium.

Cicuta Virosa

Cicuta virosa is one of the most poisonous of the enormous Umbelliferae family; it is especially lethal to horses and cattle, hence its name cowbane.

In appearance it resembles *Conium*, but its stem lacks the red blotches characteristic of *Conium maculatum*, the common hemlock. *Cicuta* is also known as water hemlock from its habitat; it is found growing on river banks, in muddy ditches, in swamps, on moist moors, at the edge of lakes or ponds. It occurs in temperate regions of the northern hemisphere.

The hollow, furrowed stem may attain a height of four feet, and has often a reddish tinge. The small white flowers are arranged in large many-rayed compound umbels; the umbellules are marked by an involucrum of small pointed bracts. The fleshy root is hollow, divided into cells by transverse partitions; it is white in colour, but exudes a yellow juice if cut into. The leaves are pennate with long stalks, the leaflets being deeply serrated and bright green in colour. The laterally compressed fruit shows five not very well marked ridges.

The root is highly poisonous, containing a soft insoluble resin in which are present the poison cicutoxin and an alkaloid, cicutine. The mother tincture is prepared from the fresh root, gathered at the beginning of flowering.

The whole plant has an odour similar to that of parsley. The root has a resemblance to parsnip; fatalities have occurred as the result of the root being eaten in mistake. Symptoms of poisoning include dizziness, drowsiness, stupor with dilated pupils; epileptiform convulsions; severe burning pain in mouth and stomach with unquenchable thirst, paralysis of tongue and dysphagia. Death is preceded by acute dyspnoea.

PHARMACOLOGY

The main affinity is with the nervous system, inducing extreme sensitivity of nerve endings in muscles, with resultant liability to spasms and convulsions, both clonic and tonic. Involvement of the brain causes first excitement, then coma. Local effects on the alimentary tract cause burning and nausea. Action on the skin tends to produce a pustular type of eruption.

PROVING

Cicuta was proved by Hahnemann, and published in *Materia Medica Pura*, Vol. VI.

APPEARANCE

The face may show pallor, with sunken eyes surrounded by a livid ring; or with excitement the face may be red and covered with sweat.

Pupils alternately dilate and contract. The eyes may show a fixed staring gaze. Eye reflexes are lost. Squint may be noticed.

Convulsions are accompanied by a variety of violent movements and contortions. Before an attack the child may be excited, singing and dancing. With cerebral involvement the subject moans, howls, gesticulates, makes odd movements and grinds teeth.

PSYCHOLOGY

In between attacks the disposition is mild, gentle and placid.

In some subjects the mind becomes blank for days, with a disordered time sense and a reversion to childhood. Places and people seem strange; there is a tendency to play with childish toys and to be violently affected by sad stories.

There may be aversion to company and a great desire for solitude. Becomes agitated, suspicious and fearful.

PHYSIOLOGY

Face and hands are usually cold.

Appetite varies; may be lacking; may feel full after the first mouthful, or hunger returns soon after a meal. Again appetite may be perverted, with a tendency to eat chalk, coal, raw potatoes and such with apparent relish.

There may be a burning thirst.

Sleep is disturbed by vivid dreams. Wakes in a profuse sweat. Apt to grind teeth in sleep.

SYMPTOMATOLOGY

General

The great characteristic of this remedy is violence; violent convulsions and violent behaviour generally. The convulsions are centripetal in distribution; they can be triggered off by such causes as dentition, meningitis, injuries to head or spine, perhaps remote. A tonic spasm may be induced by the least touch, even from loud talking in the room. Trismus or opisthotonos may be marked. Pains described as bruised and excoriating occur in various sites.

Head

Attacks of vertigo occur; objects seem to move in a circle or everything swings back and forth like a pendulum; there is a tendency to stagger and fall forward; wants to clutch some solid object for support. A stupefying headache may be frontal, one-sided or occipital. It is worse when at rest. The brain may feel loose, as if shaking about inside the skull. It is said that the head symptoms may be relieved by the passage of flatus.

Eyes

Temporary squint may result from fear, or from a knock on the head. Eyes may be inflamed, with burning pain and agglutination of lids at night. Vision may be disturbed; letters move about or are blotted out; coloured rings are seen around objects, which may appear double. Pupils are either pinpoint or widely dilated.

Respiratory System

Sneezing occurs without coryza. A raw bruised sensation is felt inside the nose. Nasal obstruction occurs with profuse mucoid discharge. The throat feels drawn together and very dry. The chest feels tight and respiration is difficult. Cough may be present with copious expectoration.

Alimentary System

Spasm of oesophagus causes dysphagia. This is especially likely to result from injury caused by swallowing a splinter of bone or other sharp object. Hiccough is both violent and noisy. Abdomen becomes taut and distended with much flatulence, colic and borborygmus.

Cardiovascular System

Palpitation occurs with intermittent pulse. The heart may feel as if it had stopped beating. Coldness is felt in the cardiac region, and elsewhere.

Urinary System
There is an irresistible urge to urinate; this may be associated with diarrhoea. Frequency may occur or retention; again there may be involuntary enuresis.

Genital System
Menses may be delayed. Puerperal convulsions continue after delivery.

Locomotor System
Stiff neck results from sudden spasm of neck muscles. Weakness in limbs is noticed after exertion. Violent jerking and spasmodic contortions occur in limbs.

Skin
Eruptions are pustular with a tendency to form thick yellow crusts. Eruptions are specially liable to occur on scalp, face (barber's itch) and at corners of mouth.

MODALITIES

Aggravation results from exposure to cold; from any jar or jolt; from even a light touch; from tobacco smoke.
Is better from warmth and at the commencement of a meal.

CLINICAL NOTES

The main indications for the use of the remedy are convulsions of particular violence and pustular eruptions. It may also be of value in cerebrospinal meningitis and in petit mal.

Cimicifuga Racemosa

SOURCE

The source of this remedy is also know as *Actaea racemosa*, black cohosh, bugbane, black snake root. It is a member of the Ranunculaceae family, a perennial herb, found in deep woods in eastern North America. There is a lack of repose about this plant. It grows to the height of some six feet; the rather wild looking array of outflung leaves are frond-like, compound, the leaflets having serrated edges; from their midst rises a tall wand-like stem bearing small white flowers at the top. The roots are thick, branched, knotty and resinous; the mother tincture is prepared from the dried roots.

The main constituents of the plant are resin, racemosin and two other crystalline principles, isoferulic acid, tannin and starch. The plant was used medicinally by Indian tribes in rheumatism, menstrual disorders, slow parturition and snakebite.

PHARMACOLOGY

An affinity with the nervous system gives rise to meningeal irritation, neuralgic pain, neuritis and generalized hypersensitivity. Hyper-excitability of muscles is also induced. Affinity with pelvic organs leads to dysfunction of ovaries and uterus.

PROVING

A proving of Cimicifuga appears in the *North American Journal of Homoeopathy*, Vol. III.

APPEARANCE

Features which may be present include the following:

Constant restless moving to and fro; cannot sit long in one spot; gets frantic and must change position.

Sudden faintness with ashy white face and cold sweat on palms.

Face pale or bluish; eyes sunken and surrounded by dark rings; forehead cold to touch; wild, scared expression.

Incessant incoherent chatter, changing rapidly from subject to subject.

PSYCHOLOGY

There is a lack of control over emotions, as over muscles. Is so restless and strung-up as to become almost frantic. There is a fear of going crazy; also fear of death. Becomes suspicious of everything, medicines included.

Seems enveloped in a black cloud of gloom. Grief and misery accompanied by much sighing alternate with tremulous joy and mirth. Moods change constantly. May be aggressively affectionate.

Actual delirium may be present with widely dilated pupils, constant muttering, and hallucinations of rats, or mice, under the bed, demons and so on. May complain of a waving sensation in the brain.

It is noticed that mental symptoms improve when physical symptoms predominate. These may be initiated by emotional stress, especially chagrin.

PHYSIOLOGY

Essentially a chilly person, never really warm.

Sleep is disturbed by restless turning about in a vain search for ease, at times from sore bruised feeling, at times from sensation of numbness. Sleep may be prevented by muscular jerkings. The insomnia may be accompanied by gloom, which drives the patient from bed to roam up and down.

SYMPTOMATOLOGY

General

Variability is a feature. Symptoms constantly change or alternate between the physical and the psychological. Neuralgic pains are shooting or like shocks. Muscle pains shift from site to site, and are accompanied by much soreness and sensation of bruisedness; the affected muscles are sore to the touch. Twitchings also occur with sudden jerky bouts of cramp, extorting cries or grunts. The cramp is brought on by movement, and relief which could be obtained by lying perfectly still is denied by the constant urge to alter position. Uterine disorders are often associated with symptoms in other sites. Left-sided symptoms predominate.

Head

A severe headache, with sensation of pressing from within outwards; feels as if the top of the head would fly off; or with every inspiration feels as if cold air was blowing on the brain; is worse from the least movement or noise, also during menstruation; is relieved by pressure and in cool fresh air. An occipital headache spreads up or down into the neck; is made worse by bending the head forwards, but relieved by retracting the head or pressing firmly on the nape of the neck. Neuralgia in the malar region is better at night but tends to recur the next morning.

Eyes
Acute pain in eyeballs often accompanies headache; is worse on moving head or eyes; relieved by pressure. There may be a sensation as if the eyeballs were being pierced by needles.

Ears
There is extreme sensitivity to the least sound. Tinnitus is also often present.

Respiratory System
Viscid mucus collects in the throat, causing hawking. A dry tickle in the larynx incites a nervous cough, made worse by any attempt to use the voice; it is worse at night. Pain in the right chest, worse from movement; may extort cries.

Alimentary System
Offensive breath. Mouth and tongue feel warm and dry. Saliva is thick and viscid. Tongue may be swollen. Pharynx is sore, especially on left side; this is worse on waking and on first attempting to swallow, but is better on repeated swallowing or towards the close of a meal. Nausea and vomiting may prove troublesome, especially in women, and in association with uterine involvement. There may be complaint of a sinking or gone feeling in the epigastrium. Colicky pains in the abdomen are relieved by bending double or by the passage of a stool. Belly pains may extend to the back and lower limbs. Diarrhoea and constipation tend to alternate.

Cardiovascular System
Anginal pain extends to finger tips on one or both sides; arm feels numb as if bound to the side; worse on effort or from violent emotion; rest affords relief. Easy palpitation on least movement. Pulse tends to be weak and irregular.

Genital System
The pelvic organs are specially liable to involvement. Various irregularities of menstruation occur. Menstrual periods may be too early, the flow too profuse with dark blood and clots. Dysmenorrhoea occurs with

irregular cramping or shooting pains; an unusual feature is that the greater the flow, the more intense the pain. Bearing-down pains occur, suggestive of uterine prolapse and associated with pain shooting into the flanks, across the lower abdomen and down the thighs. A concomitant is extreme tenderness of ovaries and uterus. Inframammary pain is often associated with pelvic disorders. The remedy may be called for in obstetrics in relation to morning sickness and nervous fidgets during pregnancy; also in threatened abortion; chills and rigors in first stage of labour; irregular labour pains; severe, almost intolerable after-pains which extend to the thighs; puerperal depression.

Urinary System
Frequency of urination is prominent with polyuria. Pressive discomfort is felt in the region of the kidneys and in the lumbar region.

Locomotor System
Muscular soreness with darting pains affects various regions, but especially the nape of the neck, the shoulders and the Achilles tendon. These pains are worse from cold and wet but relieved somewhat by continuous movement. Low back pain brought on by exposure to cold or wet or by over-strain is made worse by first movement and eased by lying flat on the back; it is accompanied by stiffness, great restlessness and pains running down the thighs, especially the left thigh. The lower extremities may be so weak and tremulous that walking is difficult. The remedy may be called for in chorea; if any part of the body is pressed on it starts to jerk; for instance, the whole of the side lain on in bed will be affected; the jerking is accompanied by soreness and by a sensation of numbness in the area involved.

MODALITIES

There is aggravation from cold and damp; on first movement after rest; during the menstrual period; at night.

There is relief from warmth in every form; in the open air; while eating a meal; also as the result of an attack of diarrhoea. The mental state is improved when walking about.

CLINICAL NOTES

The combination of pelvic disorder with psychological symptoms is a strong indication for the use of the remedy. It is also of great value in the neuromuscular sphere.

Cina

SOURCE

This remedy is a preparation of *Artemisia contra*, Tartarian southern-wood or wormseed. The Artemisiae held a prominent place among the drugs of the ancient physicians from Hippocrates to Serapion. They were recommended as febrifuge, stomachic and anthelmintic. The plant is found in Asia Minor and Turkestan. It is a hardy perennial shrub, flowering in the autumn; the upright stems carry alternate uptilted stalks bearing clusters of small flowers and short, deeply cleft leaves. The whole plant is bluish-grey in colour; when crushed it exhales an aromatic odour; the taste is bitter and reminiscent of camphor.

PHARMACOLOGY

The active principle of the plant is santonin, an active vermifuge. When used in crude dosage for this purpose it carries appreciable risk.

The drug has affinity with the central nervous system, inducing giddiness, impaired perception, coldness of surface, dilated pupils, profuse perspiration, vomiting, delirium, convulsions, coma and finally death from respiratory failure.

Other prominent effects are yellow vision, yellow vomit, urine that leaves a yellow stain. Affinity with the intestinal canal produces hyperaemia and irritation. Haematuria may result from an action on the kidneys.

PROVING

Cina was proved by Hahnemann, and reported in *Materia Medica Pura*, Vol. I.

APPEARANCE

The patient, often a child, is restless, fidgety and fretful, especially at night. Appearance is sickly, pale, with dark rings round the eyes. One cheek may be flushed and hot, the other pallid; there is circumoral pallor. The pupils are dilated; grinds teeth at night; bores finger into nose

170

and picks at nostrils till they bleed. Twitching of muscles of face and eyelids may be noticed.

The child may rise onto hands and knees at night, or lie on belly. Constant movement of the left foot may be present.

PSYCHOLOGY

Child is cross, 'ugly', averse to being touched, even looked at; turns away when approached. An infant, however, wants to be carried or jigged and rocked. The older child hits out and kicks, demands things and then hurls them away when brought; cannot be quieted, is proof against all caresses and may indulge in pitiful wailing.

The adult is touchy, quite unable to 'see the joke', obstinate as a mule; possibly obsessed by the idea of having committed a crime.

PHYSIOLOGY

The Cina subject is very chilly, and sensitive to draughts.

Is fastidious about food, desires being many and various; there is a craving for sweet things. The infant may refuse the mother's milk.

The appetite may be ravenous and insatiable, hunger returning soon after a meal.

Thirst also may be considerable.

Sleep is very restless, accompanied by jerkings, frequent swallowing, coughing or choking; there is a tendency to screaming and night terrors, accompanied by grinding of the teeth and rolling of the head from side to side on the pillow.

Yawning is frequent; trembling or shuddering accompanies the yawn.

SYMPTOMATOLOGY

General
The mental and physical picture presented gives the main indication for consideration of the remedy. Pain if present comes in shocks.

Head
Headache alternates with pain in belly. A stupefying type of headache is aggravated when walking out of doors; it is associated with giddiness which is relieved by lying down. Head and scalp are sensitive to the least touch. Symptoms of meningismus occur in association with digestive upsets.

Eyes

Eyes tire easily when reading and letters become blurred. Rubbing the eyes affords some relief. Vision may be obscured as if looking through gauze; objects appear brightly coloured, especially yellow. Pupils are dilated and touch reflex is lost. Eyebrows may twitch involuntarily. Strabismus may be present.

Respiratory System

Sneezing is violent and causes a feeling of pressure in the temples and a bursting sensation in the chest. Fluent coryza alternates with blockage; there is much burning and itching inside the nose. As a result there is constant boring of fingers into the nostrils, and epistaxis is common. A dry, suffocating, spasmodic cough accompanies the sneezing, especially in spring and autumn. It is apt to occur in sleep. It is worse at night, if taking a drink, while walking out of doors. A paroxysm may be induced by a sudden movement or even by speaking; at the end of the paroxysm a clucking sound is heard, similar to the sound produced by pouring water from a bottle. Sticky mucus in the larynx gives rise to constant hawking, especially on first rising in the morning.

Alimentary System

Vomiting and diarrhoea occur immediately after eating or drinking, the tongue remaining clean. Pinching pains occur in the abdomen, which is hot and tender to touch; pressure, however, may give relief; the infant turns onto its belly. Constipation alternates with diarrhoea, with watery stools containing shreds of white mucus. Itching at the anus is intense.

Urinary System

Frequency occurs with profuse flow. Nocturnal enuresis is common. The urine appears milky.

Locomotor System

Muscular twitchings are common, even convulsions. Shooting or cramplike pains occur in limbs, accompanied by tenderness on pressure. A bruised pain is felt in the sacrum, unaffected by movement. Burning heat may occur in the hands and spread to the whole body. Violent pains drive from bed at night, compelling the sufferer to walk about in search of relief. A sensation of being pricked by needles may be felt in the heels. Soles burn at night. Ankles are apt to 'give' in the afternoon.

Skin

Yellow discoloration is especially marked at the level of the nose, on the cheeks and in the palms of the hands. Itching is widespread, often accompanied by small painful red pimples.

MODALITIES

Aggravation from heat in summer, from least touch, at night. Is better for movement or by bending down.

CLINICAL NOTES

The remedy is indicated if round or thread worms are present. It is to be considered in the presence of chorea, convulsions, pertussis, enuresis, and fever with cold face and warm hands. Complementary remedies are Calcarea Carb., Silicea and Sulphur Iod. Liver involvement is a main indication. Complementary remedies here are Lycopodium and Mercurius Dulc.

Cinchona Officinalis

This remedy, also designated China, is derived from the bark of the quinaquina tree, whose native habitat is on the eastern slopes of the Andes. It is found growing amongst other forest trees or standing apart in solitary state at altitudes ranging from 3,000 to 9,000 feet above sea-level.

The tree belongs to the Rubiaceae or madder family, which also includes coffea and gardenia. It is tall with an upright bole reaching perhaps to a height of sixty feet. The leaves are of varying size, dark green, leathery, with a very prominent central vein and lanceolate in shape.

The slender flower stalks arise in the leaf axilla and bear a cluster of terminal cone-shaped blossoms which may be white, pink, lavender or red in colour; they have a delicate fragrance.

Just how it was discovered that the bark of this tree possessed antifebrile properties effective against that world-wide scourge, the ague, remains obscure. 'The bark' as a remedy was introduced into Europe in the seventeenth century by Jesuit priests whose colleagues were working in South America. It became known as Jesuit Powder or Peruvian Bark, and was prescribed as such or as an ingredient in secret remedies, owing to the fact that its use was decried at first by the pundits.

In 1742 Linnaeus named the tree, botanically, *Cinchona*, somewhat erroneously as it turns out, for the story that the Countess of Chinchon, wife of the Viceroy of Peru, had been cured of ague by 'the bark', which gave rise to his choice of name, has been found by recent research to be apocryphal.

However, the name was adopted and has been applied to various species of the tree with bark of different colours, pale grey, yellow, red, and affording various yields of alkaloids.

It was not till 1820 that the main alkaloid, quinine, was isolated by two French pharmacists, whereupon the demand for supplies of the bark for the production of quinine sulphate increased by leaps and bounds.

The fruit of the tree is an ovoid capsule, dark grey in colour, which splits open from the base to reveal a cluster of winged seeds. In the middle of the nineteenth century an English trader named Ledger was collecting bark and vicuna wool for export. He was living near Lake Titicaca and got wind of a very special 'tree', the location of which was a well-kept secret among the Indians. With the connivance of his Indian assistant he was, however, finally able to get hold of a consignment of seeds from this tree, and sent them home to his brother in London.

The British government refused to have anything to do with the seeds, and in the course of being traded around a Dutch buyer purchased a pound of them for about $20. From this purchase grew the huge plantations of *Cinchona ledgeriana* in Java, which before the Second World War produced some 90 per cent of the world's supply of quinine.

This variety gives a very high yield of quinine. *Cinchona calisaya* from Bolivia provides bark with a high alkaloid content. The root bark of *C. succirubra* gives a high yield of other alkaloids, namely quinidine, cinchonine and cinchonidine. *C. officinalis*, a native of Ecuador and Peru, has a pale bark and provides a lower yield of alkaloids.

It was this latter variety with which Samuel Hahnemann made his epoch-making experiment on himself. On taking a sizeable dose of 'the bark' he found himself developing typical symptoms of what was then known as the ague, the very disease the drug was reputed to cure. This experience recalled to his fertile mind the dictum of Hippocrates – 'Let likes be cured by likes' – and started him forthwith in the long series of experiments and drug trials that resulted in the introduction of homoeotherapy into practical medicine.

The scraped and cleaned quills of *Cinchona officinalis* are used at the present time in the preparation of potencies for homoeopathic use.

PHARMACOLOGY

Including quinine, the bark of various species of *Cinchona* has yielded thirty-eight alkaloids, some of which have affinity with individual organs or tissues. But in the main the pharmacology of the drug can be summed up in the statement that 'quinine is a general protoplasmic poison with a universal rather than a specific tissue affinity'.

The primary action in small doses is to stimulate, but the preponderant effect is depressant and tends to produce toxic changes evidenced by nervous sensitivity, muscular debility, retarded leucocyte activity, nausea, giddiness, headache, buzzing in ears, disturbances of vision, haemorrhage, diarrhoea, and a fever characterized by chills and sweating.

PROVING

The first pathogenesis of Cinchona appears in Hahnemann's *De Fragmenta Viribus*, and it is also in the last edition of the third volume of the *Materia Medica Pura*.

APPEARANCE

Physical features suggesting the use of the drug are pallor, sunken eyes surrounded by blue rings, a dull expression and a sickly appearance. The face may be puffy, of earthy hue, even yellowish. Other signs may include oedema, splenic enlargement, palpable liver, tympanites and very marked asthenia.

PSYCHOLOGY

The mental and emotional features probably derive in the main from the condition of extreme tiredness and weakness. There is manifest tension and irritability, aversion to company, desire for solitude, and disinclination for any mental effort. The subject is anxious and apprehensive in the extreme, and full of fears at night. Fear of animals, especially dogs and crawling insects, may be present.

There is great intolerance of noise. The sufferer is querulous, has no use for anything, is totally devoid of poise, may even feel like suicide but lacks the courage.

PHYSIOLOGY

Chilliness is very marked, with a tendency to flushes of heat and bouts of shivering.

Appetite may be voracious but digestion is weak. When hungry, sits down to a meal but appetite departs after a mouthful or two. There is aversion to butter and greasy foods, and intolerance of sour things, fish, fruit, wine and milk (especially in infants).

Thirst is variable; at times there is great thirst for water, which tends to taste bitter, but during chills and fever thirst is usually absent.

During the day there is apt to be drowsiness, often accompanied by yawning and stretching, as also by palpitations. Sleep is liable to be disturbed by vivid, distressing dreams, and is in consequence unrefreshing.

Profuse, prostrating sweats occur, especially during sleep.

SYMPTOMATOLOGY

General

Characteristic is an extreme degree of physical exhaustion often associated with progressive anaemia. The asthenia ensues as the direct outcome of fluid loss from haemorrhage, severe purging, excessive diuresis, constant seminal emissions, copious sweating or prolonged suppuration. There is a general torpor of bodily function. Pain may be severe, and induced with renewed intensity by even light touch. Twinging, tearing, cutting pains may occur anywhere in the body. Passive haemorrhages occur from any orifice of the body, often in association with congestive or inflammatory conditions. The blood tends to be dark and contain clots. Periodicity of symptoms may be a feature, with recurrence at the same time each day, or every other day, or in the autumn of the year. Fever is associated with severe chills; there is thirst before the chill, absence of thirst during the hot stage and unquenchable thirst during the succeeding sweats. There is a peculiar acuteness of all senses, with hyperaesthesia to even light touch or the impact of a current of air, especially cold air.

Head

Vertigo is accompanied by flickerings before the eyes. Headache is throbbing in type, often parietal, and accompanied by extreme sensitiveness of the scalp and even of the hair. The headache is aggravated by movement and by the jar of every step when walking, also by cold draughts, by touch and at night. Relief is obtained to some extent in a warm room and by firm pressure. The brain may feel loose and knocking against the sides of the skull.

Eyes

Transient blindness may occur, or night-blindness, as an accompaniment of the asthenia.

Ears

Tinnitus is a feature of the remedy, various buzzing, ringing, roaring or other noises. There is intolerance of noise. Deafness may occur and is apt to be progressive.

Respiratory System

Frequent epistaxis is common, and the nose-bleed may give relief to headache. A spasmodic cough is aggravated by taking food, also by laughing; it is better when sitting upright. A suffocating sensation may be experienced as if the larynx was blocked with mucus. The remedy may be called for in relation to asthma which recurs in the autumn. One author mentions a cold feeling noticed in the belly with each respiration.

Alimentary System

A bitter salty taste is complained of in the mouth. The tongue appears flabby and is often heavily coated. Toothache is aggravated by light touch, but relieved by clenching the jaws tightly. Dyspepsia occurs, associated with indifference to food and drink and a sensation of constant satiety. The stomach feels 'cold'; there is a desire for condiments and stimulants. After meals there is a sensation of weight or of a lump behind the middle of the sternum. Flatulent distension of the belly may be extreme, as tight as a drum, and this is accompanied by sour eructations and loud belchings which afford no relief. Nor does the passage of flatus give any relief. Flatulence also accompanies liver and gall-bladder complaints. Jaundice is common. A painless diarrhoea is particularly debilitating; the stools are profuse, watery, acrid, and contain undigested food particles; they are very offensive in odour, and often worse at night; in the daytime the stools usually occur only after a meal. The remedy may be indicated in cholera infantum when the child is collapsed with cold ears, nose and chin, although by then the frequent stools may have ceased.

Cardiovascular System

The heart and circulation take part in the general asthenia, with a resulting tendency to attacks of giddiness and fainting, palpitation, and possibly oedema of extremities.

Urinary System

Frequent but ineffectual urging to pass urine is accompanied by pressure in the hypogastrium. The urine is apt to be turbid, scanty, with a sediment like brick-dust.

Genital System

The menstrual periods tend to be too early and too profuse, the blood passed being black and admixed with clots. If haemorrhage occurs during the course of labour, convulsions are likely to supervene. Furthermore, convulsions during labour may be induced by exposure to a draught of cold air.

Locomotor System

Tearing pains are felt in the bones of the limbs, aggravated by any movement. The lower limbs are weak and shaky, and knees feel wobbly when walking. The limbs may feel numb, especially if subjected to pressure.

Skin

There is very characteristic hypersensitivity of the body surface to the lightest touch, which may be registered as definite pain. On the other hand, firm pressure is tolerated.

MODALITIES

There is great aggravation from contact with cold air, draughts, also from movement or the least touch. The sufferer is worse after eating, especially from eating fruit or acid things; worse also at night, especially round about midnight, and in the autumn.

Relief is afforded by warmth, drinking hot tea, by rest and firm pressure.

CLINICAL NOTES

The remedy is of special value when the symptoms have been induced by excessive or prolonged loss of body fluids. One use mentioned is the prolonged administration of the 6c potency as a prophylatic against the formation of gallstones. The remedy is said to be incompatible with Digitalis. Complementary remedies are Carbo Veg., Natrum Mur., Psorinum.

Cocculus Indicus

SOURCE

Anamirta cocculus, Indian cockle, Levant nut, fish berry, is a plant found along the coast of Malabar, in India and in Ceylon. It is a woody climber with ash-coloured corky bark; it bears pendulous panicles of small yellow flowers; the leaves are huge with long stalks, heart-shaped, eight to twelve inches long and strongly ribbed on the under-surface; the fruit is a reddish brown kidney-shaped berry about the size of a large pea.

The outer coat of the berry is thin and becomes dry, black and wrinkled; within is a hard white shell divided into two, and containing a whitish, crescent-shaped, very oily seed. The seed contains a powerful convulsant poison, picrotoxin. The drug was formerly abused by being added to beer or porter for the purpose of drugging prospective victims of robbery in low dives. A more permissible use is that of stupefying fish by throwing the entire fruits into water.

PHARMACOLOGY

The drug has affinity with the central nervous system; with the motor cells producing tonic contractions, giving way to clonic spasms and later paralysis; with the sensorium, tending to mental confusion, stupor and unconsciousness; with the vital centres in the medulla, causing respiratory and cardiovascular disorders; with the digestive tract, inducing nausea, vomiting and severe colic.

PROVING

Cocculus was proved by Hahnemann, and published in the third volume of *Materia Medica Pura*.

APPEARANCE

The general appearance is as if intoxicated. Speech is difficult; takes a long time to answer. Movements are carried out with marked deliberation. Limbs seem very stiff or even paralysed. Speech may be slurred. Has a frightened look or sits in deep reverie.

PSYCHOLOGY

Mental stupefaction; slowness of comprehension; seems stupid; cannot find the right word; cannot finish anything.

Or, possibly, great talkativeness; witty joking; desire to sing.

Time passes too quickly; cannot stand least noise or contradiction; is melancholy; sensitive to insult; easily angered.

May show lack of concern for himself while being worried about others.

In delirium sees 'something alive rolling around'; has a delusion that 'his organs are hollow and empty'.

Complaints can be brought on by anger, grief or chagrin.

PHYSIOLOGY

There is extreme aversion to food; loathes even the thought of food, though may feel hungry. Gags at the mere mention of food.

There is considerable thirst, especially for beer.

Is scared to go to sleep because of hideous dreams which occur almost as soon as he closes his eyes. Constant starting awake; unrefreshed in the morning. May become ill through loss of sleep.

Cold sweat may be noticed on one or other hand.

SYMPTOMATOLOGY

General

Prostration is a marked feature, associated with curious, hollow, all-gone sensations, often induced by emotional stress or lack of sleep.

Odd bruised or digging pains are felt; there may be undue sensitivity to the slightest touch. Twitchings and jerking movements may simulate chorea, or transient paralysis may occur.

Head

Vertigo accompanied by nausea, numbness and unsteady gait is aggravated on rising, by travel, motion, or even by looking at moving objects. Lying down affords relief. An intense occipital headache associated with nausea and vomiting is made worse by movement, cold air, eating or drinking. It is also worse after sleep. There may be difficulty in holding the head erect owing to weakness of the cervical muscles. The head may feel hollow or as if a board was strapped across the forehead. There may be painful spasms of the temporal and masseter muscles.

Eyes
Pain in the eyeballs, which feel bruised and pulled forwards. Pupils either over-large or contracted. Vision apt to be blurred with black spots before the eyes.

Ears
Tinnitus is associated with deafness, and ears feel stopped up.

Respiratory System
The sense of smell may be unusually acute. Paralytic aphonia may occur. The throat is dry and a violent tickle may be felt in the larynx at 11.30 p.m. A fatiguing cough is associated with a feeling of oppression in the chest. Various stitches, sensations of spasm and tightness may be felt in the chest.

Alimentary System
Toothache in carious teeth is only noticed when eating. Teeth become loose and gums swollen. The mouth may be dry but without thirst, and tongue coated yellow. Nausea and vomiting are prominent features and accompany most complaints. Nausea is provoked by eating, or merely by the thought or smell of food. The inclination to vomit is accompanied by a copious flow of saliva. Frequent belching leaves a bitter taste in mouth and throat. The nausea and inclination to vomit are liable to be induced by any form of travel motion, and are aggravated by any attempt to sit or rise up. Pain may be felt in the hypochondria as from a bruise. Pain in the liver region is aggravated by coughing or stooping. Various pains, burning, pinching, pulling, tearing may be felt in the belly. Flatulent colic occurs round about midnight, accompanied by an empty feeling in the stomach, or possibly as if something alive was moving about in the abdomen. Constipation may occur, with much ineffectual urging and constrictive pain in the rectum. Diarrhoea may follow drinking cold water or accompany travel sickness; it is associated with colic, passage of flatus, and possibly a sensation as if stones were rubbing together in the abdomen.

Urinary System
Frequency of urge, with copious watery urine.

Genital System
Amenorrhoea is associated with profuse leucorrhoea and extreme weakness. Dysmenorrhoea is accompanied by the head and stomach symptoms mentioned above and sensations of prostration. Menses are early, copious and prolonged.

Locomotor System

Much heaviness, stiffness, and lameness in muscles, associated with numb feelings and a tendency to tremors. An affected limb cannot be flexed when straightened out, except by forceful passive movement which may extort cries of pain. Numbness of hands alternates with tensive pain in fingers; tips of fingers sting and itch. Paroxysmal stitches occur in shoulders, arms, and forearms, especially when at rest. Shooting pains are felt in thighs. Knees creak and crack with every movement and can scarcely support the sufferer, who staggers from side to side in danger of falling.

Skin

Pruritus is severe and widespread; is noticed especially in the evening, when undressing or in bed. Miliary or papular eruptions which itch in warm atmosphere. Ulcers are extremely sensitive to any contact.

MODALITIES

Aggravation results from a number of factors: cold air; open air, touch, pressure, jar or jolt; sitting up; riding in trains or cars; passive movement, e.g. at sea; talking; eating and drinking cold things; taking coffee; smoking; loss of sleep; at menstrual period; from midnight to 2 a.m.

Some relief is obtained by lying flat and keeping quiet.

CLINICAL NOTES

The remedy is of definite value in relation to travel sickness; can be given in the 30c potency for two days before travelling and repeated en route if necessary. There is incompatibility with Causticum and Coffea.

Coffea Cruda

SOURCE

The coffee tree, which in the wild grows to a height of thirty feet, belongs to the Rubiaceae, an order which includes *Cinchona*, *Ipecacuanha* and madder. It is an evergreen, having oblong ovate shiny leaves in opposite pairs. The flowers are in axillary clusters of fragrant white star-shaped blossoms, which fade rapidly. The fruit is a red or purple berry containing two plano-convex seeds. The plant contains caffeol, caffeine and tannin. The mother tincture is prepared from the raw berries.

PHARMACOLOGY

The chief affinity, due to the caffeine content, is with the central nervous system, stimulating the mental faculties and sensory perception. The neuro-muscular system is also affected, with resulting twitching and tremors. Cardiac rate and output are increased; there is vasodilatation of peripheral vessels and a diuretic effect.

PROVING

The proving of Coffea by five persons, one of whom was Hahnemann, is recorded by Stapf in his *Beiträge*.

APPEARANCE

The face tends to be flushed, hot and dry, while hands and feet are cold.

The subject is excited, talkative, on the go; may exhibit constant quick movements. Eats and drinks hurriedly.

Tremors of the hands may be present; also convulsive grinding of teeth.

There may be an exhausted appearance and an unwillingness for conversation.

PSYCHOLOGY

The mind is unusually active; full of ideas; memory may be phenomenal with an ability to quote poetry at great length.

Is apt to labour incessantly for some good cause to the point of a 'break-down' with accompanying dullness, gloom, constant yawning and stretching, drowsiness by day and undue wakefulness at night.

Over-excitement may result from sudden emotion, especially from good news. Gloom and gaiety alternate; laughter and tears intermingle.

Pain is quite insupportable, giving rise to despair or apprehension of death.

PHYSIOLOGY

The individual may feel hot, but at the same time shiver with cold extremities.

Hunger is often excessive, but with an attack of migraine there is loathing for all food and drink.

In fever, thirst is constant, especially during the stage of sweating.

Insomnia is induced by excessive pleasure or an over-active brain; is accompanied by hypersensitivity to external stimuli, e.g. ticking of clock, rattling window, banging door and the like; there is a constant flow of ideas, going over events of the past day or over plans for the morrow. Infants become wide awake at night and want to play.

SYMPTOMATOLOGY

General

There is unusual acuity of vision, hearing, taste and touch, a state of undue excitability to all impressions. There is ability to read very small print and to hear sounds inaudible to others. Affected sites are painfully sensitive; the whole body is over-active.

Head

Unilateral headache of migraine type, comes on after waking and increases in intensity to become intolerable; there may be a feeling as if a nail was being driven into the head or as if there was a rush of blood to the head. The headache is made worse by eating, by the least noise or by movement. The sufferer wants to sit or lie quite still in the dark, or with eyes closed. Facial neuralgia is very severe, with pain extending to molar teeth, ears, forehead and scalp; cold applications give some relief, but pain recurs as the parts become warm again.

Respiratory System

Epistaxis is likely to occur. The sense of smell is exceptionally acute. Hoarseness is common on waking, accompanied by sticky mucus only dislodged with difficulty. Sore throat; the soft palate is swollen and extremely sensitive – the condition is aggravated by swallowing. A nervous tickly cough is most evident at night. The chest feels tight; breathing is shallow and heaves the chest visibly; suffocative attacks occur.

Alimentary System

Toothache is eased temporarily by holding iced water in the mouth. Nausea is associated with glairy vomit. Eructations of sour fluid occur. Bloating of the belly necessitates loosening of the clothes. Distension of the colon gives rise to pain in the right hypochondrium. Painless diarrhoea may be induced by sudden joy. Piles are associated with bleeding occurring during a normal stool.

Cardiovascular System

Violent irregularity of heart action may supervene on sudden surprise or excessive joy.

Genital System

Menstrual periods are early and prolonged. Dysmenorrhoea pain is intolerable and accompanied by the passage of large black clots. Hypersensitivity of vulva and vagina makes wearing a sanitary towel unbearable and coitus painful. Voluptuous pruritus involves the genital region. During labour and after-pains there may be inordinate fear of death.

Nervous System

Shooting pains in arms and legs are worse by movement and in afternoon and night; pressure affords relief. Hands show tremors on use.

Skin

Pruritus creates a desire to scratch, but the skin is too sensitive.

MODALITIES

Aggravation results from cold, in open air, from pungent odours, physical contact, wine, narcotics; also from strong emotion, especially if pleasurable, and at night.

Relief is obtained from warmth and when lying down.

CLINICAL NOTES

The remedy is chiefly of value in relation to insomnia and neuralgias. A complementary remedy is Aconite. Incompatibles are Causticum and Ignatia.

Colchicum Autumnale

The origin of this remedy is that delicately beautiful plant, *Colchicum autumnale*, the autumn crocus or naked maiden. The pale mauve blossom, so suggestive of a crocus, possesses a pearly white tubular quill-like stem some five to ten inches high, its base encircled by two or three membranous sheaths. The three dark green strap-like leaves may be a foot or more in length and two inches wide. The flower springs from an underground corm resembling a bulb at first sight.

The corm is, however, solid inside its two coats, not laminated. It is a node on the underground rhizome, which forms fresh nodes every year. The outer coat is dark brown in colour, the inner one reddish-yellow. The solid corm, about the size of a small walnut, is white and fleshy and contains a milky juice. It is rounded on one aspect, flattened and grooved on the other. The fruit is a large, three-valved capsule or syncarpy, containing dark brown seeds which are liberated when ripe by the bursting open of the capsule.

So much for the description of the plant and its parts. In its behaviour this plant is unique. It is indeed a member of the Liliaceae, but no other lily behaves in such an unorthodox and almost outrageous manner. The lilies are among the earliest plants to flower in the spring and are not 'naked like their strange sister, but clothed in leaves, joyful and gay'.

This plant, however, rushes into flower, or at any rate the flower suddenly comes to view above ground in the autumn, when other plants are dying. After hiding away from the sun during the normal flowering season it flaunts its lovely nakedness in the warm days of the Indian summer, devoid of leafy clothing. The leaves do not appear above ground till the following March or April, when they companion the fruit, not the flower.

The seeds, moreover, are not liberated till July, after taking an inordinately long time to ripen, fertilization having taken place in the preceding autumn. All this presents a picture of strangely distorted growth rhythm. Significantly, while this is taking place, a most virulent poison is being manufactured in the plant – an alkaloid, colchicine.

The plant therefore harbours pent-up poison. As one author writes,

'In some parts of Europe the flowers grow in such profusion that a whole meadow is filled with them. This glorious sight gives no hint of the destructive force latent in the sea of plants and blossoms. The colourful upright flowers look attractive and harmless, and children are in the habit of playing with the cheerfully-rattling seed pods during the hay harvest. Now and again it happens that a child takes out one of the seeds and swallows it, or even eats a flower.' This may have fatal results. Five grams of the seed are fatal to adults, and one and a half grams can kill a child. Murders have been committed or attempted by adding powdered Colchicum seeds to some strong alcoholic drink.

The plant was held in great renown in the thirteenth century, and from its supposed virtues in the cure of gout and rheumatism of the joints it obtained the sobriquet of Anima Articulorum, 'the soul of joints'.

The long association of the plant with gout is significant, for this malady is in itself an example of distorted metabolic rhythm, an imbalance of assimilation and elimination leading to the retention in the tissues of toxic waste products, another case of 'pent-up poison'.

This innocent-looking plant has a nauseous odour and is acrid to the taste. All its parts are poisonous, even when dried. Many fatal cases of poisoning have been recorded; it was used by the ancients for both public and secret death sentences. For medicinal purposes the corm is used and is best lifted in the spring, when a year old. The mother tincture is prepared from the juice expressed from the corm.

PHARMACOLOGY

Colchicine is a mitotic poison interfering with the formation of the chromosome spindle in the process of cell division. It is in this way cytostatic. It also disturbs the rhythm of granulocyte formation in the bone marrow, producing either leucopenia or leucocytosis. Further it possesses an anti-allergic and anti-phlogistic action, thus interfering in a deadly manner with the body's natural defences, normally manifested by inflammation. It is, moreover, a capillary poison, causing marked distension and even paralysis of the capillaries, with resulting hyper-aemia and haemorrhage. Symptoms of poisoning are instructive. One observer recorded that 'on cutting the fresh corm into slices, the acrid particles emitted from it irritated the nostrils, fauces and breath, and that the tips of the fingers with which it had been held became quite benumbed; that, applied for two minutes to the tip of the tongue, it rendered the part stiff and almost void of sensation for six hours; that less than a grain wrapped in a crumb of bread, and taken internally, produced alarming symptoms.'

The symptoms of acute poisoning usually appear in a few hours after ingestion, but may be delayed for as long as five days. A latent period is followed by a sudden and devastating 'flare-up'; the mouth and throat begin to burn; the victim suffers unendurable thirst but has difficulty in swallowing. Terrible nausea is followed by frequent and violent vomiting.

This condition lasts between twelve and twenty-four hours. Then more serious symptoms ensue, the sufferer exhibiting the typical picture of cholera, with agonizing colic which grows more and more intense and is accompanied by bloody, diarrhoeic stools. Paralysis develops, and difficulty in breathing. Death occurs in about two days unless a circulatory collapse brings an earlier release from the agony. The mind remains clear till the end.

Cushny mentions in poisoning by Colchicum, 'depression, apathy and collapse with a small rapid pulse. An early leucopenia is followed by leucocytosis'.

In the use of material doses of colchicine in the treatment of gout it is noted that the treatment 'is not effective unless early symptoms of Colchicum poisoning are produced'.

The main affinities of the plant, therefore, are seen to be: with the gastro-intestinal tract, causing severe nausea, vomiting and diarrhoea accompanied by belly cramps and collapse; with the kidneys, inducing nephritis and haematuria; with the muscular system, resulting in extreme loss of tone and consequent weakness; with serous membranes and fibrous tissues, producing irritation and rheumatic or gouty pains. Effusions may occur into pleural, pericardial, peritoneal or articular cavities, possibly haemorrhagic in character, with mucous membranes and skin, inducing redness, pricking sensations, and much burning in the mouth and throat.

PROVINGS

Colchicum was twice proved in the school of Hahnemann, first by Stapf (*Archiv*, Vol. VI) and later by Reil (*Vierteljahrschrift*, Vol. VIII).

APPEARANCE

The sufferer presents a waxy pallor of countenance. He appears exhausted and trembling; sits or lies very still, afraid to make the least movement – reminiscent of the Bryonia picture.

He may slide down in the bed from sheer weakness; may present dropsical swellings with pitting oedema or red, tender, swollen joints.

PSYCHOLOGY

The Colchicum patient is oversensitive to everything, to light, noise, any little jar or jolt and especially to odours.

Perhaps because of this hypersensitive condition the sufferer is also exceedingly irritable. The least thing annoys, nothing is right – 'there's no pleasing him...'

Again the picture may be one of absent-mindedness, forgetfulness and confusion of thought, especially in low fevers.

PHYSIOLOGY

The Colchicum subject, like the 'naked maiden' shivering in the chill mists of autumn as they dissipate the warmth of the Indian summer, is extremely chilly, feeling cold even when close to the fire. There may, however, be occasional flushes of heat.

The reactions to food are peculiar, normal appetite being deranged. An extraordinary aversion to all kinds of food is associated with intense nausea. This latter is excited by the sight, smell, even mention or thought of food; the smell of food or cooking is sufficient to induce gagging, retching, vomiting and perhaps fainting. As a result the very idea of food becomes repugnant and all food may be refused.

Thirst varies considerably. It may be excessive or entirely absent.

Insomnia is common and loss of sleep tends to produce an extreme degree of exhaustion and debility.

Sweating is prominent, at times of the cold clammy variety. If the perspiration is suppressed, perhaps by being in a cold draught, semi-paresis of the limbs may supervene.

SYMPTOMATOLOGY

General

Colchicum illnesses are acute and grave, but they are in essence an exacerbation of a smouldering internal disorder, underground as it were, which flares up into sudden obvious activity, possibly accompanied by effusion or by deposition of waste products in the tissues. Pains are intolerable owing to the acuteness of all sensations. The hypersensitivity is, moreoever, associated with a grave lack of reactivity, leading to low states, as met with in typhoid or other fevers. Extreme exhaustion is a prominent feature, the patient being too weak even to raise head from pillow – the withered blossom can no longer cope with its altered surroundings and withdraws into relative inertia below ground. Hydrops of serous cavities or anasarca, local or general, may develop.

Head

Headaches are 'rheumatic' in type, often spreading to the nape of the neck, aggravated by stooping; and in the afternoon and evening, also by any mental exertion. They are associated with sensitiveness of the scalp; in fact the whole skull feels sore and bruised.

Eyes

With headache the pupils tend to be unequal and vision dimmed. There is a liability to iritis in association with rheumatic symptoms. Styes or ulcers may be present on the lids. Lachrymation is common and the tears excoriate the skin.

Respiratory System

The sense of smell is abnormally acute, even to the detection of odours unperceived by others. Smells are apt to cause revulsion, even nausea and fainting. Tingling and tickling sensations may be complained of in nose and throat and trachea. The latter may give rise to a tiresome dry cough.

Alimentary System

Teeth are very sensitive; hurt when clenching the jaws. Gums recede and teeth become loose. One prominent feature mentioned already is a deadly nausea, associated with violent bilious vomiting and leading to extreme prostration. The nausea and vomiting are made much worse by any attempt to sit up, a symptom reminiscent of Bryonia. Burning may cause distress in the pit of the stomach, but sometimes an icy cold feeling is present in this region. The belly becomes extremely distended and tympanitic, with much flatulence and soreness to touch. Spasmodic pains occur, colicky, burning, griping pains, causing the sufferer to bend double in search of relief. Any movement or taking food increases the suffering. Diarrhoea, or actual dysentery, may occur, especially in the autumn; the stools are extremely painful, frequent and may be passed involuntarily. They are jelly-like or putrid, dark, blood-stained and contain mucous shreds. Rectal prolapse may occur in association with much tenesmus and anal spasm. The remedy may be called for in the 'typhoid state' – dilated pupils, cold sweat on brow, head falls back weakly on pillow if he attempts to raise it, lower jaw sagging widely, face cadaveric, tongue protruded with hesitant difficulty, aphonia, cold breath, restlessness, cramps in legs, nausea, vomiting and retching. But in spite of this conglomeration of severe symptoms the patient shows little concern over his condition and none of the fear of death so prominent in the Arsenicum Alb. sufferer.

Cardiovascular System

Palpitation occurs with a sensation of oppression behind the sternum, especially at night and when lying on the left side. Anginal pains may be present, dyspnoea on slight exertion and 'cardiac anxiety'. The pains in the region of the heart may be violent, cutting or stinging in type, and palpitation may be so severe that the heart's impulse can be heard at a distance. The chest feels as if 'tightly bandaged'. In low fevers the heart action becomes weak with a thready pulse, low blood pressure and threatened collapse. In rheumatic illness, subacute or chronic pericarditis may develop with or without effusion.

Nervous System

Paraesthesia – pins and needles – occurs in wrists, hands, fingers and under the nails, and this is especially noticed when grasping something. Neuralgic pains are described, affecting usually one side of the face, with a tendency to spread to the head and the ears.

Urinary System

Quite severe symptoms are recorded arising from inflammatory lesions of the urinary tract. Painful, scalding urination, oliguria, anuria, albuminuria, haematuria, nephritis, anasarca with pitting oedema.

Locomotor System

The remedy may be of service in connection with rheumatic affections of the fibro-muscular tissues and also in arthritic lesions. The pains of a shooting, tearing type are more superficially felt when the weather is warm, but in cold weather they affect the deep tissues and the bones. Moreover, these pains may start on the left side and later extend to the right, as is the case with Lachesis symptoms. Pains in the muscles are accompanied by a bruised sensation and often by twitchings. They may especially affect the nape and the muscles of the chest. Pains in the arms may so paralyse the limb that it becomes impossible to grasp quite small objects. Redness, heat, swelling, with sharp sticking pains affect the small joints of hands and feet, especially the big toes. These pains are apt to shift from joint to joint, to be worse from both cold and warmth, especially damp cold. They are aggravated by the least touch or jar, which induces a fear of being approached, similar to that associated with Arnica. The least movement augments the pain and the sufferer is apt to become intensely irritable.

MODALITIES

Aggravation results from exposure to cold and damp, especially cold rains in autumn. Extreme heat in mid-summer is also not well tolerated. There is aggravation also from the least movement or even from being touched, owing to hpyersensitivity.

Warmth, being well wrapped-up, and rest afford relief. The delicate flower of the autumn crocus unfolds on still sunny days in the warmth of the Indian summer.

CLINICAL NOTES

Colchicum has been often employed in low potency, mother tincture or 3x, especially in the treatment of gout, but higher potencies are also efficacious.

It is essentially called for in acute and severe conditions as instanced above, and especially when the sufferer is extremely weak, extremely chilly, extemely sensitive and extremely irritable.

Related remedies are Arsenicum Alb., Cantharis, Colocynthis, Veratrum Alb., Cactus Grandiflorus and Bryonia.

After misuse of Colchicum, Spigelia can be used as an antidote.

Colocynthis

SOURCE

The source of this remedy is a gourd, *Cucumis colocynthis*, also known as bitter cucumber or bitter apple. The fruit, however, is much more like an orange in colour and size. The plant is a member of the Cucurbitaceae family, to which *Bryonia dioica* also belongs. It is a trailing plant, not seeking firm attachment like Bryony, but twisting and twining in a much more active and restless manner.

The white annual branched root strikes deep into the ground. The angular hispid stem bears long stalked palmate leaves, also hairy, a fine green on the upper aspect and rough and pale below. A filiform tendril arises opposite each leaf stalk. The five-petalled star-shaped flower arises from the axilla of the leaf and has a short stalk; its colour is yellow with greenish veins. The pollen-bearing organs and the seed vessels are on separate flowers.

The fruit is a greenish-yellow globose berry, almost obscenely large in relation to the quite small flower from which it arises. It has a thin but solid rind and contains a white spongy pulp in which are embedded smooth, oval, yellowish-orange seeds. The fruit varies in size from two to four inches in diameter. It has an intensely bitter taste, which is retained in the mother tincture when prepared from the pulp.

This plant develops a most powerful purgative in the bloated pulp-filled belly of the fruit. Its cathartic action is mainly due to a glucoside, colocynthin, which possesses toxic properties. Resins and an alkaloid are also present and possess purgative powers.

The twisting and twining habits of growth are exemplified in the sufferer from poisoning with the pulp of the berry, who will be found writhing in agony and doubled up with excruciating colic. The bristly stem and prickly leaves, not to mention the separation of the sexes on different flowers, suggest an irascible, irritable, unsociable nature.

PHARMACOLOGY

In moderate doses the drug acts as a purge and was employed extensively by both Arabian and Greek physicians for this purpose in dropsy, lethargy and mania. It was also used to induce abortion. Its chief habitat is in the countries bordering the Eastern Mediterranean.

In large doses it causes violent inflammatory lesions of the intestinal tract leading to gangrene and death, the liver and genito-urinary organs being also involved.

The acute irritant effect on the gastro-intestinal canal results in nausea, vomiting, violent purging and severe griping pains. An affinity with the nervous system is manifested in paroxysmal neuralgia in various sites. Renal inflammation has occurred as the result of inhalation of the powdered pulp during its manufacture.

PROVING

There is a pathogenesis of Colocynthis in the sixth volume of Hahnemann's *Materia Medica Pura.*

APPEARANCE

The Colocynthis patient presents a mixed picture of anger and anguish. The face tends to be dark red and distorted with pain. The sufferer will be writhing in agony or doubled up with pain, possibly pressing some hard object into the belly in search of relief. He is quite unable to keep still. He may be speechless with rage or, possibly, screaming with agony. The child lies on its belly or in a doubled-up posture.

PSYCHOLOGY

Extreme irritability is the predominant feature in this sphere. A tendency to flare up over the least thing, to be easily upset by trifles. Friends irritate; he wants to be left alone; is disinclined to talk. The child is inclined to be naughty and to take offence very readily.

It should be noted that complaints induced or precipitated by grief, anger, indignation or chagrin may well respond to this remedy. The sequence of events may start from emotional disturbance of endocrine activity, leading to autonomic imbalance, altered tone in plain muscle of gut and also of blood-vessel walls, and ensuing disorders of rhythm and function.

PHYSIOLOGY

The Colocynthis subject is on the chilly side and is sensitive to cold, especially damp cold.

There may be a disinclination for food, but not nearly to the extreme degree manifested by Colchicum patients.

There is a constant desire to drink fluids, which taste good at the time but leave a flat taste behind in the mouth. The skin is often hot and dry. Sweat, if present, may smell like urine.

Sleep is apt to be disturbed by vivid dreams or may be difficult. When asleep there is a tendency to lie on the back with one hand beneath the head.

SYMPTOMATOLOGY

General

All pains are paroxysmal, coming on in waves of agony. Both onset and relief are abrupt, a characteristic also of the pains of Belladonna, Kali Bich. and Kalmia. The pains, moreover, are often accompanied by faintness and weakness; actual syncope may occur, or the sufferer may be too weak to speak. The tearing, violent neuralgic pains are so severe that the victim must keep moving. While movement may not give much relief the pains are nevertheless much worse if he keeps at rest. Firm pressure affords some easement and local heat may help. The typical pains may be brought on by a fit of anger or as the result of a quarrel or grave annoyance. 'Getting mad' induces the pain, and the severity of the pains makes him madder still – so much so that he gets angry with sympathizers and desires to be left alone. The pains are often left-sided.

Head

Giddiness is noticed when turning the head sharply, especially on turning it to the left. The remedy has an important sphere in facial neuralgias affecting various regions, supra-orbital, infra-orbital and mandibular, and usually one-sided. The pain comes on in waves and may be relieved somewhat by pressure and heat. Mag. Phos. is another remedy of service in facial pain, especially when on the right side.

Eyes

Sharp boring pains are recorded, with relief from pressure. A sensation on stooping as if the eye would fall out. Quivering of the right upper lid.

Ears

Itching deep in the ear is relieved by boring the finger into the external auditory canal. Sounds tend to re-echo in the ears.

Respiratory System

Fluent coryza occurs in the morning, without sneezing. A dry, teasing cough is accompanied by oppressive tightness in the chest. Stitches may be felt in the muscles of the thorax, between the shoulder-blades, or in one or other scapular region. Smoking tobacco immediately excites a persistent cough.

Alimentary System
It is in this sphere that the remedy really comes into its own. The taste in the mouth is often very bitter. There is a sore, very red tongue and the tongue feels 'burnt' or 'scalded'. It may, however, be heavily coated white. Teeth are sore, as if the nerve of the tooth had been put on the stretch, especially the teeth of the lower jaw. An extreme degree of flatulent distension in the belly is associated with violent, paroxysmal, cutting, griping colic – as if 'guts were being ground between stones', or as if 'stomach was grasped by the fingers of a powerful hand'. The pains are made worse by eating or drinking even the smallest amounts. They are often accompanied by nausea and vomiting, diarrhoea and the passage of vast quantities of flatus. Kent points out, 'The vomiting of Colocynthis is different from that of most other remedies. Nausea does not appear at first, but when the pain becomes sufficiently intense, nausea and vomiting begin, the contents of the stomach are ejected and the patient continues to retch until the severity of the suffering decreases. The colic of infants is relieved by lying on the stomach, but as soon as the position is changed they begin to scream again.' Although the pain is relieved or eased at first by firm pressure, later on the belly becomes so sensitive that even touch is not tolerated. Temporary relief is afforded by local heat, by violent movement, by passage of flatus or a stool, by drinking coffee, by smoking. Rectal urging is common, and stools tend to be copious, fluid, spluttery, frothy and saffron-yellow in colour, and have a musty or mouldy odour. The stools may be dysenteric in character with severe tenesmus, or jelly-like. Taking even the least amount of food or drink precipitates a further bowel action.

Genital System
Drawing pains may be felt in testicles and spermatic cords. Priapism may be troublesome. Severe, tense, penetrating pain may be felt in the left ovary, doubling the sufferer up, and accompanied by intense agitation.

Urinary System
Renal colic is associated with copious reddish-brown urine showing a flocculent sediment. A frequent, often ineffectual urge to urinate is accompanied by scalding micturition and associated with pressure in the hypogastrium and colicky pains in the belly. Urine may be scanty, quickly becoming thick, gelatinous and sticky when passed, and having an intensely offensive odour.

Nervous System
Frightful pains, neuralgic in type, occur in the spine, limbs, head, ovaries. They are often brought on by anger or rage, are shooting or

lancinating in character and may be associated with numbness. Trigeminal neuralgia may occur in association with gastro-enteritis. Sciatica is a special indication if the symptoms agree. It is usually left-sided with cramp-like pains, worse at rest. The pain extends from the loin downwards into the thigh and may be accompanied by a sensation as if 'the hip is fixed in iron clamps'. The pain is aggravated by extending the limb and at night. It is eased to some extent by lying on the affected side, by drawing the limb up or by moving about.

Locomotor System

Pains and stiffness afflict the muscles, especially in the nape and cervical region, the upper dorsum, the right shoulder region and the palms. The pains are vice-like, made worse by movement, and possibly accompanied by formication and numbness. They are eased by warmth and also by the passage of flatus. These tearing stitches in muscles are possibly due to local spasm or perhaps to local vaso-spasm. A symptom mentioned is a cramping pain in the right thigh when walking, as if the psoas muscle were too short. On standing still the pain ceases, only to return on a further attempt to walk. Such sudden unaccountable spasms do occur at odd times and in odd sites; it might be that Colocynthis would give relief.

Skin

There is mention of pruritus affecting the whole surface of the body, accompanied by great restlessness. This is especially noticed in the evening and in bed, when it may be followed by sweating. Widespread desquamation may occur.

MODALITIES

Aggravation is caused by cold wind, damp cold, eating raw fruit, drinking iced water when hot; also by rage or indignation; by suppressed sweat; by repose; around the hour of 4 p.m.

Relief is felt to some extent by bending double, by hard pressure, and from locally applied heat.

CLINICAL NOTES

The 200c and higher potencies are often extremely effective. Hahnemann states that the action of Colocynthis is of long duration.

Lower potencies are frequently employed on the Continent, mainly 2x to 4x.

A complementary remedy is Causticum. Opium is listed as an antidote.

Conium Maculatum

SOURCE

Conium maculatum, common hemlock, spotted hemlock, poison hemlock or herb Bennet is the famous plant associated for all time with the death by poison of Socrates. It was indeed widely used by both Greeks and Romans for both judicial and criminal homicide. It was also employed medicinally in various ways, notably in the treatment of tumours, especially those affecting the breast.

The plant is the only member of the very large family of Umbelliferae which possesses a smooth spotted stem. It is a biennial, flowering in June and July, and widely distributed in the northern hemisphere. It is found growing in hedges, orchards, on waste ground and rubbish-heaps, often close to human settlements where the soil contains more than the usual amount of nitrogen.

The root is conical, fleshy, often forked, with sparse rootlets; it is pale in colour, sweetish in taste and has an unpleasant odour.

The stem is distinctive in that it is very freely marked with reddish or brownish purple spots and blotches, rather suggestive of the eruption of a malignant fever. It is upright, three to six feet in height, rounded, smooth, hollow, shiny and much-branched.

The large spreading, deeply-cleft leaves resemble those of parsley at first sight, and have been eaten in mistake with fatal results. The taste of the leaves is bitter and sharp. Their colour is a deep shining green and the leaf stalks are sheathed at the base.

The multi-rayed umbels bear small white flowers of five petals. At the bases of the secondary umbels and at the junction of the main umbel with its stem there are three collars of small pointed bracts.

The seeds are ovoid, somewhat flattened, showing five thick wavy ridges on the outer aspect. They have been utilized in mistake for anise seeds, which they resemble, with dire results.

The whole plant exhales a foetid odour when bruised, reminiscent of mouse urine; fruit, leaves and root are all poisonous. The plant contains a number of alkaloids, the most important of which is coniine (alpha-propyl piperidine); this, unlike the majority of alkaloids, is volatile and is responsible for the repulsive odour. It possesses an action on peripheral

199

ganglia similar to that of nicotine.

The mother tincture is prepared from the fresh plant when in flower. If the fruit alone is used, it should be gathered while still green from plants of second-year growth.

PHARMACOLOGY

The plant has a special affinity with the motor elements, leading first to stiffness and spasticity of voluntary muscle, followed by progressive paralysis, spreading from below upwards. Other effects are nausea, vomiting, salivation; also headache, dilation of the pupils and inhibition of glandular activity. Delirium and stupor may occur, but usually the mind remains clear and respiration ceases while the heart is still beating.

Dr J. H. Bennett records the case of a man who ate a large quantity of hemlock in mistake for parsley. Soon afterwards there was loss of power in the lower limbs but he apparently suffered no pain. In attempting to walk he staggered about as if drunk; at length his limbs refused to support him and he fell down.

On being raised, his legs dragged behind him, and when his arms were lifted up they fell like inert masses and remained immovable. There was complete paralysis of both upper and lower extremities within two hours after he had taken the poison. There was loss of the power of deglutition and a partial paralysis of sensation, but no convulsions, only slight occasional motions of the left leg; the pupils were fixed.

Three hours after eating the hemlock respiratory movements ceased, and death took place in three and a quarter hours, evidently due to gradual asphyxia from paralysis of the muscles of respiration. The intellect was perfectly clear until shortly before death. This account closely parallels the description by Plato in the *Phaedo* of the death of Socrates.

PROVING

Conium is one of the medicines of the *Materia Medica Pura*. Its pathogenesis appears in the fourth volume.

APPEARANCE

The face may appear red and flushed or present a palish livid hue. Tremblings, twitchings, jerkings may be evident, and a tendency to pick at nostrils and fingers till they bleed.

Paralytic weakness is manifested by clumsy movements and staggering gait.

PSYCHOLOGY

Mentally the Conium subject seems dull, unable to make sustained mental effort. There is a disinclination for any application to business or other tasks; wants just to play around and idle. There is aversion to company, probably from an unwillingness to make the effort of conversation, but on the other hand there is a dread of being left alone.

There seems a sort of passive indifference; it is too much trouble to think. Great anguish of mind may supervene, even melancholia; this tends to recur every second week. Depression is marked before the start of the menstrual period. This state of affairs may ensue as the result of excessive grief, mental overstrain or suppression of menses.

PHYSIOLOGY

Chilliness is a feature of the subject's make-up, even flatus or stools seem cold when passed. Numbness is also often complained of.

Appetite is poor, with aversion to bread. Quite small amounts of alcohol may cause excitement, trembling, and a feeling of weakness and prostration. There may be a craving for salt, sour things and coffee. There is a distaste for milk.

Although irresistibly drowsy during the day, may lie awake on going to bed, till midnight. Sleep is disturbed by frightful dreams, even nightmares. Sweats are heavy, especially when falling off to sleep or merely on closing the eyes.

SYMPTOMATOLOGY

General

Pains when present are cutting, stabbing, knife-like and often accompanied by numbness. Tumours, enlarged lymph nodes or glands, even injured parts tend to become indurated and feel stony hard.

Head

Giddiness is a prominent feature, especially noticed on turning the head quickly, when turning over in bed or on rising from sitting. There is a sensation as if the bed was turning in a circle, and a desire to hold the head perfectly still. The face may feel hot, or a cobweb sensation may be felt on the right cheek. A sick headache is liable to accrue from looking at moving objects, the result of weakness in the ocular muscles; relief is obtained by lying quite still with the eyes closed. Stabbing pains may be felt in the occipital region, synchronizing with the pulse beat. A bursting headache may be present on waking in the morning.

Eyes

Extreme photophobia and excessive lachrymation may occur, out of all proportion to the obvious signs of pathological changes in the eye. Pricking and burning pains are felt in the eyes and objects appear red or rainbow-coloured, or maybe striped, doubled, or blurred. Paresis of lids causes ptosis.

Ears

Tearing or shooting pains occur in and around the ears, chiefly noticed when walking out of doors. There is a tendency to the accumulation of wax, which may be the colour of red blood. Tinnitus may be troublesome, a variety of noises being described.

Respiratory System

Nasal symptoms are various, including twitching and itching of the nostrils and a distinct tendency to frequent epistaxis which may be associated with bouts of sneezing. A very persistent cough is provoked by constant tickling and scraping in the throat. It may be suffocating or paroxysmal in nature and is worse in bed, especially on first lying down, and is aggravated also by taking a deep breath. It compels the sufferer to sit up and hold onto the chest with both hands when coughing. Sputum is scanty and expectoration difficult, so that the phlegm is usually swallowed. Dyspnoea is noticed on effort, and especially on walking; it may be accompanied by a sensation of tightness or violent pains in the chest. The remedy may prove of value in some types of asthma, also in whooping-cough.

Alimentary System

Dysphagia associated with a feeling of a lump in the throat may result from neuromuscular incoordination. This may cause frequent involuntary attempts at swallowing. The tongue may feel stiff and swollen and may 'burn' at the tip. Belching may be persistent and noisy, the eructations tasting of food; pyrosis, nausea and vomiting may occur, associated with the sensation of a tight band across the hypochondrium. Cutting, cramping pains occur in the belly, which is tender to touch. There is much bloating, even on waking in the morning, and noisy borborygmi. Constipation tends to give trouble every second day. There is much ineffectual urging and much straining at stool. The passage of a hard stool is followed by sudden tremulous weakness, palpitation, even fainting. Flatus is discharged with difficulty and feels cold as passed. Diarrhoea may alternate with constipation. In old people chronic painless diarrhoea may supervene, and stools may be involuntary.

Lymphatic and Glandular Systems

Breasts become swollen before the menstrual period, with associated soreness and sharp pains. Mammary tumours tend to be of stony hardness and show increase in size before the periods. Enlargements of salivary glands or of lymph nodes also tend to be notably hard.

Urinary System

Great pressure may be felt in the bladder, associated with frequency and interrupted urination – urine flows in fits and starts. Cutting pains are felt at the neck of the bladder; burning and shooting pain may be felt in the urethra during and after the passage of urine.

Genital System

In the male, impotence is associated with increased libido. Testicles become enlarged and feel hard. In women menstruation is delayed in onset and shortened in duration. Preceding the period there is pruritus of vulva, and swelling of breasts which become heavy, hard and painful. During the period uterine cramps occur, and abundant, milky, acid leucorrhoea follows the period for about ten days. The period can be abruptly cut short if the hands are placed in cold water.

Nervous System

The remedy may be called for in chorea, epilepsy, mania and delirium tremens. Paralytic weakness occurs in the lower limbs, associated with tremors, spreading from below upwards. The limbs are cold, stiff and clumsy, with a tendency to fall forward.

Skin

Pruritic patches in varying sites. Yellow discoloration of palms and nails. Urticarial weals and spots may appear after violent exercise. Dry, scaly crescentic patchy eruptions come and go in any site. Petechial spots tend to 'burn'.

MODALITIES

Aggravation is mostly from physical causes: when standing still, sitting at rest, turning in bed; from touch, jar or jolt, or pressure of tight clothing. There is also aggravation after meals, at night when lying with the head low, and both before and during the menstrual period.

The subject feels better in the dark, from warmth, when moving about, walking briskly, and by allowing the limbs to hang down.

CLINICAL NOTES

Conium is of special value in old age when the vital powers of the body are failing. It has frequently to be preceded by other remedies. It is said to be a long-acting remedy. It has been employed in relation to the scirrhous type of malignant tumour.

Cuprum Metallicum

SOURCE

The metal copper gets its name from Cyprus, the island sacred to Venus. Its ores manifest an amazing range of vivid colours, blues, greens, reds, purples. The metal itself when burnished glows like gold. It burns with a shining blue-green flame tinged at the tip with red. It is a very active metal with a great capacity for absorbing water and transforming it into form and colour.

Next to iron, copper is perhaps the most useful metal in the world. Millions of miles of copper wire and cable carry electric current and transmit messages from one end of the earth to the other. Alloyed with zinc the metal forms brass. Alloyed with tin it forms bronze. Copper was indeed the first metal used by man as he emerged from the Stone Age.

Copper is an essential constituent of the body, but in trace quantities. Poisoning hazards may however derive from copper contamination of fumes, dust or air in connection with smelting, from the use of the metal in welding, in the preparation of alloys, in the electrical and building industries, in the manufacture of inks, paints, and agricultural products such as fungicides and pesticides.

For use as a remedy, triturations are made of dry powdered copper up to the third centesimal potency, when it becomes soluble in water or alcohol. Further potencies are then prepared by succussion.

PHARMACOLOGY

The metal acts as an irritant throughout the whole length of the intestinal tract, causing severe nausea, burning, vomiting and purging. Affinity with the nervous system produces first spasms and convulsions, and later paralysis. Copper dust if inhaled involves the lining of the air passages, resulting in laryngitis, bronchitis, and possibly asthma.

PROVING

Cuprum Met. was proved by Hahnemann and published in the third edition of his *Chronic Diseases*.

APPEARANCE

The face tends to be reddish or red and white in patches. Jerking occurs in the limbs, starting in toes and fingers. In the presence of convulsions the lips and limbs acquire a bluish tinge. A characteristic feature is forcible flexion of the thumbs into the palms. Eyelids may show snapping movements. Speech may be impaired and stammering, owing to partial paralysis of the tongue. There are long pauses before replying.

PSYCHOLOGY

Emotional instability is prominent; 'flies off the handle' moods vary – sullen, loquacious, malicious, morose, often with fixed ideas, possibly a terror of death. The spoiled child, tricky, changeable, disorderly, dissatisfied. Sudden urge to injure, to scream, to run away, to escape. Tendency to shrink from people; aptitude for mimicry. Wild-eyed, maniacal fits of rage; or may lie like someone dead, blue and rigid.

PHYSIOLOGY

Is excessively chilly, yet thirsty for cold water. Gluttony may alternate with anorexia. Sleep is deep; twitching and jerking occur in sleep with audible borborygmi. Sweats occur at night and are profuse.

SYMPTOMATOLOGY

General

Violence characterizes all symptoms. Paroxysms of cramp or actual convulsions recur at intervals and are followed by extreme mental and physical exhaustion. Spasms can be triggered off by vexation or fright, or are associated with uraemia or other form of toxaemia, resulting perhaps from suppressed eruptions. Nervous prostration affects young people. Exhaustion may derive from loss of sleep or be brought on by undue effort, either mental or physical. Both onset and cessation of the cramps are abrupt. Periodicity is a feature, and symptoms tend to be left-sided.

Head

Severe headache is accompanied by spasmodic vomiting of all food and fluids ingested. Throbbing headache occurs in the region of the frontal sinuses; some relief is obtained by lying down with the head warmly wrapped. Giddiness accompanies various ailments, with a tendency for the head to fall forward on the chest. There may be a feeling as if cold water was being poured onto the head.

Eyes

Snapping of lids has been mentioned. There may be rapid rotation of the eyeballs. Inflammation may occur in the orbital tissues or in the lachrymal gland. Violent itching in eyes towards evening. A bruised pain is felt in the orbit on moving the eye.

Ears

There is mention of itching in the ears; of something hard pressing on the ear; boring pain in and behind the ear.

Respiratory System

Throat feels very dry, accompanying violent thirst. Voice persistently hoarse. A dry cough, paroxysmal in type, is associated with redness or cyanosis of face; is often worse from 11 p.m. to 1 a.m. The cough, which may have a gurgling sound, is aggravated by contact with cold air, but relieved by taking a drink of cold water. Whooping cough results in a cataleptic state – face blue, finger nails discoloured, eyes turned up, apnoea and insensibility, till it seems the child will never breathe again. Cold water relieves the spasm. Frightful asthmatic attacks cause the sufferer to clutch frantically at the air, totally unable to speak or swallow. In pneumonia sudden suffocative attacks occur, with coldness of surface, great prostration and cold clammy sweat. Acute constriction may be felt in the region of the xiphisternum; possibly a sensation as if transfixed with a knife or as if a lump in that spot was squeezing the life out of him and he must die. Any serious interference with respiration, the basis of life, is likely to be accompanied by a fear of impending dissolution.

Alimentary System

Saliva is thick and sticky. A peculiar metallic taste may be noticed in the mouth. The tongue is pale, moist, paralytic. The gums may be ulcerated, with a dark green or purple line at the tooth margin. Dysphagia occurs from spasm of the oesophagus, accompanied by a gurgling sound when swallowing. Nausea and anorexia of nervous origin may be severe. Abdomen is tender, stony hard, hot and very sensitive to touch. Horrible colic may be present, associated with hiccough. Colic is relieved immediately after passage of stool. Diarrhoea is profuse, violent, painful, associated with cramps and frequent urge to stool. Cholera calling for the remedy is accompanied by very severe cramps; the stools are fluid, green and contain blood. If icy coldness and dryness are the prominent features, Camphor is indicated; copious sweating, purging and vomiting call for Veratrum Alb. Intractable vomiting may be relieved by a drink of cold water.

Cardiovascular System
The remedy may be indicated in angina pectoris. Pulse is changeable, small, soft.

Urinary System
Urgency of urination with scanty amount passed. Scalding shooting pain in urethra during and after urination. Nocturnal enuresis.

Genital System
Crampy dysmenorrhoea before or during menstrual period. Cramps may also be associated with amenorrhoea. Convulsions accompany eclampsia or occur in the puerperium, often preceded by loss of vision.

Nervous System
In a typical epileptic seizure the subject falls with a shriek, jaws are clenched, face distorted, eyes turned upwards, lips blue, thumbs acutely flexed in clenched fists and the surface of body covered in cold sweat. At the same time there is incontinence of both urine and faeces. The attacks often occur at night or at the time of the new moon and tend to recur at regular intervals, possibly at the menstrual period.

Locomotor System
Cramp is a prominent feature, especially at night, forcing the subject to get out of bed and walk up and down for relief.

Skin
Dry itching eruptions occur, such as psoriasis. Tetters with yellow scabs may be located at the flexures of joints. Itching is aggravated by heat and is worse at night in bed. Miliary rashes may also occur.

MODALITIES

There is aggravation from cold air, cold wind; from touch or pressure; before the menstrual period; in evening and at night; at the new moon.
    Curiously enough is better by taking cold drinks. Sweats also give relief.

CLINICAL NOTES

Lesions accompanied by cramp or convulsion provide the main indications for the remedy. It has been found of value in meningitis. Calcarea Carb. is a complementary remedy.

Drosera Rotundifolia

SOURCE

Drosera rotundifolia is a queer and interesting plant found growing in bogs and damp ground. It rejoices in a variety of local names – round-leafed sundew, red-rot, youth wort, moorgrass, oreille du diable. It presents a circle of low-lying cup-shaped leaves somewhat like salt-spoons with short thick handles for stalks; these leaves are fleshy, greenish-red in colour, and their margins and upper surfaces are covered with a menacing array of tentacle-like hairs. The tips of the hairs are club-shaped and secrete drops of sticky fluid; this is most abundant when the sun is at its height, giving the appearance of dew-drops. Any luckless fly alighting on the leaf in search of refreshment is quickly entrapped by infolding of the marginal hairs, and duly digested for the nourishment of the plant. Slender stalks arise from the centre of the leaf rosette, two to six inches in height, bearing at the tip a cluster of small white flowers. The juice of the plant is bitter, acrid, caustic and odourless; it contains both citric and malic acids. The mother tincture is prepared from the active fresh plant.

PHARMACOLOGY

There appears to be an affinity with the lymphatic system, pleura, synovial membrane, larynx and shafts of long bones, inducing an inflammatory reaction and a susceptibility to tuberculous changes in the parts affected.

PROVING

Drosera was proved by Hahnemann, and recorded in *Materia Medica Pura*, Vol.VI.

APPEARANCE

Pallor and emaciation may be observed.

There is stiffness, lameness and evident reluctance to active movement. Despite this there is an uneasy restlessness when lying down, owing to discomfort and a 'hard-bed feeling'. Supports the affected part with the hands, especially when coughing.

Drosera Rotundifolia

PSYCHOLOGY

The subject may be suspicious, silent, reserved, and unduly irritable over trifles. Is restless, uneasy, often with delusions of persecution. There is fear of solitude, of ghosts; dreads the night.

Possibly an inclination of suicide by drowning.

PHYSIOLOGY

The subject is always too cold; chilly even in bed; shivers and shudders when at rest. The head and face may be hot and the rest of the body cold.

There is a distaste for acid things and for pork. Thirst is marked in the hot stage of fevers.

Sleep is interrupted by starting awake in fright. Tends to snore in sleep.

Perspires profusely, especially at night.

SYMPTOMATOLOGY

General

A feeling of bruised soreness all over is accompanied by hypersensitivity to all stimuli and considerable weakness. Spasms, flashes of heat, stitching or shooting pains occur. There is a tendency to cramping, constricting sensations in throat, oesophagus, abdomen, and hands when grasping an object. Is easily exhausted.

Head

Vertigo is worse when out of doors, with a tendency to fall to the left. A pressive or stabbing headache is worse on moving the eyes; some relief is obtained by holding the head firmly between the hands. Headaches may be associated with a stuffed-up feeling and accompanied by nausea, which is worse in the morning; it is aggravated by heat and by stooping. A curious symptom is coldness of the left side of the face, with stinging pains associated with dry heat on the right side.

Eyes

Outward-shooting pains are felt in the eyeballs, especially on stooping. Vision may be dim with a sensation of gauze before the eyes. Eye dazzle may be troublesome.

Ears

Shooting and squeezing pains are felt in the ears, worse when swallowing. Tinnitus is described with buzzing, roaring or humming noises.

Respiratory System
Epistaxis occurs, especially in the evening. Fluent coryza is accompanied by much sneezing. Blood is seen on handkerchief on blowing the nose. There is much burning and scraping with stitching pains in the throat, which may appear dark red or purple. A crawling or tickling sensation in the larynx is associated with pallor and paresis of the vocal cords, redness of the mucosa over the arytenoids, and a measure of aphonia; the voice is low and husky; there is yellow slimy sputum. The hoarseness is associated with attacks of suffocation when talking or coughing. A violent tickling cough comes on in paroxysms and is accompanied by choking, vomiting and cold sweats; it is worse on first lying down – infants start coughing as soon as the head touches the pillow; it is worse also after midnight, especially about 2 a.m., also from talking, eating food, or drinking cold fluids. The patient often holds onto the chest for support when coughing. Sputum is yellow, blood-streaked or purulent, and has a bitter or foul taste.

Alimentary System
Shooting pains are felt in the teeth after taking hot drinks. Ulcers occur on tongue and palate. Food tastes bitter, especially bread. Hiccough, waterbrash, gagging and vomiting may occur. Dysenteric stools are accompanied by cutting pains; passage of stool is followed by pain in abdomen and lumbar region.

Lymphatic System
This is an important sphere for the remedy, especially in relation to tuberculous adenitis, including tabes mesenterica.

Urinary System
Frequency of urination, but only scanty quantities passed.

Genital System
Menses are delayed or absent. Leucorrhoea is accompanied by pains similar to those of parturition.

Locomotor System
Widespread muscle pains with stiffness and shivering when at rest. Pain of gnawing or stinging character is felt in long bones, especially close to joints; it is worse when at rest and relieved by movement. The remedy may be considered in rheumatic affections, also in tuberculosis of bones or joints.

Drosera Rotundifolia

MODALITIES

There is aggravation when lying down; on drinking; when singing or laughing; towards evening and in the second half of the night.

Is better in the open and when walking or active in any way.

CLINICAL NOTES

The remedy is of signal value in whooping cough and any cough that is essentially paroxysmal in type. As mentioned, it can be of service in dealing with tuberculosis of larynx, lymph nodes and other tissues. It is strongly indicated if there is a family history of tuberculosis, or a history of previous tuberculous trouble or contact with cases of active disease. High potencies should be avoided in treating active tuberculosis.

Dulcamara

SOURCE

Solanum dulcamara, the woody nightshade, belongs to the same family as *Belladonna* (deadly nightshade), *Solanum nigrum* (garden night-shade), *Capsicum*, *Hyoscyamus*, *Mandragora* and *Stramonium* (thorn-apple).

The plant grows in damp and shady places, its woody stem giving place to slender branches which climb and trail restlessly over shrubs and hedgerows by twining around any available support. This urge to keep moving is characteristic also of the Dulcamara patient.

The star-shaped flowers are very striking with their five pointed purple petals surrounding a central cone of golden stamens. The flowers continue to bloom throughout the summer months; they are borne on branching stalks which always point in the opposite direction to the corresponding leaves. The leaves are dark green with short stalks, and the upper ones have three lobes, the central one being large with two much smaller lobes at the base.

Clusters of ovoid berries form the fruit, dangling from slender stalks which show a distinct kink, and turning from green to bright scarlet. The berries are shiny, without any down, and in fact have a watery, almost translucent look. They are poisonous and have caused death in children.

The juice of the stem and leaves is intensely bitter when first chewed but afterwards leaves a sweet taste in the mouth, as the action of the saliva produces sugar. Hence the old name Amaradulcis, or bittersweet. The mother tincture is prepared from the young green shoots and leaves when the plant begins to flower.

PHARMACOLOGY

Symptoms of poisoning by the berries are described as 'hard griping pains in the bowels followed by unconsciousness and spasms. Theselatter are tetanic and accompanied by hot, dry skin, trismus, loud rattling breathing and, possibly, death.'

Besides the steroid alkaloid solanine, or rather the very similar solaceine, the plant contains a mixture of saponines, called dulcamarine.

213

The plant also contains mucin and tannins, and the ash contains a considerable amount of silicic acid.

The tissue affinities are widespread, namely with mucous membranes, glands, muscles, kidneys and skin, giving rise to inflammatory changes, catarrh and a tendency to interstitial haemorrhage. There is also an action on the central nervous system, inducing at first tetanic spasm with trismus and, later, paralysis, coma and death.

PROVING

Dulcamara was proved by Hahnemann, and appears in the *Materia Medica Pura*.

APPEARANCE

The skin tends to be dry, delicate and very sensitive to cold. It may show a sickly pallor, or the face and hands may have a dusky, purplish hue.

Lips are apt to twitch in cold air, and the mouth may be drawn to one side.

The general appearance may suggest emaciation or there may be puffy swelling of the limbs.

PSYCHOLOGY

The mental state is restless, irritable, even confused, with difficulty in finding the right word when speaking. There may be an impatient desire for something which, when obtained, is not wanted after all. There is a compelling urge to keep constantly on the move.

PHYSIOLOGY

A chilly feeling all over may be accompanied by a sensation as if 'the hair was bristling'.

Appetite is curious; a sensation of hunger may be accompanied by repugnance towards all food. Easy satiety also may be noticed when taking a meal.

An insatiable burning thirst may be present for cold drinks.

Drowsiness and much yawning are common in the daytime, but sleep at night is apt to be disturbed by frightful dreams or by inability to stay long in one position.

Perspiration is often excessive and offensive in odour.

SYMPTOMATOLOGY

General

Dulcamara pains are described as tearing, shooting or drawing in type, and are relieved by movement. Paralyses may occur in various sites and the affected parts feel icy cold. There may be unilateral spasms. A feature of the remedy is a tendency to alternation of symptoms. Catarrhal or asthmatic conditions alternate with skin eruptions or with rheumatic manifestations. Symptoms are often left-sided.

Head

Vertigo is often associated with trembling and a liability to fall. Things go black before the eyes. A galaxy of headache types are described under this remedy. Headache may be associated with much heaviness, mental confusion and nausea, all made worse by movement, talking or walking – a contrary modality to that usually encountered with this remedy. Headache may be located to one particular spot, as if it were being pressed on firmly by a blunt instrument. A rheumatic type of headache is accompanied by stiffness in the nape and a feeling as if the neck was broken. Headache may be associated with dry coryza, but quick relief is obtained from fluent discharge – in fact as soon as the flow starts. Facial neuralgia may occur after exposure to wet or cold. Eczema of scalp with thick brown crusts is aggravated at the onset of cold weather and in wet weather; it tends to improve in summer.

Eyes

Catarrhal ophthalmia is accompanied by thick yellow discharge; the eyes become very red. Colds tend to settle in eyes. Dimness of vision may be noticed when reading, as if looking through a layer of gauze. Eyelids tend to twitch when weather becomes damp or cold.

Ears

Pricking or squeezing pains are felt in the ear. Earache in children associated with nausea persists all night, preventing sleep, but lets up quickly in the morning.

Respiratory System

The nose becomes acutely congested and stuffed up in rainy weather. There is at times a curious sensitivity to the odour of new-mown grass or drying weeds. Nasal catarrh is characterized by a thick, yellow mucoid discharge and possibly crusts of dried blood. The catarrh is worse in a cold room and out of doors; is better in the warm, and the sufferer wants to keep the nose warmly covered. Entrance into a cold room sets off a bout of sneezing, accompanied by pain in the nasal bones and a free flow of watery discharge. This reaction may be contrasted with Allium Cepa and Nux Vomica; in both these sneezing starts in a warm room and is relieved in the open air. Concomitants of catarrh may be herpes labialis, the presence of pimples inside the nostrils, epistaxis of hot bright red blood. Post-nasal discharge is common, with a tendency to downward spread and involvement of the chest, evidenced by oppressed breathing, respiration clogged by mucus, various pains in chest, especially behind the sternum, and possibly sharp darting pain in the left chest. A paroxysmal type of cough develops, accompanied by expectoration of tasteless mucus sometimes streaked with blood. The cough is worse in wet weather, by taking a deep breath, as soon as lying down, after meals. Rather curiously it is also aggravated in a warm room and better in the open air. Winter coughs tend to clear up in the summer.

Alimentary System
Pimples and ulcers occur in the mouth. A curious stiffness and discomfort of the tongue and the jaw muscles produces a sensation of paresis and makes speech difficult. Cracking in the temporo-mandibular joint is noticed on opening the mouth. Salivation is excessive, the saliva being sticky, soap-like and having a foul odour. This also causes much spitting or frequent swallowing and a tendency to keep scraping the throat. Considerable nausea is associated with a positive disgust for food in any form. Nausea and vomiting may accompany the passage of a stool. Great distension of the belly is likely after meals, accompanied by much belching, the eructations tasting of food. Pinching or shooting pains are described at or in the region of the umbilicus; also stitches in various parts of the abdomen with definite tenderness at the affected site.

Diarrhoea results from suppressed eruptions or from becoming chilled when hot; the stools are slimy and green or yellow; the condition tends to become chronic unless treated with Dulcamara. The stools are preceded by pains around the navel, and borborygmi. The pains are relieved by the passage of the stool but the patient is left very exhausted and weak. The diarrhoea is liable to occur in the autumn when hot days are followed by cold nights. Another feature associated with this remedy is a tendency to much ineffectual urging to stool, from similar causes, as the result of rectal catarrh; only a little frothy mucus is passed.

Lymphatic and Glandular Systems
In cold wet weather the cervical, axillary and inguinal lymph nodes may become swollen.

Genital System

An urticarial rash is apt to appear on the face before the menstrual periods, which are late and usually heavy.

Urinary System

Urgent urination, even loss of sphincter control, results from getting chilled. The urine contains muco-pus, appears turbid and may stain linen. The remedy may be called for in acute or chronic nephritis associated with generalized oedema.

Locomotor System

The remedy is often of value in complaints resulting from exposure to cold and wet. These include stiff neck, digging pains in the back beside the spine or in the loin above the iliac crest. Severe pains occur in the thighs, which are worse when sitting still and in the evening, and relieved by walking about. Limbs become terribly heavy, perhaps with an icy cold feeling. Fingers go stiff and can hardly be moved. Limbs feel paralysed and useless. Cramps occur in both upper and lower extremities. Inflamed joints are painful, red, swollen and tender to touch. Here too movement gives relief, and the sufferer keeps changing position. Rheumatic symptoms are apt to alternate with diarrhoea.

Skin

A great variety of eruptions are described under this remedy, notably herpetic, but also miliary or urticarial. Although brought on by cold, the eruption is often aggravated by warmth and is worse at night. Itching and pricking occur in various sites, sometimes without any eruption; this tends to be worse on exposure to cold air, e.g. when undressing. Scratching gives no relief. Crusting eruptions occur on head and face, e.g. crusta lactea of infants. Ulcers may occur, of spreading and very chronic type, possibly becoming phagedenic. Another indication is in relation to warts which are fleshy, large and smooth in type, occurring especially on hands, fingers and face. Circinate herpetic eruptions occur on scalp and face, especially in children.

MODALITIES

There is aggravation from every change in weather, warm to cold, dry to wet, and especially sudden change as when a hot sultry day is followed by a cold night. Aggravation is also noticed to result from proximity to water or damp surroundings.   Is worse when at rest, when lying on the back, when stooping; towards evening, during the night, during the wane of the moon and in the autumn.

Relief is obtained by warmth, in dry even-temperatured weather; also by frequent changes of posture or by keeping on the move. Feels better when standing erect or when lying on one or other side.

CLINICAL NOTES

The outstanding indication for the use of this remedy is the aetiological factor in the case. It is of value in complaints arising from contact with damp surroundings, proximity to water, getting wet or becoming chilled when hot; in illness brought on by change of weather from a hot dry spell to cold and wet, especially perhaps in autumn.

Complementary remedies are Baryta Carb. and Natrum Sulph. The remedy should not be given in sequence either before or after Acetic Acid, Belladonna or Lachesis.

Gelsemium Sempervirens

SOURCE

Gelsemium sempervirens, *Gelsemium nitidum*, yellow jasmine, false jasmine, Carolina jasmine, is one of the most beautiful native plants of North America. It is found growing in rich moist soils, by the side of streams, along the seacoast from Virginia to the south of Florida and extending into Mexico.

Despite its local names the plant is not in any way related to the true jasmines, but belongs to the Loganaceae, a family which also includes *Curare, Ignatia, Nux vomica* and *Spigelia*.

The plant is a woody climber, manifesting a need for support – something to hold onto or be held up by. Its twining purplish stem often attains great heights as it ascends lofty trees and festoons from one tree to another.

The plant contains a milky juice, and bears opposite, shiny, evergreen lance-shaped leaves. The flowers form axillary clusters of one to five large, funnel-shaped, very fragrant yellow blossoms. The fruit is composed of two separable jointed pods enclosing numerous flat-winged seeds. The stem often runs underground for a considerable distance, and it is from the bark of this rhizome, together with fresh roots the size of a goose-quill, that the mother tincture is prepared.

The plant has a bitter taste and is highly poisonous. The taste derives from alkaloids present mostly in the bark. There are two main alkaloids. Gelseminine is amorphous, yellow in colour, bitter and poisonous, readily soluble in ether and in alcohol. Gelsemine is colourless, odourless, intensely bitter and forms crystalline salts. It is sparingly soluble in water, but readily forms a hydrochloride which is completely soluble. A further alkaloid, gelsemicine, has a depressant effect on motor neurones and is highly toxic.

PHARMACOLOGY

Lethal doses of the drug kill by its action on the respiratory centre in the medulla. Shortly after administration, respiration is slowed and finally arrested altogether.

219

Toxic doses produce a sensation of languor, relaxation and muscular weakness, which may progress to a degree of actual paralysis. The expression becomes anxious, the temperature subnormal, the skin cold and clammy, and the pulse rapid and feeble.

Ptosis of the upper eyelids, dropping of the lower jaw, medial squint, double vision and dilation of the pupil all ensue as the result of loss of muscle tone. Respiration becomes slow and feeble, shallow and irregular, and death may follow in periods differing from one to seven and a half hours. Arrest of the heart occurs almost simultaneously with failure of the respiration.

Interesting accidental provings of the plant have resulted from its use to give a kick to watered-down bootleg alcohol. The drinker experiences a pleasant but short-lived initial effect, being possessed by a total freedom from desire and euphoric happiness. But catastrophic symptoms soon follow, ending in collapse. The victim is overcome by a sudden, terrible weakness; he begins to tremble, his movements become jerky, his heart fails, and he is seized with a deadly anxiety that sobers him up completely. Actual convulsions have been met with, the victim manifesting spasms and opisthotonos, similar to those seen with poisoning by nux vomica or strychnine.

The tissue affinities of the drug are thus mainly with the nervous system: with the central nervous system, producing depression of the motor areas of the cord and consequent muscular weakness, paralysis and relaxation of sphincters; with the respiratory centre, leading to failure of respiration; with sympathetic ganglia, causing depression and passive hyperaemia, both venous and arterial; with mucous membranes, also, tending to catarrhal inflammatory states.

PROVING

Gelsemium was first introduced into homoeopathic practice by Dr Hale, who with Dr Douglass published a monograph on its properties in 1862.

APPEARANCE

The Gelsemium visage acquires a suffused red or purplish hue, owing to venous stasis, and the patient looks drowsy, even besotted. The upper lids droop over dilated pupils and there is a glassy look in the eye.

Quivering may be seen in the lid muscles as also in the tongue, and speech may be difficult and thick. The lower jaw may be dropped and tend to wobble sideways.

Muscular weakness is evidenced by loss of power in the limbs or ocular muscles, and limbs feel so heavy they can scarcely be moved at all. If out of bed, the gait is staggering. The neck muscles may show rigidity.

Another prominent feature is the tendency to tremors and twitching. Tremulousness of the hands is especially noticeable when attempting to lift a cup to the mouth. There may be violent and generalized trembling, so much so that the patient desires to be sat on or held firmly to control the shaking.

The lips tend to be very dry, even cracked. The saliva acquires a yellow hue. The tongue is coated yellowish white and the breath is foetid.

The pulse becomes weak, soft, frequent and difficult to detect.

PSYCHOLOGY

The mind seems paralysed. The sufferer becomes listless, indolent, wants to be left alone, may even be apathetic. There is aversion to noise or bright light, but a tendency to become scared in the dark and demand a light.

Depression is prominent, even with fear of death (respiratory weakness may account for this, the function of respiration being essential to life).

There is a great disinclination for any sort of effort, probably secondary to hypoxia of tissues. Associated is an overwhelming desire to lie down.

Actual fear may be present, fear of the dark, and also fear of falling – the child will clutch the nurse or the sides of the cot, lest it fall or stumble.

Another characteristic of the drug is a nervous restlessness and apprehension, especially before any kind of ordeal or the undertaking of some new responsibility. This reminds one of a similar feature of Argentum Nit., but Gelsemium probably lacks the tense agitation of this remedy. Rather is the nervous reaction manifested by trembling and weakness about the knees, and a tendency to go cold and experience a hollow empty feeling, relieved by moving about.

Suicidal tendencies are mentioned, with the urge to jump from a height. Such causal factors as undue excitement, sudden fright, bad news, apprehensive anticipation or chagrin may precipitate or induce a Gelsemium type of psychosomatic disorder.

221

PHYSIOLOGY

The thermal reactions are somewhat contradictory. In a hot room there is discomfort, the subject feeling hot and sticky and distressed from lack of oxygen to assist respiration, but at the same time there is a complaint of shivers of cold up and down the spine – not actual shuddering, but a sensation as if somebody was running a cold hand or spilling a trickle of cold water down the back. Again, face and head may be hot while the extremities are cold.

With regard to appetite there is often a gnawing type of hunger – a horrible empty sensation without any real desire for food.

Lack of thirst is an important characteristic, and there may be even a dread of fluids.

Although drowsy by day, sleep at night tends to be disturbed, with a liability to wake with a jerk and a feeling of having fallen out of bed.

Sweats may be profuse and exhausting, but do tend to give relief to pains and aches.

SYMPTOMATOLOGY

General

The picture presented is one of loss of muscle tone associated with great lassitude and listlessness, and a not surprising aversion to making any kind of effort. The symptoms in fever are of the influenza type – slow onset, vague aches and pains, chills up and down the spine, great weariness in body and limbs, head heavy and dull, muscles sore and feeling bruised. The regions especially involved are the shoulders and the lower extremities. Fever tends to be remittent or intermittent.

Head

Vertigo with this remedy seems to start from the occiput, causes a feeling of intoxication and unsteadiness, as if would fall. Gelsemium is an important headache remedy and several varieties of headache are described. A headache of sudden onset associated with dizziness, blurred vision and staggering gait is worse in the morning, aggravated by any sudden movement and when walking. Relief is obtained by lying down with the head raised on pillows. A violent throbbing occipital headache is worse when standing up and better by lying quite still. It is also relieved by the passage of copious amounts of pale urine. There is a tendency for the headache to spread from the nape to the forehead, above the eyes, and to be accompanied by great heaviness of head and eyes, soreness of scalp, and stiffness of neck muscles. There may be a feeling as if the head was 'bound by a tight band'. A neuralgic type of headache in the frontal region is associated with nausea and aggravated by vomiting. By contrast, a bilious headache accompanying menstruation is relieved by vomiting. A menopausal headache occurs in association with drowsiness, giddiness, and blurring of vision. The headaches are usually aggravated by warmth or by hot local applications. The remedy may be called for in meningitis when there is extreme tenderness to the least touch in the occipital region and definite rigidity of the neck.

Eyes
Eye symptoms accompany other manifestations of illness, as mentioned in connection with headache. Not only dimness of vision, but other disturbances such as double vision, nystagmus, ptosis, and soreness of eyeballs, aggravated by moving the eyes, may occur.

Respiratory System
Coryza appearing some days after exposure is associated with severe sneezing in the early morning, accompanied by profuse flow of scalding watery discharge in nose and throat, with concomitant soreness of nostrils and alae nasi. There is also often a feeling of extreme blockage at the root of the nose, and epistaxis is not uncommon. With sore throat the parts look red, puffy and congested; swallowing is acutely painful and pain shoots from the tonsil to the ear; swallowing may even become quite difficult, with a feeling of constriction or of a 'lump stuck in the throat'. There may be actual paresis of the muscles of deglutition with resulting regurgitation of fluids through the nose. Aphonia occurs, either nervous or catarrhal in origin. A violent, spasmodic, frequent cough is accompanied by soreness in the chest and a tendency to spasm of the glottis. A cough often occurs in the spring at the onset of warm weather. Sudden alarming dyspnoea is described, accompanied by a sensation of suffocation and extremely shallow respirations, with ensuing extreme restlessness due to oxygen lack, and incessant demands for more air.

Alimentary System
Perhaps the main feature in this sphere is the tendency to nervous diarrhoea from emotional stress or apprehensive anxiety. The stools are painless, even involuntary. Similar symptoms are found under Argentum Nit., but in this case are associated with great excitement and agitation. The Gelsemium patient is 'all of a dither'; the Argentum Nit. patient is 'all keyed up'. There may be anal troubles, spasticity of the sphincter muscles so that even a soft stool is passed with difficulty, or on the other hand actual paresis with patulous anus and incontinence of faeces. The stools tend to be yellow in colour.

Cardiovascular System

The general asthenia may involve the heart muscle, and produces a curious feeling associated with palpitation, namely that the sufferer 'has got to move about or the heart will stop altogether'. With Digitalis the reverse is the case. Here the sufferer must keep still and dare not move lest the heart stop beating.

Urinary System

Nervous polyuria occurs, presumably due to increased renal bloodflow. Paresis of the bladder may occur, leading to distension and overflow.

Genital System

The remedy may be called for when dysmenorrhoea is associated with pains which shoot up the back and down into the thighs, often accompanied by giddiness and faint feelings. It may be needed in relation to threatened abortion resulting from fright or from apprehension. Its use is mentioned both in connection with rigid os in protracted labour and in the condition of complete uterine atony. Sensations of heaviness of the uterus, or as if the organ was being squeezed by a band, are also mentioned.

Nervous System

The remedy may be indicated in various paralytic conditions, e.g. diplopia and post-diphtheritic paralysis of palate. It is of undoubted value in relation to peripheral neuritis with loss of muscular power, either single muscles or muscle groups being affected. Numbness and tingling may occur, made worse on attempting to grasp something.

Locomotor System

Apart from heaviness, neuralgic and rheumatic pains in the limbs, the remedy has a sphere of usefulness in relation to occupational neuro-muscular affections due to overuse of some particular muscle group, such as writer's or violinist's cramp.

MODALITIES

Aggravation of symptoms results from being in a hot room or from direct sunlight. They are worse also in wet weather and fog and before a thunderstorm, and if feverish, are aggravated by a cold draught. Furthermore symptoms are always aggravated by dwelling on them. The worst time of the day is 10 a.m.

Some relief is obtained however in the open air, from continued movement (if the effort can be made), from stimulants, as the result of sweating, and after passing a large quantity of pale urine.

CLINICAL NOTES

Gelsemium has proved of signal value in many cases of influenza, in paralytic nervous disorders of sudden onset, in virus toxaemias, in measles. The 200c is a useful potency in relation to apprehension before ordeal. The remedy can be used prophylactically in influenza epidemics of characteristic type – three doses of 30c in twenty four hours and one dose a week later.

Graphites

SOURCE

This remedy is prepared from powdered graphite, black lead or plumbago, a mineral carbon containing traces of iron. Rather surprisingly, considering its medicinally inert source, the remedy in potency has a very wide range of therapeutic usefulness. Hahnemann obtained his preparations from 'the purest black-lead taken from a fine English pencil'.

PHARMACOLOGY

An affinity with skin and nails leads to malnutrition and a variety of skin eruptions; an affinity with connective tissue tends to fibrosis and also the deposition of adipose material. Other affinities are with mucous membranes and lymph nodes, inducing inflammatory or hypertrophic lesions.

PROVING

A pathogenesis of Graphites appeared in the first volume of Hahnemann's *Chronic Diseases*.

APPEARANCE

The usual picture is of a gross, obese, but at the same time poorly-nourished individual with a pale puffy look reminiscent of Calcarea Carb. The face is described as having a pale, waxy, sickly hue.

Children appear flabby and florid, often with seborrhoeic scalp and unhealthy eyelids. Adults look anaemic with pale lips and a tendency to easy flushing.

The skin is thickened, dry and liable to show cracks or fissures, especially at the fingertips and mucocutaneous junctions. Nails are likely to be thickened, dark in colour and fissured.

PSYCHOLOGY

The sphere of the emotions is profoundly affected under this remedy, especially in the case of adults.

Children are 'not at all awed in the presence of the doctor; prowl around manhandling charts, instruments, anything within reach, and ignoring parental admonitions'.

The adult is anxious, restless, apprehensive, full of fearful forebodings which cannot be stilled; regards himself as unlucky and ill-used.

Is weepy, sad, despondent, full of self-pity, at times preoccupied with thoughts of death. Gets rattled with the children; dreads and avoids mental effort; is affected by music, even to tears; weeps on least pretext or for no reason at all.

Moods vary; often quite cheerful in the morning but shows agitation, impatience, irritability, especially over trifles, in the late afternoon and evening.

Is extremely irresolute and quite unable to make a decision.

Thought processes are sluggish and memory is poor, especially for recent events. There is utter lack of zest for any form of activity, and this may almost take the form of catalepsy.

There is a desire for solitude because is annoyed by everybody. May get really mad and fly into a rage, but is also easily consoled.

PHYSIOLOGY

The Graphites subject is extremely chilly and sensitive to the least draught of cold air, but also averse to great heat and feels oppressed in a hot stuffy atmosphere. Craves air, like Carbo Veg. and Pulsatilla. Feels cold both indoors and in the open, and desires to be warmly clad. The face may be flushed and hot, with at the same time icy cold hands and feet.

The appetite is often ravenous with a constant urge to eat, for a feeling of ease rather than from genuine hunger. There is desire for beer, acid drinks and cold fluids – which may disagree. There is distaste for sweets, meat, salt, fish, cooked foods. Fat cannot be taken with impunity; sweets may cause nausea.

There is a violent thirst in the morning with a dry mouth. This is in contrast to Pulsatilla with its characteristic lack of thirst.

Drowsiness by day is followed by sleeplessness at night, often accompanied by pulsations all over the body, especially in the first part of the night. Keeps constantly waking and feels unrefreshed in the morning.

Sweats readily on least exertion; night sweats are very profuse; the sweat stains linen yellow; foot sweats are offensive.

227

SYMPTOMATOLOGY

General

There is a tendency to the sudden onset of weakness and exhaustion, with a desire to lie down. Dropsical conditions may develop. Offensive odour of breath, sweat and discharges is noticeable. There is a great liability to skin eruptions, small pimples which come and go and are often worse during menstruation, or moist eruptions with a viscid discharge. Pains may be burning in nature, or complaint may be made of numb sensations. Symptoms tend to be left-sided.

Head

A sensation may be felt of cobwebs on the face or forehead, unaltered by attempts to brush them off. This rather curious symptom is shared also by Alumina, Baryta Carb. and Borax. Alopecia is common, in shiny bald patches. Scalp is itchy and there is much scurf which disappears on washing the hair. Eczema occurs on the scalp with massive dirty crusts which mat the hair; the scalp is sore and tender to the touch. Sebaceous cysts may be present. Vertigo occurs readily on looking upwards, or when rising from stooping. It causes a feeling as if would fall forward and is accompanied by a desire to lie down for relief. A unilateral headache is described with tearing pain extending to teeth and neck; it is present on waking and is accompanied by nausea and a desire to vomit; the head feels numb and torpid, as if the contents of the skull were made of pith. A constrictive pain occurs in the occiput extending to the nape, and the neck feels 'broken'. Headaches are aggravated in a warm room and better in the open air. There may be a surge of blood to the head region accompanied by faintness and possibly epistaxis. A burning spot is felt on the vertex.

Eyes

Excessive lachrymation is accompanied by extreme photophobia in bright sunlight or intense artificial light. Inflammation of the lids is associated with fissures at the lateral canthi. Fissures at the medial canthi point to Zinc. Edges of the lids are pale and thickened, in contrast to Sulphur blepharitis with red rims. The lids often show cracks covered with scales; they tend to adhere with dried discharge on the eyelashes. Styes may be present. Cysts occur on the lid border. The lids feel heavy. Conjunctivitis is associated with a thin acrid discharge from eyes and nose. Dacryocystitis may occur with intense itching. Vision may be disturbed at the menstrual period. Zigzags may be seen before the eyes. Acute eye conditions often call for Pulsatilla; in chronic conditions Graphites is indicated.

Ears

Deafness occurs, associated with tinnitus. Often hears better in a noise, e.g. of traffic. May notice his own voice, or the sound of his own footsteps, reverberating in his ears. (Causticum shares this last symptom). Ears 'crackle' on moving the jaws or on swallowing. Chronic otitis media is associated with a thin offensive discharge. Eczema may be present on and behind the external ear with a very sticky type of discharge.

Respiratory System

Nose is often sore inside, and blowing the nose is painful. Nose is often red, and nostrils are fissured with formation of crusts. Nose becomes obstructed with badly-smelling mucus. Eczema occurs on alae nasi and upper lip. The sense of smell is affected variously; it may be very acute so that the scent of flowers is unbearable; it may be lost altogether; or odours may be imagined. Acute sneezing with fluent coryza may occur, or chronic rhinitis with dryness of mucosa and formation of crusts, clinkers and cracks. A chronic sore throat is described with a choking feeling as from a lump in the throat which causes a constant desire to swallow, but attempts to do so only increase the distress. Spasmodic asthma attacks wake from sleep, and the chest feels narrow and constricted; taking some food affords relief. Paroxysms of coughing occur, ending in copious expectoration of white viscid mucus.

Alimentary System

Burning blisters occur on the edges and tip of the tongue. There is a bad taste in the mouth as if eggs had been eaten. The gums burn, sting and recede. Cracks form at the corners of the mouth, possibly with ulceration. The tongue is whitish, sore, often ulcerated. Salivation may be inopportune; dribbles during sleep, but in spite of this the mouth is very dry on waking. Stomach pain occurs some hours after taking food; it is gnawing or colicky and accompanied by heartburn and eructations, which are sour or rancid and taste of food previously ingested. The pain is relieved by taking food or drink, especially warm milk. It is also better by lying down. Food is sometimes vomited soon after being taken. There may be a feeling of nausea, worse in the morning and also worse at the menstrual period. With an acute attack of pain the patient may experience a very horrible, sudden sensation of extreme weakness – as if about to pass out. This may, of course, be due to haemorrhage with accompanying haematemesis or subsequent melaena. When treated with this remedy, duodenal ulcers revealed by X-rays are often shown in subsequent X-rays to be well healed. Acute attacks of heartburn are at times accompanied by a feeling of intense heat in stomach and throat, causing a desire for cold drinks. As a rule, however, cold food and cold fluids aggravate the symptoms.

Great distension of the abdomen may be present and associated with much belching, which does not relieve the bloating. Vomiting gives relief. A good deal of flatus is passed and is offensive in odour. By comparison the flatus passed in a Lycopodium case is odourless. Constipation occurs, the stools being large, hard, knotty and covered with mucus, or in hard lumps connected by threads of viscid mucus. There may also be attacks of diarrhoea with fluid, brown, ill-digested and very offensive stools. Piles burn and sting. Anal fissure may be present, causing sharp pains after stool or on sitting. The anus may be sore and sensitive to touch. Pruritus ani is worse at night. The liver may be congested, swollen, hard and sore, accompanied by a sense of weight in the right hypochondrium. A burning sensation is felt in the left hypochondrium if attempting to lie on that side.

Lymphatic and Glandular Systems
Cervical and other lymph nodes become enlarged and painful. Breasts become large and hard, especially during the menstrual period. Indurations are felt in the breast, often resulting from previous sepsis. Pain may be felt in the left breast at the menstrual period. Nipples become cracked and sore. Secretion of milk may occur before or during the menstrual period.

Cardiovascular System
Sudden 'shocks' are felt in the heart, associated with a feeling of constriction, palpitation and strong pulsations all over the body. Oedema of feet and legs may be present.

Urinary System
Urine is turbid with a sediment either white or red in colour; on standing an iridescent film forms on the surface. An urgent desire to urinate may occur soon after emptying the bladder. The urine may be passed drop by drop. Nocturia is frequent, or enuresis may occur at night.

Genital System
Disturbances of sexual function may occur in the male. Menstrual periods may be accompanied by hoarseness of voice, with or without nasal coryza and cough. The period may be delayed and the flow scanty and pale. It is liable to be associated with belching and gastric distress relieved by taking food. Severe pruritus vulvae may precede the period.

Leucorrhoea occurs both before and after the period; the flow is profuse, milky, white, excoriating and comes in gushes both during the day and at night. Pain may be felt in the uterus when reaching up to grasp something at a height. Pain may be felt in the left ovary when taking a deep breath, when coughing or on pressure over the left iliac fossa.

Nervous System
Limbs easily 'go to sleep' with complaint of numbness, dead feeling and coldness of fingers and forearms. Muscular weakness may progress to virtual paralysis with a cataleptic condition – is conscious but unable to move or speak.

Locomotor System
Pain may be felt in the nape, extending to the shoulders. Lumbo-sacral region is subject to pulling, shooting, burning pains which are worse before midnight and also tend to be worse during or after the menstrual period. Pain in the lumbar region may be described as a sensation as if the spine were broken. Pain may be felt in sacrum and coccyx while urinating. Shooting pains may occur in the limbs, accompanied by a paralysed feeling, especially affecting the left upper limb.

Skin
The skin is unhealthy; wounds and scratches tend to become septic and take a long time to heal. Oozy, moist eruptions exude a thick, glutinous, viscid, honey-coloured fluid; the areas most likely to be affected are flexures, the dorsal aspect of hands and forearms, the external auditory canal, and behind the external ear, face and chin. Similar eruptions may occur at the orifices and on the external genitals. Cracks and fissures itch and bleed and are painful; these are liable to occur at the tips of the fingers, the nipples, the angles of the mouth, the vulva, the anus and between the toes. Itching is severe, worse at night, from heat and contact with water; it is relieved by cold. This is in contrast to the pruritus of Petroleum and Psorinum, which is aggravated in cold weather. Unaffected areas of skin are dry and rough. Old scars tend to burn; palms likewise. Skin of hands is tense and hard and liable to form cracks in winter. Psoriasis may be present on the palms. Nails become brittle, cracked, distorted, thickened and may blacken and fall off. Indolent ulcers have an indurated base and a very offensive discharge. Smarting soreness may be felt in the groins and perineum. Feet perspire and the skin between the toes exfoliates. Recurrent herpes affects especially the anal region and the external genitalia.

MODALITIES

There is aggravation from cold, cold drinks, damp in all forms; also from the heat of the bed and if over-heated by exertion. Is worse also when lying on the left side; before and during the menstrual period; at night, especially before midnight.

Feels better when warmly wrapped up, but must have plenty of air; is better also when resting and in the dark.

CLINICAL NOTES

This remedy acts deeply and is especially suited to chronic conditions. Its 'acute' remedy is Pulsatilla. Complementary remedies are Causticum, Hepar Sulph., Lycopodium, Sulphur.

It is of special value in peptic ulcer, and various skin affections. May be helpful in the resorption of scar tissue. It follows well after Calc. Carb in the obesity of adolescence.

Helleborus Niger

SOURCE

Helleborus niger, the Christmas rose, is probably the most ancient member of that primitive family of plants, the Ranunculaceae. Disregarding blatantly the normal annual plant rhythm of dying and becoming, this beautiful plant blooms amid the snows of winter. Moreover it shows no unseemly haste, no panic of growth, but usually takes from five to seven years before it blooms at all.

Few plants are more elegant; the large cup-shaped flowers, white with a tinge of blush-colour, contrast finely with the ample dark and shining foliage. The whiteness of the flower suggests a waxen tablet on which is painted a succession of brilliant hues, ranging from the vivid vermilion of dawn to a deep shade of rose. Again, the flowers after fertilization do not wither but persist and turn green, thus revealing their true nature as sepals, not petals. Inside each flower are not only the nectaries (petals) but also a cluster of almost a hundred stamens arranged round a central group of seven to ten pistils. The flower gives off a delicate scent.

The flower stem is erect, smooth, fleshy and succulent-looking, and rises to a height of six to eight inches from a circle of ground leaves. The leaves of the plant also are in no hurry, taking many years to develop and become full-grown; as they gradually increase in size they divide more and more into long blade-like fingers, deep green in colour, with a shiny surface and small notches in the distal half. Only when the leaves are fully developed do the flowers open.

Both flower stems and leaf stems are often shaded pink, whereas the root stock is dark brown or black, possessing numerous rootlets and having the appearance when lifted of a large multi-legged insect.

The plant is found in most parts of Europe and favours rocky or wooded sites on the slopes of limestone mountains.

The mother tincture is prepared from the fresh root, dug up during the winter months.

Paracelsus extolled the virtues of this herb in relation to gout, epilepsy, jaundice, apoplexy and dropsy. Philosophers of old drank an infusion of the plant before engaging in intense and prolonged meditation. Here too there is the suggestion of longevity of effect rather than sudden impatient

233

activity, a feature of the Aconite picture. Medicinally the drug has been found especially effective in torpid, phlegmatic types.

PHARMACOLOGY

The powdered root has a bitter-sweet sharp taste; if inhaled it causes violent sneezing. Its toxic effects are due to the presence of two crystalline glucosides. One of these, helleborin, has a burning acrid taste and possesses narcotic properties; the other, helleborein, has a sweetish taste and is a cardiac poison somewhat similar in its effects to digitalis. It is also a drastic purgative.

Symptoms of poisoning include salivation, nausea, repeated vomiting, difficulty in swallowing, pains in the belly, diarrhoea, blood-streaked stools, cramps in the calf muscles, pallor, vertigo, photophobia, tinnitus and interference with vision. Later symptoms are delirium, sobbing, feeble irregular pulse, dyspnoea, somnolence, convulsions and death.

The prominent feature of more chronic poisoning is related to disturbance in the sphere of the body fluids. The tendency is for displacement of fluid to the upper pole of the body as evidenced by hydrocephalus, exudative meningoencephalitis and other effects of derangement of the normal flow of fluid in the region of the choroid plexus; such disturbances tend to produce stupor and sluggishness of responses. Other aspects of disturbance of fluid balance in the body are seen in the development of pleural effusion, ascites and anasarca, the latter possibly in association with renal dysfunction and oliguria.

PROVING

The proving of Helleborus Niger appears in the third volume of Hahnemann's *Materia Medica Pura*.

APPEARANCE

The picture presented by a patient requiring this drug may include the following features: eyes turned upwards, pupils wide and non-reactive, or unequal; pallor and cold sweat on forehead; sooty appearance of nostrils. Head burrows into pillow, or is thrown from side to side; lies on back with limbs drawn up; chewing movements of the jaws with wrinkling of the brow; automatic movements – continuous movement of one arm or leg, while the other limbs lie as if paralysed; very slow answers in response to questions; possibly a stuporous state accompanied by involuntary cries and groans; bad breath; picks at lips which are dry, cracked and peeling.

PSYCHOLOGY

Mental processes are so sluggish that the subject feels utterly stupid. Unable to memorize anything, whether what has just been read or what he was intending to say.

There is a tendency to melancholy and despair, especially after debilitating illness such as typhoid fever or in amenorrhoea setting in after menstruation has just started. There is no wailing or wringing of hands, as with Aurum Met., but the subject just sits around in apathetic silence. Attempts at consolation are resented and only make matters worse.

There is great aversion to making any effort and the sufferer is very easily angered. Odd ideas may be entertained, which become fixed and obsessive.

PHYSIOLOGY

Hunger may be voracious; intense thirst for cold water which is gulped down greedily. The recipient may bite the spoon without being aware of it. Sleep is stuporous. Dreams are anxious and confused, and not remembered.

SYMPTOMATOLOGY

General

Stupefaction in greater or lesser degree is the hallmark of this remedy. There is a peculiar type of virtual imbecility, and an extremely sluggish type of response both in mind and muscle. The will seems to lose full control over the muscles; any object held in the hand is apt to be dropped if attention is diverted. Another feature is a widespread sensation of numbness.

Head

A stupefying type of headache occurs in the occipital region or the nape of the neck, accompanied by numbness and aggravated by any movement of the head. There may be a feeling as if the contents of the skull were being extruded through forehead and orbits. Vertigo is associated with nausea and vomiting, and is made worse by stooping. Marked retraction of the head may be present.

Eyes

Severe pain may occur in the eyes, or a feeling of great heaviness. Twitching of the lids may cause distress.

Respiratory System

Violent sneezing has been recorded in provers, especially in the morning. Dyspnoea may be present with a dry hacking cough, worse at night with gagging. Pleural effusion may occur.

Alimentary System

The mouth, and palate especially, are very dry, or salivation may be increased. The tongue is apt to be swollen and feel numb. Aphthous ulcers may be present. Abdominal symptoms include nausea, distaste for any kind of food, flatulent rumbling, and possibly ascites. Watery diarrhoea is associated with tenesmus and the stools contain jelly-like mucus. Stools may be passed involuntarily, or days may pass without a stool as the result of the atonic state of the bowels.

Cardiovascular System

The heart muscle may partake of the general muscular weakness and cause palpitations associated with anxiety. General circulatory atonia gives rise to decidedly subnormal temperatures. There may be a quite sudden onset of widespread anasarca or effusion into a serous cavity.

Urinary System

Retention of urine may occur, possibly with distension and overflow. Again, in the presence of kidney involvement, only scanty amounts of urine are passed, often dark in colour with a sediment resembling coffee-grounds. Albuminuria may be present.

Nervous System

Meningitic conditions are often accompanied by exudative inflammation. Hydrocephalus may be present. Convulsions are associated with extreme coldness of the body, apart from the head, which is hot. Delirium, if present, is not wild or violent but of the low muttering variety, possibly accompanied by hallucinations.

Locomotor System

Quite apart from the tendency to muscular weakness, almost paresis, a variety of twitchings, pinchings, tearing or shooting pains have been recorded in the dorsum and limbs, in many instances involving articulations.

Skin

Pallor is marked. Angioneurotic oedema may occur, but is likely to be less acute and more persistent than the type associated with Apis.

Helleborus Niger

MODALITIES

There is aggravation from contact with cold air, from uncovering, from exertion, from 4 p.m. to 8 p.m. and during the night.

The sufferer feels better from warmth and being well wrapped up, also when lying quietly at rest and undisturbed.

CLINICAL NOTES

The main sphere of usefulness of this remedy is in acute inflammatory conditions of the brain and spinal cord and their membranes. A further indication is in dropsical states of sluggish type.

Hepar Sulphuris Calcareum

SOURCE

This rather curious but eminently effective remedy is prepared from Liver of Sulphur, an impure form of calcium sulphide. The crude product was obtained according to Hahnemann's directions from a 'mixture of equal parts of finely powdered oyster shells and quite pure Flowers of Sulphur kept for ten minutes at white heat'.

PHARMACOLOGY

From the homoeopathic point of view this substance possesses a remarkable affinity with the nervous system, producing an extreme degree of hypersensitivity and overexcitability of both mind and body. It also affects the respiratory and alimentary mucous membrane, causing a profuse catarrhal type of inflammation. There is also an affinity with skin and with lymphatic nodes, producing a liability to easy suppuration from slight cause.

PROVING

A pathogenesis of Hepar Sulph. appears in the fourth volume of Hahnemann's *Materia Medica Pura*.

APPEARANCE

The skin of the face often has a yellowish tinge. The general appearance tends to be scrawny, even scrofulous, with enlarged lymph nodes in various sites.

A crack may be present in the centre of the lower lip. Chaps and deep cracks occur on hands and feet.

The skin has an unhealthy look and festering sores may be present. An unpleasant body odour is common. Any discharges present will have a foul smell. This is sometimes likened to old cheese. The Hepar subject tends to speak rapidly and also to drink hurriedly.

PSYCHOLOGY

The sufferer is immoderately sensitive to touch, pain, people, surroundings. Pain is quite intolerable and may be felt so intensely as to cause fainting or rigors; this too, whether the cause of the anguish is physical or psychological.

The subject is excessively irritable, touchy, quarrelsome and extremely difficult to get on with; gets furious over mere trifles; wants constant change but is never satisfied; is impossible to please. Is often sad and disconsolate, especially in the evening; may even become suicidal. On the other hand he may become impetuous, impulsive, feeling an urge to violence.

Memory is poor, with a liability to forget words and localities.

PHYSIOLOGY

The Hepar subject is essentially a chilly mortal, sensitive to the least draught of cold air; cannot bear to be uncovered; wants to be warmly wrapped, even in a warm room and in summer; likes especially to have the head warmly covered; enjoys a heated atmosphere.

There is craving for vinegar, pickles, alcohol, condiments, but aversion to fat foods. Faint feeling with hunger occurs in mid-morning. Thirst may be violent.

Drowsiness is common in the day time, accompanied by much yawning, but sleeplessness is likely in the latter part of the night.

Sweats tends to be profuse, especially at night; are often sour or offensive in odour and afford no relief to symptoms. The Hepar subject sweats easily on the least provocation.

SYMPTOMATOLOGY

General

Pains are excessive and of a peculiar sticking character, sometimes described as a splinter piercing the flesh. The sensibility to touch is most marked, and inflamed parts feel bruised or sore 'like a boil'. The contact of a hand or a dressing is resented strongly. There is a great liability to sepsis; any small injury tends to suppurate. Symptoms show periodicity with seasonal recurrence. Laterality is usually right-sided. There may be complaint of a sensation of wind blowing on some part of the body.

Head Region

The scalp is very sensitive; even combing the hair may be quite painful. The head too is sensitive to the least cold. A severe hemicrania may occur with a sensation of a plug or a nail being thrust into the skull. Neuralgia may afflict the right side of the face, accompanied by tenderness of the bones to touch. A boring or bursting headache is described, located at the root of the nose. This is aggravated by the weight of the hat, but curiously enough relieved by tight bandaging. Headache is apt to be increased by shaking the head or when riding. An ache is mentioned at the right aspect of the occiput, spreading to nape, shoulders and throat. A moist, itching, burning eruption may occur on the scalp.

Eyes

Various eye conditions may call for this remedy – conjunctivitis with profuse sticky purulent discharge; corneal ulcer; iritis resulting in hypopyon; extreme photophobia. The eyes are sensitive to least touch or to any impact of cold air. Eyeballs are painful and feel as if pulled back into the head. Vision is affected, objects appearing red or too large.

Ears

Otitis media is associated with very offensive sanious discharge. The remedy is called for in threatened mastoiditis. Scurfy eruptions occur on and behind the external ear. Pustules or boils may be present in the external auditory canal.

Respiratory System

The sense of smell is very acute. Sneezing occurs on least contact with cold air and the nose becomes blocked. There is a great liability to catch fresh cold from the slightest exposure. A well-established coryza is apt to be accompanied by painful swelling of the nose, especially the alae, and a boring pain at the root of the nose. Sinus infection may call for the remedy, as well as ozaena with loss of sense of smell and a foul sanious nasal discharge. The remedy may be appropriate in some cases of hay fever. Sore throat is associated with pain radiating to the ears on swallowing. Hot drinks afford relief. A 'fish-bone sensation' may be noticed in the throat. Tonsils may be enlarged and septic. Catarrh of larynx is common with great sensitivity to cold, especially dry cold, and loss of voice is usual. Quinsy is liable to accompany infection of tonsils. Post-nasal discharge with much hawking of mucus is also frequent. A noisy cough is aggravated by the slightest breath of cold air, by exposure to cold wind or even by uncovering an arm or foot. A hot drink gives relief. Bronchitis is accompanied by a rattling cough with a tendency to suffocative bouts, when the sufferer has to rise up and bend the head backwards for relief. There is much mucus, which is only raised with difficulty, and efforts at expectoration are apt to cause nausea and sweating. Purulent pneumonitis is accompanied by free expectoration of offensive sputum and a paroxysmal cough, especially on first lying down at night. The remedy may be indicated in empyema.

Alimentary System

Swelling of the upper lip may occur, and there is also a tendency to the formation of a crack in the centre of the lower lip. Gums become painful and bleed readily. Ulcers form on soft palate and roof of mouth. Salivation may be profuse. The tip of the tongue feels sore and is very painful. Belching is frequent, but without any special taste in the eructations or odour. Bloating occurs with the necessity to loosen the clothing. Gastric upsets occur easily, often accompanied by nausea and vomiting. Periumbilical griping is associated with flatulence, and the belly may be tense and tympanitic. Liver involvement is associated with pain in the right hypochondrium, aggravated by walking, coughing, breathing and even light pressure. Jaundice may be present. Rectal urging is accompanied by slow and straining passage of a scanty, soft stool. Chronic diarrhoea is associated with painless, white or clay-coloured stools, sour, undigested, foetid in odour. The diarrhoea is worse during the day, especially after taking a meal.

Lymphatic and Glandular Systems

Involvement of lymph nodes is apt to be accompanied by rapid suppuration. By comparison the inflammatory process with Silica is slow and insidious.

Urinary System

Dysuria is accompanied by delay in starting the act of urination, and the flow is slow and intermittent. Inadequate emptying of the bladder results. The urine may show an oily film on the surface if left to stand.

Genital System

Fig warts may develop on the male genitalia, with a very offensive odour. Suppuration may occur in the inguinal lymph nodes. Pruritus vulvae may be present. Labial abscess may occur. Leucorrhoea is very offensive in odour.

Locomotor System

Rheumatic pains and stiffness are much worse in cold weather, both dry and wet. There may be swelling of the finger joints. Tremor of hands may occur when writing, or of knees when walking. Cramps occur in thighs or calves, especially in the second part of the night, after midnight. Soreness and tenderness of the soles of the feet is especially noticed when walking on an uneven surface. Joints seem weak, leading to easy dislocations. Pain in the nail of the great toe is noticed on the least amount of pressure.

Skin

There is a liability to the formation of chaps and cracks, and to eruptions of pimples, pustules and boils, Wounds easily become septic. Ulcers may form of indolent type, and are serpiginous, shallow and so sensitive that the sufferer cannot bear contact of dressings or even impact of cold air. The discharges are of foul odour. Moist eruptions occur, especially at flexures, associated with unpleasant odour and much itching, which is worse in the morning. The remedy may be indicated in acne, especially if the eruption is pustular. Ulcers are often ringed with small pimples, and may be haemorrhagic or gummatous. Chronic or recurrent urticaria is also mentioned.

MODALITIES

There is aggravation from cold, even cool air, from cold dry winds, from draughts, from cold food or fluids. Aggravation also from light touch, from pressure, when lying on the affected side; this becomes unbearably painful, causing the sufferer to turn over. Symptoms are worse in the morning and again in the evening, and are also worse in winter.

The patient feels relief from warmth, and also in wet weather, especially warm wet weather, a feature shared with Causticum and Nux Vomica (compare Silica, worse in wet weather). There is some relief too after a meal.

CLINICAL NOTES

In the incipient stage of inflammation the 30c or 200c may abort the process. If suppuration is inevitable, lower potencies such as 3x will be of value. After incision of an abscess the 30c will encourage resolution.

Hepar follows well after Belladonna, and in respiratory affections may be called for in sequence to Aconite or Spongia.

Hyoscyamus Niger

SOURCE

This plant is the hairy henbane, also known as hog's bean and stinking Roger. As its names imply it is a plant with a somewhat sinister reputation, which is shared by other poisonous members of the Solanacae – *Belladonna*, *Stramonium* and *Mandragora*.

It is a shrubby herb growing to the height of two to four feet. The gay funnel-shaped flowers are yellowish in colour and veined with purple; they are quite large and striking in appearance with an exceedingly dark purple centre, like the pupil of an eye.

The leaves are of two kinds. Those appearing first spread out from the crown of the root, lying flat on the ground like a rosette. These leaves are ovate, more or less sharply toothed, with acute points, and may exceed a foot in length; they are greyish-green in colour and freely covered with sticky hairs. The stem and calices of the flowers are also hairy, suggesting hostility.

These leaves die off at the approach of winter and the flower stem appears the following spring. The stem leaves occur alternately along the stem which they encircle at the base. They are pale green in colour, with a broad conspicuous mid-rib, and are covered on both aspects with soft glandular hairs which secrete a resinous substance that gives the fresh leaves a nasty, sticky, clammy feel.

The fruit is a hard capsule which opens transversely by a lid and contains numerous small seeds. The underground portion consists of a large, brownish, freely branching root, from which the flower stem pushes up in the spring. Owing to its appearance the root has been eaten in mistake for parsnip or chicory, with disastrous results.

The whole plant has a heavy, oppressive, nauseous odour. It is well described by Schenk: 'Black henbane grows on rubbish dumps and wherever the ground is covered with human garbage. We have only to look at this three-feet tall plant with its grey leaves and yellowish flowers veined with purple to see that it is a typical poisonous plant. Sombre, luxuriant, sticky, evil-smelling and covered with close hairs, this sinister-looking herb seems to live exclusively on human refuse, on the corpses in the cemetary or the offal that lies around human dwellings. Black henbane seems to suck up and retain within it all the poisonous matter from its habitat.'

Even the fruit capsule with its clamped-down lid and poisonous contents exemplifies bottled-up banefulness. Nor does the age-long history of the plant belie its appearance.

Used extensively in classical times as a medicine, Pliny nevertheless has this to say of its possibilities: 'For mine own part I hold it to be a dangerous medicine, and not to be used but with great heed and discretion. For this is certainly knowne, that if one take in drinke more than four leaves thereof, it will put him beside himself.'

The plant is widely distributed in Central and South Europe and further east in Siberia and India. It has been found in sixty British counties. The mother tincture is prepared from the whole plant, gathered in May, June or July.

PHARMACOLOGY

The plant contains two main toxic alkaloids, the crystalline hyoscyamine and the amorphous hyoscine, also known as scopolamine. These toxic principles are not destroyed by boiling or drying.

The main affinity of the plant is with the realm of the psyche and with certain areas of the central nervous system. The hyoscine component is credited with producing a sedative, narcotic, antispasmodic effect, and the psychological disturbance is ascribed to the hyoscyamine/atropine element.

That the psyche is profoundly affected is quite evident from the numerous instances of poisoning by the plant.

Henslow tells how 'The whole of the inmates of a monastery were poisoned by using the root instead of chicory. They had such hallucinations that the establishment resembled a lunatic asylum. They rang the bell for matins at midnight; and those who attended were unable to read, or read what was not in the book.'

Sir Hans Sloane records the case of four children who ate some of the capsules in mistake for filbert nuts and exhibited all the symptoms of narcotic poisoning, continuing for two days and nights in a profound sleep. This was an instance of the sedative, narcotic properties of the plant. It is interesting to note in this connection that during the Middle Ages a sponge saturated with the juice of the plant was held under the nose of those about to undergo an operation.

But a very extreme form of hallucinatory madness with associated muscular ataxia is also an effect of henbane poisoning. This was exemplified in a striking manner by a gallant experiment carried out by

Schenk himself. He describes his personal experience as the result of inhaling the fumes from roasted henbane seeds thus:

'To comprehend the power of black henbane the reader must picture the following condition. The ears become deaf, the eyes almost blind; they see in a haze only the bulk of objects, whose contours are blurred. The sufferer is slowly cut off from the outside world and sinks irretrievably into himself and his own inner world.

'The room dances; the floor, the walls and the ceiling tilt slowly to the right and then back to the left. But the victim has no sense of moving himself, although obviously he is staggering about in a stationary room.

'Now image followed upon image; they were shattered fragments of the real world. I saw them within the area of my own eyes. My uninhibited hilarity quickly vanished, making way for a feeling of amazement that everything I saw appeared completely topsy-turvy.

'Although I could hardly walk, or even stand up, I was seized by a raging impulse to move. Since my feet seemed welded to the floor I could only clutch and grasp at things with my hands and tear them to pieces.

'I was flung into a flaring drunkenness, a witches' cauldron of madness. Above my head water was flowing, dark and blood-red. The sky was filled with whole herds of animals. Fluid formless creatures emerged from the darkness. I heard words but they were all wrong and nonsensical, and yet possessed for me some hidden meaning.

'My teeth were clenched and a dizzy rage took possession of me. I know that I trembled with horror, but I also knew that I was permeated by a peculiar sense of well-being, connected with the crazy sensation that my feet were growing lighter, expanding and breaking loose from my body. This sensation of bodily dissolution is typical of henbane poisoning.

'As the delusions come to an end they are replaced by the consciousness of pain and nausea. Sight, hearing, smell and touch do not obey the will and seem to be going their own ways.'

Truly a psychosomatic pandemonium, with complete loss of rational control, both physical and psychological. With Belladonna there is turmoil in the circulation and a definitely belligerent type of delirium. Here there is utter tumult in the realm of thought and subjective sensation, liable as in the case of Belladonna to merge into somnolence and insensibility.

PROVING

The proving of Hyoscyamus Niger, by Hahnemann, is in the fourth volume of *Materia Medica Pura*.

APPEARANCE

The physical features of the Hyoscyamus patient are similar in many respects to those exhibited by Belladonna subjects, but there are some dissimilarities.

The eyes sparkle, look red and injected, not so 'staring' as is the case with Belladonna. The pupils are dilated and insensible.

The face tends to be pale, rather than blazing or dusky red as in Belladonna patients.

Muscular twitching is common, from eyes to toes, or clonic spasms may occur with coarse angular jerks which throw the body about.

There is a tendency to bump into things with wild wide-open eyes, or stagger about in a drunken manner. The hands show incessant movements, picking, clutching or performing mimetic gestures.

Speech is irrational and incoherent and may show a slant towards lewdness. Short abrupt answers are given to imaginary questions, or the sufferer may lapse into hysterical aphonia.

A persistent endeavour to throw off all covering and clothing may be a feature – probably the result of an extreme degree of hyperaesthesia coupled with loss of rational control.

Physical asthenia may be marked; the sufferer slides down in the bed with sagging lower jaw. The tongue becomes so dry that it rattles in the mouth and has the appearance of burnt leather. It is protruded and retracted with the utmost difficulty and great tremulousness.

PSYCHOLOGY

The mental disturbance associated with Hyoscyamus is extreme and diverse. The sufferer may be raving at one moment and at the next in a stupor – as one author puts it, 'deprived of all his senses, just sits on the bed like a statue'. Fear is prominent; fear of solitude; fear of running water; fear of being poisoned or of having been poisoned. Delusions of this type may progress to a veritable persecution complex with confirmed paranoia.

The exact form which these delusions and hallucinations take varies from one individual to another and, as with dreams, may assume protean shapes even in the same individual. One may manifest scruples of conscience and wallow in self-reproach; another may 'curse and swear and make a fearful racket about quite imaginary grievances' or 'make disclosures in subjects about which he would normally be silent and reserved'. Hilarity is replaced by abysmal gloom.

PHYSIOLOGY

Hyoscyamus lacks the heat of Belladonna and its subject is made worse by cold in any form. Warmth affords relief. Hunger tends to be ravenous and thirst excessive.

Sleep is troubled and restless with much twitching, talking or crying out and waking in terror. Extreme drowsiness alternates with wakefulness, and sleep may depart for hours on end.

Debilitating sweats may occur during sleep and be cold and sour-smelling.

SYMPTOMATOLOGY

General

Although the rages of Hyoscyamus may be accompanied by great strength, marked debility and prostration are prominent features with many states. Haemorrhages also may occur, especially from the nose.

Head Region

Headache is liable to be accompanied by giddiness, tinnitus and visual disturbance. There may be a complaint that 'the brain seems to shake and sway in the skull when walking'. A gnawing pain in scalp, vertex and nape is aggravated by touch and by any movement of the head. This is similar to the Belladonna headache which is made worse by the least jar or jolt.

Eyes

Spasms occur in the ocular muscles, leading to squinting or rolling movements of the eyes. Photophobia is marked and vision is disturbed. Sparks may be seen before the eyes, objects appear very sharply outlined, assume a red colour, and small objects may look enormously enlarged.

Respiratory System

Catarrh of the larynx and trachea may be present with accumulation of mucus and hoarseness of the voice. A dry teasing cough is aggravated by eating, drinking, talking or singing, also by lying down, and at night, especially after midnight. It is better when sitting up. A paroxysmal cough which shakes the whole body is also described.

Alimentary System

The tongue is tremulous and catches on the teeth when protruded. It feels numb or as if burnt. Paresis of muscles of deglutition may cause difficulty in swallowing, and fluids may regurgitate through the nose or get into the trachea. Nausea, vomiting, cramping or cutting pains in the abdomen are described, or the belly may be blown up like a drum. An accompaniment of these troubles is excessive tenderness of the epigastrium or the abdomen to the least touch. Constipation with total absence of call to stool may alternate with frequent urge and the passage of scanty stools. Stools may be passed while urinating. Involuntary diarrhoea may eventuate with passage of mushy, blood-streaked, foul stools of typhoid type.

Urinary System

Frequent urination with passage of only small quantities may alternate with infrequency and passage of large amounts of clear urine. Enuresis is common.

Nervous System

The Hyoscyamus convulsions come on suddenly, often during sleep. They may be preceded by gnawing hunger. There are sudden starts and twitchings with angular movements, purple discolorations of the face, frothing at the mouth, a wild look in the eyes with squinting, grinding of teeth and uttering of shrieking cries. The fit is accompanied by involuntary urination and followed by drowsiness and snoring.

Locomotor System

Tremulousness in the limbs may cause distress. Cramps are common in the lower limbs, especially in the toes, and noticed when walking.

MODALITIES

Aggravation is noticed after eating, when lying down, from touch or contact; also during the menstrual period. Symptoms are worse at night, especially after midnight.

Some relief is obtained by sitting up, by movement or walking about.

CLINICAL NOTES

Hyoscyamus finds its main application in maniacal states, puerperal mania, delirium tremens, coma vigil and similar conditions. It is indicated when convulsions come on with suddenness and great violence in strong vigorous subjects.

Hypericum Perforatum

SOURCE

Hypericum perforatum, St John's wort, is found growing in open woods and hedge banks. The plant is a perennial with short runners. The stems show a ridge on either side and attain a height of one and a half feet. The leaves are smooth, devoid of hairs and sessile, placed in opposite pairs; they are deep green in colour, rather narrow and curiously appear to be perforated when looked at against the light. These 'perforations' are actually translucent areas, secretory cavities containing minute oil glands. The flowers seen in summer and autumn have five bright yellow pointed petals, which are about twice the length of the five green sepals.

When crushed the flowers, leaves and stems emit a curious, almost resinous scent; this persists in the mother tincture (prepared from the whole fresh plant). The plant if injured exudes a reddish brown juice, suggestive of blood; this may account for its original use by the ancients as a vulnerary.

Gerrard wrote of it thus: 'A most precious remedie for deep wounds and those that are thorow the bodie or any wound made with a venomed weapon.'

Thus Culpeper, some 250 years ago: 'St John's Wort is a singular wound herb as any other whatsoever, either for inward wound, hurts or bruises, to be boiled in wine and drunk or prepared into an ointment, bathe or lotion outwardly.'

It was used by Ambroise Paré. It was said also to be one of the blessed herbs which protect poor folk from the 'horrid charms of wizard seer, whose potent spells could hold in dreadful thrall the labouring moon'. Anthony Ascham wrote: 'The virtue of it is thus, if it be put in a man's house then shall come no wicked spirit therein.' Tournefort in his *Compleat Herbal*, 1731, recommended the plant 'to be put into one's Hat, to be laid under one's pillow in the Night and to be strewed up and down the House.'

There were indeed many herbs endowed in popular imagination with the power of warding off witches, but the most efficacious of them all was St John's Wort, which the French call 'All-Holy' and the Irish 'Mary's Glory'. It was the *fuga daemonium* or 'flight of the devil'. The hanging of herbs in the house was practised more particularly on the eve of the feast of St John the Baptist.

The peculiar colour of the juice as mentioned above is due to the presence of a red pigment, hypericin, which causes photosensitization in white animals or those with little protective pigment in skin or hair. This oversensitivity to light can result in liver dysfunction with or without jaundice, necrosis and sloughing of non-pigmented areas of skin, leaving ulcerated patches which heal slowly and produce hairless scars.

PHARMACOLOGY

The affinity of the plant is essentially with the nervous system, causing hyperaemia and hypersensitivity, especially sensitivity to light. Involvement of nerve sheaths and meninges gives rise to stitchy, tearing pains, also to pricking and crawling sensations.

PROVING

A proving of Hypericum, by Dr G.F. Mueller, is recorded in the fifth and sixth volumes of *Hygeia*.

APPEARANCE

The expression may be one of suffering due to severe pain at the time of, or persisting after, an injury.

PSYCHOLOGY

The chief feature in this realm appears to be severe depression following an injury which probably involves either central or peripheral nervous tissue. Impairment of memory and a tendency to make mistakes in writing are also mentioned.

PHYSIOLOGY

There may be a craving for wine. Desire for warm drinks is recorded; also intense thirst in association with trembling.

Drowsiness may be marked. Limbs jerk when going to sleep; may talk in sleep or wake in a state of excitement at about 4 a.m. Feels very weary on first waking but is better by noon.

The scalp perspires, especially in the morning on waking from sleep.

SYMPTOMATOLOGY

General

Pains typically shoot centrally from the part involved. There is excessive soreness and tenderness of affected areas, and extreme sensitivity to touch. Pains are stitching and darting in character and tend to come and go.

Head

Vertigo is accompanied by a sensation as if the head became suddenly elongated upwards like a Welsh hat; this is worse at night. A throbbing headache is located on the vertex and associated with a curious feeling of being lifted high up in the air. Accompanying the sensation is anxiety, a fear of falling from this height. A headache of this type is liable to ensue from a fall on the buttocks or onto the sole of the feet. Headache or neuralgic pains extend into the zygoma and cheek. The head may feel as if touched by an ice-cold hand. Twitching of the facial muscles may be present. Pain occurs across the bridge of the nose. Sticking pains may be felt in eye or ear.

Respiratory System

Hoarseness is accompanied by scraping and roughness in the throat. Stitches, burning and tightness, especially in left side of chest, are aggravated by movement. A frequent dry hacking cough may be present. Asthma is worse in foggy weather and from any change in weather. It is associated with a sensitive spine and better for profuse perspiration or free expectoration.

Alimentary System

Lips are dry; there is a taste of blood in the mouth. The tongue is coated white at the base and clean at the tip. Ulcers in the mouth are very sensitive. Toothache is better by lying on the affected side and keeping still. There is a sensation of a lump in the stomach. Diarrhoea drives from bed in early morning. Dull pressive pain occurs in rectum with urge to stool. Piles are tender, sore and tend to bleed.

Nervous System

Neuritis is associated with tingling, burning pain and numbness. Feet feel as if pricked by needles. Convulsions occur after a head injury.

Genital System

Menstrual periods may be delayed. A tight sensation is felt in the pelvis.

Locomotor System

There is much jerking and twitching of muscles. Pain is felt especially in tips of fingers and toes. Joints feel bruised. There is great sensitivity of nape, back and along the spine, and any movement extorts cries. Violent pains make it almost impossible to stoop or walk. Pain is felt on rising from sitting posture. Pains in limbs are accompanied by weakness and trembling. The left arm or left leg is often affected, associated with numbness and better for being rubbed.

Skin

Eczema occurs on hands and face; itching is severe. Herpes zoster may occur. An urticarial rash may be present on hands with smarting pain. Scars are painful. Bunions and corns are accompanied by excruciating pain.

MODALITIES

There is aggravation in cold air, in damp weather, especially if foggy; before a storm; from touch, movement; from 6 p.m.to 10 p.m.; in the dark.

Feels better when keeping still; by bending the head back.

CLINICAL NOTES

Undoubtedly the outstanding use of the remedy is in lacerated or punctured wounds involving nerves. In the wounds caused by sharp objects, by bites of cats or rats or other rodents, Ledum is probably first choice, to be followed by Hypericum if pains shoot up the limb. These two remedies are said to be prophylactic in relation to tetanus and could well be given in addition to Tetanus Toxoid when this is available.

The remedy is indicated in injuries to head and spine with concussion, injuries to coccyx, and affections of nerves.

Ignatia Amara

SOURCE

This remedy is prepared from the so called St Ignatius bean, fruit of the *Strychnos ignatia* plant, a member of the Loganiaceae group.

The plant is a tall, woody, climbing shrub found in the Philippines. The ovate glabrous leaves are in opposite pairs; white tubular flowers give rise to a large pyriform berry about 10cm in diameter, which contains up to twenty-four pebble-like seeds embedded in a bitter pulp.

The seeds are heavy, hard, somewhat pyramidal in shape with flattish sides and roughly 20mm by 15mm in size. The colour is greyish or reddish black, the surface smooth with few or no hairs, and if fractured the endosperm is seen to be translucent and to enclose an irregular hollow cavity in which is an oblong embryo. The seeds are inodorous but intensely bitter in taste. One characteristic of the Ignatia subject is intense bitterness of spirit.

The seeds, which are used for preparation of the mother tincture, contain proportionately more strychnine than those of Nux Vomica. The powdered seeds contain 2.5 to 3 per cent of strychnine and brucine.

PHARMACOLOGY

Owing to the high strychnine content – up to two-thirds of the total alkaloids of Ignatia represent strychnine – the symptoms of poisoning are similar to those of Nux Vomica. The affinity for the central nervous system induces a state of hypersensitivity, which leads to muscular irritability and emotional unreliability. Severe dyspnoea and an unbearable feeling of anxiety precede tetanic spasms, which are followed by extreme exhaustion and paralysis.

Despite the similarity of alkaloidal content, the two remedies Nux Vomica and Ignatia are quite distinct from the point of view of total symptom picture and constitutional type. This demonstrates the importance therapeutically of employing potencies of whole natural products rather than using isolated alkaloids.

PROVING

Ignatia was fully proved by Hahnemann himself, and he published his results in the third edition of the second volume of *Materia Medica Pura*.

APPEARANCE

Whereas irritability is a chief characteristic of Nux Vomica, instability is a prominent feature of Ignatia. This is shown physically in various ways. Frequent changes of colour are noticed in the face, deadly pallor contrasting with easy flushing at the least emotion. Facial grimacing is common or actual spasmodic tic affecting different muscle groups. Involuntary laughter alternates with much sighing and yawning.

Movements tend to be hurried and awkward, and tremulousness may be evident. There is a tendency to let the head hang forward, to clench the teeth and bite the side of the tongue or the inside of the cheek. May become aphonic and speak in a whisper. Cracked bleeding lips, hot knees and cold nose are also mentioned.

PSYCHOLOGY

It is in the emotional sphere that Ignatia presents a most typical picture differing from that of Nux Vomica. Unlike the explosive irascible Nux type, always ready for a scrap or an argument, the Ignatia subject avoids controversy, does not stick up for herself, and retires into her shell to nurse her injured feelings in silence.

The tension is there, but whereas with Nux it is obvious and uninhibited, leading to rows, rampagings and ruthlessness, with Ignatia it is inward, pent up and occult, giving rise to sighs, sobbing and self-pity. Nux blows up. Ignatia bottles up.

With Ignatia, moods are changeable and contradictory; laughter and tears alternate or mingle; desire for solitude gives place to a longing for company and affection. The child is at first rude and rebellious, then relents and becomes docile.

The Ignatia subject broods on injuries, real or imagined, but does not break out into violence, hates sympathy and feels misunderstood; is very sensitive to blame and strongly resents contradiction, is hyper-conscientious; liable to causeless fears.

May be morose and so absorbed in her dismal thoughts that it is impossible to get her to talk or to cheer up. On the other hand she may be so 'hurried' that she makes mistakes in speech, in writing, in doing things, and finds herself constantly obliged to make reparation for these silly mistakes. She may be constantly pursued by some fixed idea which obtrudes itself in conversation.

There is inability to stand pain or noise and a tendency to be easily upset by trifles, as well as by the smell of tobacco smoke.

PHYSIOLOGY

The Ignatia appetite is paradoxical, with aversion to ordinary diet, warm food and meat, but a craving for indigestible or exotic comestibles. Sometimes there is an insatiable hunger for bread or for sour things.

There may be a surprising absence of thirst with fever, but thirst ensues during the period of chilliness.

Sleep is so light that it may be disturbed even by the striking of a clock at a distance. Jerking of the limbs when falling off to sleep is a symptom shared with Belladonna, Hypericum and Lycopodium. Excessive dreaming is common; may dream all night on one theme. The child may whimper in his sleep.

Sweating may occur on the face while eating, a symptom noted also under Chamomilla, Natrum Mur. and Sulphuric Acid.

SYMPTOMATOLOGY

General

As regards aetiology, the Ignatia syndrome may be induced by various kinds of emotional stress – shock, grief, resentment, and especially the 'injured feeling'. Chilliness may occur, even to the point of actual 'gooseflesh', but is relieved at once by warmth. Flushes of heat are accompanied by a feeling of imminent perspiration. Pains appear and disappear with equal abruptness. Pain is often felt in quite small circumscribed areas. Symptoms tend to be curiously unpredictable and contradictory. For instance, although there is hypersensitivity to pain there is relief from firm pressure on the painful part; an empty feeling in the stomach is not relieved by taking food, although in general the act of eating ameliorates; with a severe sore throat relief is felt by swallowing solids; although hot with fever, desires to be well covered; the face is red despite chill; a tickle in the throat is made worse, not relieved, by coughing.

Head

In this region a great variety of symptoms are recorded. The head is apt to feel hot and heavy, and is held in a forward-hanging position. It may feel hollow, or muzzy and confused, possibly accompanied by actual

vertigo causing swaying or staggering. Headache may extend to the eyes
or the root of the nose, and be associated with fiery zigzags in front of the
eyes and blurring of vision. This type of headache is relieved by vomiting
but aggravated by movement. Headache may also be induced by strong
odours or by contact with tobacco smoke. In general the Ignatia
headache is made worse by talking and by any extra effort or excessive
emotion, and is ameliorated by stooping forward, by lying on the same
side as the pain, and after passing a large quantity of pale, limpid urine.

Eyes
Among the eye symptoms mentioned under the remedy are quivering of
lid muscles, ocular neuralgia, agglutination of lids after sleep, and patchy
scotoma.

Ears
The only ear symptoms of note are itching in the external auditory
meatus, and tinnitus increased by mental worry.

Respiratory System
Ignatia is associated with severe and distressing throat symptoms. These
are probably secondary to tension in the muscles of the region. There is a
most unpleasant and persistent choky plugged sensation, sometimes
described as 'a ball rising up in the throat'. A constant soreness in the
throat may be present, made worse by dry swallow or by drinking fluids,
but oddly enough relieved when swallowing solids and also by belching.
The remedy may be called for with ulcerative tonsillitis. Hysterical
aphonia and laryngismus stridulus are also mentioned. The irritable,
tickly cough of Ignatia is associated with a sensation as if there were some
dust or fumes in the trachea. Moreover coughing merely aggravates the
cough. Shooting pains may occur in the chest with a tight oppressed
feeling which provokes a constant desire to take a deep breath.

Alimentary System
There may be complaints of shooting pains in the lips, or of the inner
surface of the lower lip feeling raw and sore. A bitter taste is often
noticed in the mouth, a physical symptom perhaps associated with
bitterness of spirit. Salivation is apt to be excessive. Stitches occur in the
palate and extend to the ear. The Ignatia toothache is worse when not
eating. Gastric complaints are pyrosis, regurgitation of food and
hiccough, which is aggravated by taking food and by tobacco smoke. A
meal may be interrupted by vomiting and continued forthwith. A sinking
feeling is experienced in the epigastrium associated with a desire to take

a deep breath for relief. Cutting pains occur in the belly, and borborygmi cause embarrassment. As with Nux Vomica there is a tendency to much ineffectual urging to stool. When constipated, the passage of a soft stool is more painful than a hard stool. Piles are less painful when walking about than when sitting still. Rectal symptoms include proctalgia, anal spasm, prolapsus recti, and a sensation as if a packet of needles was present in the rectum. Painless urgent diarrhoea may occur as the result of emotional upset.

Cardiovascular System
In this sphere the variability of Ignatia is manifested in attacks of palpitation, with a very variable, rapidly altering pulse. Also the blood pressure levels tend to show much variation at different times.

Urinary System
An irresistible urge to pass water may be accompanied by inability to do so, owing to spasm of the sphincter muscle, as with retention of urine after labour. Often large quantities of pale lemon-coloured urine are passed.

Genital System
As would be expected, Ignatia is associated with psychogenic disturbance of hormonal balance evidenced by menstrual irregularities. The menses tend to be very dark, offensive and containing clots. Colicky dysmenorrhoea occurs, relieved by pressure, by lying down and also by change of position.

Nervous System
In this sphere the remedy is related to epileptic attacks precipitated by fright or by punishment, especially in children. It is also to be considered in connection with muscular twitchings and tics, with chorea in children and manifestations of hysteria.

Locomotor System
Among the symptoms mentioned in this sphere may be noted: stiff neck; quivering in deltoid muscle; sharp cutting pains in lower back extending to the thighs; sacral pain, worse on lying down; cramps in lower limbs associated with numbness and tingling. Also a form of sciatic pain of intermittent character, the attacks being preceded by coldness and shivering; it is worse in cold weather and at night, and during the paroxysm the sufferer is driven from bed to walk the floor in search of relief.

Skin

Disturbances of sensation occur, such as formication and numbness, but especially pruritus. This latter is aggravated by becoming heated, also in the open air; scratching affords relief but the itching then starts up in some other site.

MODALITIES

There is aggravation from cold, from eating sweets, from taking coffee or alcohol, and to a marked degree from contact with tobacco smoke, or any strong odour. Other sources of aggravation are yawning, pressure on non-painful areas, and any emotional upset.

Conversely, relief is obtained by warmth, while eating, by change of position, by pressure on the painful part; in other words, by activity which distracts from preoccupation with herself.

CLINICAL NOTES

Ignatia is not considered to be a deeply-acting remedy. It is certainly of great value in many psychosomatic disorders. It is complementary to Natrum Mur. and Sepia, and can be antidoted, if necessary, by Chamomilla or Pulsatilla.

In *Typologie* by Leon Vannier there is a pertinent passage on the therapeutic value of the remedy, which can be roughly translated as follows:

'Ignatia diminishes the sensitiveness of the individual, gets rid of the tendency to air-swallowing and the paradoxical and contradictory manifestations which baffle the doctor.

'The patient is submitted to endless examinations; the blood is analysed, also the urine; the basal metabolism is estimated, the stools examined, X-ray examinations are carried out.

'All are reported normal. 'There's nothing the matter with you' the patient is told. 'You can stop worrying. All your symptoms are just 'nerves' – meagre consolation for the sufferer! Ignatia rapidly deals with the situation.'

Iodum

The oceans are the main reservoir of iodine, as they also are of salt – Natrum Mur. – a remedy which shares many characteristics with Iodum. This is probably due to the chlorine element in the salt.

Iodine is the heaviest of the halogens. When isolated and purified it appears in crystalline form as dark bluish-grey flakes having a metallic lustre. These crystals give off a violet-coloured irritant vapour which has a peculiar, somewhat pungent odour and a rather metallic taste.

Formerly iodine salts were extracted from the ashes of slowly-burned seaweed; more recently it has been obtained from iodate salts found in Chile in association with saltpetre. Homoeopathic preparations are made from the 1 per cent tincture, which has a yellowish-brown colour. The colour of a saturated solution in chloroform is a deep violet.

PHARMACOLOGY

The tissue affinities of iodine are widespread throughout the body. Minute amounts of the element increase the rate of oxidation of proteins, carbohydrates and fats, and stimulate the secretory activity of the thyroid gland, the gonads, the adrenals and the breasts. In greater dosage an opposite effect is produced. This results in glandular atrophy, irritant lesions of mucous membranes and skin, inflammation and swelling of lymph nodes. More rarely, tissue proliferation occurs with the formation of gummatous nodules or cholesterol lesions in the walls of arteries.

In sensitive subjects, symptoms of iodism may be provoked by quite small doses, with acute involvement of the mucosa of the respiratory passages, the conjunctiva, the frontal sinuses, the throat and bronchial tubes. Such symptoms may result from the employment of iodine preparations for diagnostic purposes and are both distressing and alarming. Involvement of the larynx has on occasion necessitated tracheotomy.

There is a special affinity with the thyroid gland. Iodine deficiency in the food can induce symptoms of goitre. On the other hand, many cases of hyperthyroidism are benefited by small doses of iodine. Optimal absorption of iodine is thus essential for the proper function of the thyroid gland.

PROVING

Iodine was discovered in 1812, and a proving of it appears in the first edition of Hahnemann's *Chronic Diseases*.

APPEARANCE

The Iodum subject is often dark-haired, dark-eyed, dark-skinned. The face tends to be flushed, the expression anxious, the appearance excited and tremulous. Facial twitching may occur. The eyes may look widely open and staring. The subject is usually thin, even emaciated in appearance, with enlarged lymph nodes. The child looks like a 'little old person'. The thyroid gland may be enlarged.

Speech is careful with attention to accuracy in describing symptoms.

PSYCHOLOGY

The Iodum subject is restless, apprehensive, preoccupied, anxious, even anguished, and expects the worst. Is excessively impatient, never still, never sits down, must be doing something all the time, must hurry, and in consequence is easily tired.

There is a tendency to impulsiveness, impulse to do something violent, even to kill.

Again, the Iodum person may be zealous, literary, over-careful, exigent, intense.

PHYSIOLOGY

The Iodum subject is essentially a warm-blooded type, wants a cool place to move, think and work in, and prefers light clothing.

Appetite is typically voracious, and if meals are delayed he feels anxious and irritable and complains of a nagging sensation in the stomach. Despite, however, eating heartily he remains thin or actually loses weight – a characteristic shared by Natrum Mur. There may also be bouts of anorexia. There is a special fondness for meat, also for alcohol. Thirst may be excessive.

There is a liability to sudden profuse hot sweats; the sweat is said to stain linen blue. Foot sweats are acrid.

Agitation tends to interfere with sleep, which is often uneasy or dream-haunted.

SYMPTOMATOLOGY

General

Iodine has a profound effect on body metabolism, evidenced by extreme weakness, dyspnoea on ascending stairs, palpitations, pulsations, flushes, sweats, trembling and agitation. A striking characteristic of the element is that its effect may be in either of two opposite directions, e.g. excessive hunger or complete loss of appetite; hyperplasia of tissues or atrophy of the same tissues. This, however, is not surprising when it is realized that the balance between hyperactivity and hypoactivity in bodily processes is a very delicate one, and that it may easily be influenced in either direction by such an active agent as the halogen iodine.

Head

The Iodum vertigo is made worse by stooping, and is accompanied by hot flushes, throbbing in the head, buzzing in the ears, deafness, palpitations and fainting. Headache is often associated with arteriosclerosis. A left-sided headache is accompanied by a sensation as of a 'tape tied tightly round the skull'. There is a liability to sudden rush of blood to the head.

Eyes

Exophthalmos may be present. Pain and heat are felt in the eyes. Pupils tend to be large. Lids may be oedematous. Lachrymation is excoriating. Nystagmus may be noticed.

Ears

The remedy may be called for in relation to tinnitus and deafness resulting from involvement of the Eustachian tube.

Respiratory System

Pain may be felt at the root of the nose, in association with sinus involvement. Nasal catarrh is accompanied by much sneezing and profuse, hot, watery discharge which excoriates; this is worse on going into the open. In a warm room the nose becomes obstructed by sudden congestion and swelling of the lining mucosa. Inflammation of tonsils and palate may be accompanied by the formation of a greyish-white exudate. Oedema of the glottis may occur with alarming suddenness. A dry, suffocating cough is most exhausting, and often associated with gagging, retching and a frontal headache. There is much tickling and itching in the air passages, aggravated in a warm room and when lying down. Rapid shallow breathing and dyspnoea occur on exertion.

261

Alimentary System

Gums tend to be spongy, sore and bleed easily. Salivation is excessive, accompanied by a salty or soapy taste in the mouth. Aphthae occur in the buccal mucosa and on the tongue. Foetor oris is noticed, especially on waking in the morning. There is much belching, empty eructations occurring from morning till night, as if 'every morsel swallowed turned to gas'. The belly is blown up, with loud borborygmi. The liver or spleen may be enlarged, sore and hard. Jaundice may be present. An exhausting diarrhoea may occur from nervousness or as the result of taking some special food, especially milk; the stools tend to be pale, frothy and fatty. The diarrhoea is worse in the morning. Constipation may also occur with clay-like stools, only passed with difficulty.

Cardiovascular System

Pulsations and palpitations are liable to occur on least exertion, with surgings of blood towards the head and dyspnoea. Precordial distress may enforce constant change of position in search of ease. The heart may feel as if 'squeezed by a hand' or 'gripped in an iron vice'. The remedy may be of value in relation to pericarditis or cardiac hypertrophy exhibiting the foregoing symptoms.

Lymphatic System

The breasts may show induration or atrophy. They may feel very heavy, as if they would 'drop off'. Lymph nodes may be enlarged and indurated in any area. Various affections of the thyroid gland.

Urinary System

Incontinence of urine occurs in old men, probably associated with prostatic hypertrophy. Urination is frequent, with polyuria. Urine may be dark, strong-smelling and, if allowed to stand, an iridescent film forms on the surface.

Genital System

Swelling and induration of testes occurs, especially affecting the right side. Also atrophy may supervene with resulting impotence. The remedy may be called for in relation to hydrocele. Ovarian troubles are associated with a wedge-like pain extending towards the uterus or downwards into the thigh. The menstrual periods tend to be too early and too prolonged. Chronic leucorrhoea occurs with an acrid excoriating discharge.

Locomotor System

Violent pains occur in the joints at night, unaccompanied by any swelling. With chronic arthritis the joints become enlarged and deformed.

Skin

Various eruptions may occur, usually of dry type. Boils are of a peculiarly hard type with very little pus formation.

MODALITIES

There is aggravation from heat, in a warm room, if too warmly clad, when the weather is humid. Feels worse when fasting, or if unoccupied, but also from exertion, such as climbing stairs. Chronologically is worse at night, especially from 3 to 4 a.m.

Is better in cold air, by washing in cold water, when eating, and when fully occupied, or when walking out of doors.

CLINICAL NOTES

In hyperthyroidism high potencies are of value. Dr Tyler suggested giving Iodum CM on four successive nights at the wane of the moon. In ovarian troubles low potencies have been found to be effective.

With cardiovascular lesions the metallic salts, Aurum Iod. or Baryta Iod., may be preferable. Sulphur Iod. may be indicated in relation to acne or boils.

The remedy is said to be inadvisable in treating tuberculous lymphadenitis.

Ipecacuanha

SOURCE

The source of this remedy is the dried root of the perennial plant *Cephaelis ipecacuanha*, one of the Rubiaceae family, of which *Cinchona* is also a member. It occurs as a low straggling shrub, found principally in the forests of the Matto Grosso and Minas Geraes provinces of Brazil, growing in the rich, moist forest humus.

The brownish underground portion consists of a slender rhizome bearing wiry roots covered with little annular discs, and more slender smooth rootlets. The rhizome arches upwards and becomes continuous with a short, green aerial stem, five to nine inches in height. This bears pairs of large, petiolate, entire leaves with stipules at their base; the leaves are some three to four inches long, shaped like the head of a spear, bright green above and whitish green underneath. They are relatively few in number. The flowers are rather insignificant, white in colour and aggregated in a solitary head. This has a short round downy stalk which tends to droop with the weight of the flower head. The fruit is a cluster of purple berries, each containing two plano-convex seeds.

The plant as a whole is described as bitter, acrid and nauseating to the taste, and possessing a peculiar odour which may cause sneezing or even asthma in sensitive subjects. The roots together with portions of the rhizome are gathered from wild or cultivated plants from January to late March, dried in the sun and packed in bales made from hide.

There is a record in 1648 of the wide use of the drug in Brazil for the treatment of dysentery and it was introduced into France for the same purpose in 1672. In subsequent years the drug became used for a great variety of ills and was combined with opium and potassium sulphate in the popular remedy known as Dover's Powder.

PHARMACOLOGY

There are a number of alkaloids in the root of the plant, the most important being emetine (60 per cent) and cephaeline; other constituents include a glycoside, an acid, starch and calcium oxalate. The expectorant, emetic, diaphoretic and germicidal actions of the plant are attributed mainly to the presence of the above-mentioned alkaloids.

It has been observed that the smallest quantity of the powdered root in the air of a room is sufficient to induce in a sensitive individual considerable swelling and injection of the conjuctiva and nasal mucous membrance, with resulting lachrymation, sneezing, salivation, bronchial catarrh and asthmatic respiration.

When applied to the skin as a liniment the drug produces redness, itching and occasionally a pustular eruption.

When large doses of emetine are injected hypodermically the toxic effect of the drug is revealed in severe nausea, vomiting and purging, with blood in the stools, and collapse. This indicates that the drug is excreted by the mucous membrane of the gut, inducing irritation and inflammation in the process, and dealing with any amoebae present at the same time.

Toxic symptoms have also been observed following over-large dosage with the fluid extract of the drug, evidenced by severe vomiting, intermittent convulsions, apnoea, and the passage of bright red blood per rectum. A fatal issue has been recorded in children.

A poisonous action on the heart muscle has also been observed both as acute and cumulative effects. Deaths following the emetine treatment of dysentery have occurred, especially among white children in the East. It is recognized that emetine is a general protoplasmic poison tending to produce degenerative changes in liver, heart muscle, kidneys and muscle elsewhere.

The main tissue affinities of the plant thus appear to be with: (a) the mucous lining and musculature of the digestive and respiratory tracts, giving rise to increased secretions and spasm; (b) the vomiting centre in the medulla, inducing via the pneumogastric nerve a very persistent nausea with or without vomiting; (c) heart and liver, causing degenerative changes; and (d) the skin, producing erythema and blister formation.

PROVING

There is a pathogenesis of Ipecacuanha in the third volume of *Materia Medica Pura*.

APPEARANCE

Pallor predominates, and a typical facies nauseatica may be present with down-turned corners of mouth and well-defined nasolabial furrow. This is especially likely to be observed in children and will call to mind two other remedies, Aethusa Cynapium and Antimonium Tart.

In fever, however, the face may be flushed and bright red. Alternatively, if there is much gagging and choking, the face will become suffused and dark red owing to obstruction of the venous return from the head and face.

Again, if owing to lung involvement there is impaired aeration and consequent hypoxia, the facial hue will be cyanotic, associated with blue lips and nails.

The pupils tend to be large, and a gummy exudate accumulates at the lateral canthi.

Rather surprisingly the tongue usually remains clean.

Speech is affected in that the child tends to 'go dumb'. The adult becomes glum and not a word is spoken.

Movements are awkward and clumsy with a tendency to bump into the furniture. Shuddering may be prominent.

PSYCHOLOGY

The Ipecacuanha subject manifests extreme impatience, and is described as being full of desires which are vague and ill-defined. This leads to discontent and a tendency to be scornful of anything and everything.

Children wail and scream continuously; adults are sulky and ill-humoured all day long. Everything is repugnant – a psychological nausea and disgust.

There is a great sensitivity to noise, especially music played loudly.

The remedy may be called for when illness has been brought on by vexation and bottled-up displeasure.

PHYSIOLOGY

Excessive chilliness is the rule; there is no warmth in the body at all; the slightest cold is unbearable. Feels cold shudders as if from a fright or in terror; actual rigors may occur.

Appetite is seriously affected; anorexia is accompanied by aversion from all food, and this is associated with a deathly nausea which nothing relieves.

A prominent feature may be thirstlessness, when the opposite might be expected.

Sleep is restless and disturbed by vivid dreams, the content of which is not remembered. There is a tendency to sudden starting awake with a jerk.

Ipecacuanha

SYMPTOMATOLOGY

General

The special feature of this remedy is that all complaints are accompanied by nausea, also very often by shuddering, yawning and malaise. The onset of the illness is sudden, and progress rapid; this is in contrast with Antimonium Tart., which is characterized by a gradual onset of symptoms.

Pains are associated with a bruised sensation, and sudden exhaustion is common. Absence of marked thirst would distinguish here from the exhaustion so characteristic of Arsenicum Alb. Fever is accompanied by severe pain between the shoulders and a sensation as if the back would break. Haemorrhages are prominent in connection with the remedy, occurring from any mucous surface, associated with nausea, a sinking sensation, even actual syncope. The bleeding is of oozing type with intermittent gushes of bright red blood.

Head

An occipital headache is described, associated with a bruised or crushed feeling in the bones of the skull, as if 'something pierced through the skull from vertex to face, teeth or root of tongue'. The whole head aches. Hemicrania is accompanied by pallor, deadly nausea and blue rings round the eyes, vomiting may be so intractable that not even a sip of water can be retained. Prostration occurs in spells, again differing from that associated with Arsenicum Alb., which is continuous. A bursting type of headache may occur, similar to that associated with Ptelea and Veratrum Alb.

Eyes

Various eye symptoms are listed, notably neuralgic pains in the eye, spasm of the lids with gush of tears when the spasm relaxes; the spasm accompanies sudden severe inflammation with photophobia.

Respiratory System

Acute coryza is accompanied by much sneezing and either blockage of the nose or profuse discharge of blood-stained mucus. Copious epistaxis of bright red blood may occur. There is a tendency to downward spread. A dry, teasing cough results from a very persistent tickle in the larynx or all the way down the air passages. Sudden, suffocative spasmodic cough is associated with severe dyspnoea, much wheezing and rattling in the chest, accompanied by gagging and vomiting. The chest feels oppressively tight and the sufferer has to sit up in order to breathe. The child is apt to become apnoeic while coughing, turn pale or blue, and go quite stiff. The adult may suffer from moist asthma and stand for hours beside the open window in search of oxygen. An indication for the remedy is bronchiolitis of rapid onset in infants with great accumulation of mucus in the chest, which is full of bubbling rales; cough is spasmodic, dyspnoea acute, and phlegm is vomited. If the cough lessens but the condition worsens, owing to progressive weakness and loss of expulsive power, and the lungs are still clogged with mucus, it is advisable to switch to Antimonium Tart. in frequent doses till an adequate cough reflex is restored. Should pneumonic changes supervene, a switch to Phosphorus would be called for, and possibly then to Sulphur, if the response is inadequate. The remedy may be called for in whooping cough, if associated with epistaxis, red visage, gagging and vomiting and lack of thirst. It also has a sphere of usefulness in relation to emphysema and asthmatic bronchitis in old people, especially when the condition is aggravated by damp or by a sudden change in the weather. Indicated also in haemoptysis with bright red blood, which wells up without effort and is increased by the least exertion.

Alimentary System
Toothache is mentioned with a sensation as if the tooth was being pulled out. Very characteristic is a combination of nausea with persistent vomiting which does not, however, relieve the nausea. This is accompanied by an abundant flow of watery saliva. The tongue remains clean and may even look pale. Antimonium Crud. may present a somewhat similar picture, but the tongue will be thickly coated and milky-white as if it had been whitewashed. The condition may occur after over-indulgence in rich food, or it may accompany chronic gastritis. Severe haematemesis may demand the remedy. Cutting or pinching pains occur in and below the epigastrium; the pains pass from left to right and are so severe that the sufferer cannot stir or breathe till the pain passes off; vomiting and prostration are concomitants. Flatulent colicky pains may be felt in the region of the umbilicus, and a sensation as if 'the bowels were grasped by a hand' or as if 'the stomach was hanging down'. The abdomen may be distended, tympanitic and tender to touch. Dysenteric symptoms are accompanied by an almost continuous urge to stool, and awful tenesmus; nausea and vomiting are prominent and may even be the first symptom. The stools are slimy and usually contain blood. Choleraic diarrhoea in infants is characterized by stools which are grass-green in colour or foamy and fermented in appearance, like molasses. The child passes copious amounts of greenish slime.

Nervous System

The remedy may be called for in connection with cerebro-spinal meningitis associated with vomiting of everything ingested, a red raw tongue, severe convulsions especially affecting the left side, and possibly opisthotonos. The face is red and flushed.

Urinary System

Shooting pains are felt in the loin, associated with haematuria. There is a frequent urge to urinate, and bright red blood and small clots are passed. The urine appears turbid with a sediment like brick dust. Distress is felt in the whole length of the urinary tract, and nausea and vomiting are likely concomitants.

Genital System

Here the most prominent indication is bleeding. This may be a menorrhagia after taking cold or after a shock, or some other form of uterine haemorrhage, showing a steady flow of bright red blood, or intermittent gushes with oozing in between. The bleeding is accompanied by nausea, faintness, and by air hunger if excessive. Another indication is in threatened abortion, with pinching pains around the umbilicus; the pains tend to fly from left to right and nausea is present.

Locomotor System

Pains are felt in bones as if bruised, and tingling may be noticed in the joints which feel 'dislocated' or as if the part had 'gone to sleep'.

Skin

Pruritus occurs in association with nausea. The itching is especially violent in arms and thighs; the sufferer must scratch till vomiting ensues, and this affords some relief.

MODALITIES

As would be expected, there is aggravation in cold weather, but great heat is also resented. While dry weather is uncongenial there is also an adverse reaction to hot moist winds. Taking food causes aggravation, especially eating veal or pork.

While contact is resented, firm pressure may give relief. Feels better in the open or when at rest with the eyes closed.

CLINICAL NOTES

The 200c potency has been found effective in both haemorrhage and asthma. Complementary remedies are Arsenicum Alb. and Cuprum Met.

Kali Bichromicum

SOURCE

The remedy is prepared from the bichromate of potash, obtained from chromium iron ore. It is a chemical widely used in the dyeing of fabrics, staining of wood, photography, and in electric batteries. It is a powerful oxidising substance and a corrosive irritant poison.

PHARMACOLOGY

There is a strong affinity with skin, mucous membranes and periarticular tissues. The effect is to produce irritation and inflammation. The mucosal irritation is accompanied by the secretion of thick ropy or stringy discharges, or by the formation of adherent fibrinous exudates and 'false membranes'.

PROVING

Kali Bichromicum was first proved in England by Dr Drysdale, and published in the *British Journal of Homoeopathy*, 1846.

APPEARANCE

Children are fat and chubby; adults likely to be stout, of sallow complexion and light hair.

Yellowness is in evidence; yellow sclerotics, yellow discharges, yellow vomit, yellow exudates resembling wash-leather.

In chronic conditions the subject may be emaciated, even cachectic.

PSYCHOLOGY

The subject is usually ill-tempered, low-spirited, listless. There is aversion to meeting strangers; misanthropic. Memory is poor with a tendency to the vanishing of thought. Aversion to making any kind of effort may be a feature.

PHYSIOLOGY

Is chilly and likes to be well wrapped up, but is apt to suffer from a change to warm weather.

As to appetite, there is often a desire for beer or acid drinks, and possibly a distaste for meat. Intolerance may be present for potatoes, starchy foods and coffee.

May sweat on the back when straining at stool.

Drowsiness is accompanied by prostration – can hardly write a letter. Is apt to wake with a start about 2 a.m., feeling nauseated, hot and sweaty; may also have a rapid pulse, palpitation and dyspnoea. Wakes unrefreshed.

SYMPTOMATOLOGY

General

The pains associated with this remedy are sharp, often burning; they tend to shoot and shift rapidly from site to site; they come on with suddenness and pass off with abruptness. Sometimes pain is limited to an area so small that it can be covered by the tip of a finger.

Extremely characteristic of the remedy is the type of discharges; these are ropy and sticky and can be pulled out into strings. Sometimes the mucous secretions are lumpy and jelly-like rather than stringy. Again, there is a tendency to the formation of adherent exudate on mucous surfaces. Another feature peculiar to the remedy is an alternation of symptoms or a periodic recurrence. Rheumatic symptoms may appear when catarrhal symptoms clear up; rheumatic symptoms may improve with the advent of gastric upset or diarrhoea. Rheumatic symptoms are apt to recur in spring, and dysentery in early summer.

Head

A headache of migraine type is preceded by blindness, which improves as the headache increases; it is accompanied by nausea and vomiting and aggravated by light, noise, walking, stooping, and is worse at night. The sufferer is forced to lie down in a darkened room. Severe pain may be felt at the root of the nose in association with sinusitis; it is worse at 9 a.m. An intense headache may be felt in quite a small spot. Pain also may be located in the malar bones.

Eyes

Eye affections become chronic, such as an indolent type of corneal ulcer which is rather surprisingly not accompanied by much pain, photophobia

271

or lachrymation. Eyes may burn and itch; lid margins are red and swollen. Vision may be disturbed by bright spots and various colours before the eyes. Conjunctivitis with much heat and redness and a great desire to rub the eyes on account of itching. Chronic eye affections of various kinds.

Ears

Earache is associated with stinging pain which shoots up into the head and down into the neck; it may be accompanied by swelling of the regional lymph nodes and parotid gland. Chronic otitis media is associated with a stringy, yellow purulent discharge of offensive odour. An itching eczematous eruption may be present on the external ear.

Respiratory System

Post-nasal catarrh occurs, with production of stringy mucus in the nasopharynx and much hawking of ropy or lumpy discharge. There may be complaint of the sensation of a hair on the back of the tongue. Rhinitis, both acute and chronic, accompanied by thick yellow viscid mucus which may block the nasal passages. Actual ozaena may be present with the discharge of green plugs or clinkers. Perforating ulcer of the septum may develop. Sore throat is associated with a swollen oedematous uvula. Follicular tonsillitis occurs, or ulceration of tonsils, with 'wash-leather' exudate. Perforating ulcers may be present in fauces or on palate. The soreness of the throat may be relieved by swallowing hot fluids. The remedy may be required in membranous croup. A brassy cough is associated with dyspnoea and gagging in the endeavour to get rid of tough stringy sputum; it is worse on waking in the morning; it is accompanied by irritation deep to the lower part of the sternum and pain extending from mid-sternum through to the back. The cough is aggravated by both eating and drinking and also by uncovering; it is eased by warmth and by lying down. It is better in warm weather and worse in winter. After sputum has been raised there is a desire to blow the nose. A paroxysm of coughing may occur during a meal with total loss of food ingested. Pressure and heaviness is felt in the chest; wakens with this sensation at night and is better after rising. Asthmatic attacks occur at 3 to 4 a.m., compelling the sufferer to sit up and lean forward, head on arms crossed over knees; relief is obtained by bringing up stringy mucus.

Alimentary System

The mouth is dry; the tongue is glazed, smooth or cracked and fissured and, possibly, coated with yellow at the base. Pain is felt at the root of the tongue when it is pushed forward. Much bitter, viscid or frothy saliva may accumulate in the mouth. Pyorrhoea alveolaris is common, with foetor oris. The stomach is upset by the mildest food; gastritis is associated with neuralgic or blinding headache, yellow vomit; food ingested may be gulped up unchanged. The symptoms are aggravated by taking food. Soreness and tenderness may be noticed at a small spot to the left of the xiphisternum. Repletion may be felt after only a few mouthfuls of food. Food seems to lie like a load in the stomach. Heartburn comes on immediately, or quite soon after a meal, and the pain may extend to the back. Nausea is very sudden in onset. Nausea and vomiting of drunkards; the vomiting recurs at every attempt to eat or drink. A sensation of coldness may be felt in stomach and bowels with much soreness. Peptic or malignant ulcer may be present. Belching may be a feature, affording a measure of relief. The stomach may swell, especially in the evening, with concomitant discomfort causing the clothes round the waist to be loosened. Pain in the liver region extends to the shoulder. Gallstones may be present. Constipation may be present associated with debility, coated tongue, headache and coldness of extremities. Stools are hard; rectal prolapse and protruding, very painful piles are a likely accompaniment; a plug sensation may be felt at the anus, so painful as to make sitting almost unbearable. Morning diarrhoea is aggravated by drinking beer. Dysentery recurs in spring or early summer; the symptoms are worse in the morning, with gelatinous blood-stained stools, followed by tenesmus. Stools may be clay-coloured and passed unawares.

Cardiovascular System
A cold feeling or sensation of pressure may be felt in the cardiac region. Pricking pain is felt at the apex of the heart.

Urinary System
During and after urination burning is felt in the urethra. Residual drop sensation may be felt in the fossa navicularis. Constant urge to urinate is present by day, and frequency at night. There may be a ropy discharge from the urethra.

Genital System
Stitches in the prostate gland when walking may compel the sufferer to stand still. Libido is lost. Constrictive pains may be felt at the root of the penis. Penetrating ulcers may occur on the external genitals. Uterine prolapse may occur in hot weather. A yellow ropy or lumpy vaginal

discharge may be present. The remedy may be called for in vomiting of pregnancy. During lactation the milk may become stringy.

Locomotor System

Rheumatic pains wander from site to site; may specially affect fingers and wrists; involved joints are red, hot and swollen, or may crack and creak on movement. The rheumatic symptoms may alternate with attacks of respiratory catarrh or gastric symptoms. Bones all over the body may feel bruised; actual caries may be present. A sensation as if something cracks across the sacrum may be noticed when stooping. Pain in the coccyx is relieved by passage of urine. Sciatic pain is aggravated by heat and relieved by movement.

Skin

Eruptions may be morbilliform, papular or pustular. Ulcers are circular, deep and punched out; the edges may be ragged; healed ulcers show a depressed scar.

MODALITIES

Aggravation results from exposure to cold air, cold winds, even open air; is worse in wet weather and when snow is melting. Is worse also from touch, when stooping, on undressing. The chronological aggravation is from 2 a.m. to 5 a.m. and is worse usually after waking from sleep. Spring and autumn also are adverse seasons.

Better from warmth, especially when tucked up warm in bed; movement affords relief, also firm pressure. Usually better in summer, but the sudden onset of hot weather may have an adverse effect, especially on rheumatic conditions.

CLINICAL NOTES

The remedy is of great value in nasopharyngeal catarrh. It should be considered in peptic ulcer, in diphtheria, and in advanced syphilis.

Complementary remedies are Arsenicum Alb., Phosphorus and Psorinum.

Kali Carbonicum

SOURCE

Kalium carbonicum is potash, the carbonate of potassium. The salt derives its name from its ancient source, plant ash, called in Arabic 'al kaljun'.

Unlike sodium, which occurs chiefly in the oceans linked to chlorine as sodium chloride, common salt, potassium in the form of various salts is found in soil and plants. In the body as in nature sodium is predominant in the fluids. Potassium on the other hand is an important constituent of colloid material, of the humus of the soil, of the cell-substance of the body.

PHARMACOLOGY

For an understanding of disturbed potassium metabolism it is necessary to review the function of the element in the living body.

There is a fundamental balance between the two elements, sodium and potassium, as also between their main accessories calcium and magnesium. This vital equilibrium maintains the tone of living tissues. It results from the co-operation of these elements with anions such as chloride, carbonate, phosphate and sulphate in balancing opposite charges.

Although potassium is chiefly a component of the intracellular colloids, it moves about freely and at great speed in the body, adjusting itself to the prevailing needs of cells and organs. For instance, during muscular activity the potassium concentration in the blood rises, to fall again during rest.

When there is serious depletion of sodium chloride, as in severe haemorrhage, in shock, or as the result of excessive vomiting, potassium migrates from the cells into the circulation. Such conditions are associated with marked muscular weakness, the consequence of potassium deficiency in the muscle cells and resulting loss of tone.

Potassium is a radioactive element emitting beta rays, negative electrons, from the atom nucleus. The rate of electron emission is only about one thousandth of that of uranium, but potassium is an

275

indispensable agent in cell processes and in this sphere its radioactivity may not be without significance.

This is thought to be specially the case in relation to functions which are distinguished by automatism and rhythmicity. It is known, for instance, that Kali Carb. has a definite affinity with the heart muscle and with the smooth muscle of organ ducts and blood vessels.

Muscle cells are rich in their potassium content, the element being indispensable for their function of contractility, that is so long as the potassium is within the cell. Of all the alkali ions, however, the most damaging to muscle cells, if present in excess on the outside of the cells, is this same element. The provings of Kali Carb. show a tendency to marked muscle weakness, manifesting thus a further affinity with striated muscle.

There appears to be a reciprocal relation between the impulses of the vagus and those of potassium. The element stimulates the vagus, and stimulation of the vagus activates the flow of potassium ions. Kali Carb. in potency may well act as a stimulus to a delicately poised equilibrium through the vegetative nerve transmitter.

Potassium acts generally in a parasympathetic way, tending towards depression, decrease of skeletal and cardiac muscle tone and also disturbance of rhythm. Excess of potassium, however, causes increased tone and active contractions in plain muscle of intestines, bronchi, uterus and arterioles.

Potassium is also necessary for normal conductivity in sensory nerves. Disorders of potassium flow in peripheral nerves are likely to be manifested as pains, especially the sharp, stabbing, stitching pains associated with the provings of Kali Carb.

Potassium appears to be no less essential for the normal transmission of impulses in the central nervous system. Excess of potassium, however, may depress or even paralyse the vital centres. Complete absence of potassium also results in depression. In other words, potassium must be present in optimal relation to other ions. The proper balance must be maintained if disturbance of vital processes is to be avoided.

The main affinities of Kali Carb. are therefore seen to be with the nervous system, both central and peripheral, tending to depression and hypotonus; with the heart, leading to myasthenia and disturbance of rhythm; with the smooth muscle of organ ducts, giving rise to increased tone and active spasm; with mucous membranes producing irritation, ulceration and necrosis.

PROVING

Hahnemann published a proving of Kali Carbonicum in the first edition of his *Chronic Diseases*.

APPEARANCE

The picture presented is of a chilly, shivery, restless individual whose disquietude makes interrogation difficult and tedious. This may be due to such a state of weariness that even carrying on a conversation is too much of an effort.

The sufferer appears not only weary but also full of woe, and may weep while recounting symptoms, a feature shared with Medorrhinum, Pulsatilla, Sepia and Streptococcinum.

Bag-like swellings may be present between the eyebrows and upper lids. Puffiness of the upper lid may be noticed – compare puffiness of both lids (Apis) and puffiness of lower lid (Arsenicum Alb.). Doughy oedematous swellings may be found in various sites.

The skin is often of a dry, milky white appearance; the nose may be red and show brawny swelling.

There is a tendency to jump and cry out if startled by a sudden noise or if touched unawares. The least touch is resented, especially on the soles of the feet, and the subject is excessively ticklish.

PSYCHOLOGY

The worn-out state results in an extremely irritable and touchy individual who complains of being 'all on edge', 'strung up', unable to cope.

Is averse to solitude; wants company but not sympathy. At times may appear witty and whimsical, but is inclined to be at variance with everybody and everything. Is both uninterested and uninteresting, both weary and wearisome.

There is hypersensitivity to noise. A loud noise, or a sudden shock, or bad news is apt to cause a queer feeling 'in the stomach'. A fit of actual trembling – 'all of a quiver' – may ensue on a scare or an emotional upset.

Fear is common, fear of the future, of death, of ghosts.

The state of mental and physical asthenia tends to produce a crotchety chronic, full of complaints.

PHYSIOLOGY

The Kali Carb. subject is always cold, often actually to the point of shivering. The chilliness is aggravated by eating, or by any activity which throws extra strain on the feeble circulation. There is a tendency to catch cold on every exposure to cold air and, in consequence, a dread of being out of doors; a well-heated room is much appreciated. Hands and feet are nearly always icy cold.

Appetite is poor with positive repugnance towards food, especially brown bread. There may be a desire for sour things which temporarily titillate the depressed appetite. There is often intolerance of milk.

Thirst is variable, but there is often an entire inability to perspire, even in great heat. Conversely, when debility is extreme, sweating may occur on least pretext, especially at night. Sweats tends to be cold and clammy, and may be circumscribed in area.

Drowsiness is common during the daytime, especially during meals, but the nights are disturbed by anxious horrible dreams and a tendency to wake in the small hours and stay awake.

SYMPTOMATOLOGY

General

In the main this is a right-sided remedy. The sensitivity to cold is so great that coldness is felt as actual pain; it'hurts'. Pains seem to derive from altered biochemical conditions in nerves, to stagnation rather than to inflammation. They are described as peculiar, stitching, stabbing or cutting, and may occur independently of movement, while sitting or lying at rest. The pains are accompanied by a feeling of coldness in the affected part, although the actual pain may be burning in character. The pains may be so severe and sudden as to extort a cry, and are made worse by cold, touch, pressure and by lying on the painful part. Warmth gives some relief. The pains tend to be located in muscle or in connective tissues, and also to shift from one spot to another. If the pain in one spot is eased by warmth, fresh pain is likely to start up somewhere else. There is a liability to puffy swelling in various sites as the result of localized oedema. Symptoms are commonly accompanied by rapid emaciation, cardiac weakness and easy exhaustion. Iron deficiency anaemia may be present.

Head

Owing to the circulatory hypotonia, vertigo in various forms is common. It may occur even while sitting still. Burning pain may occur in the region of the frontal sinuses, or neuralgic pains in scalp, eyes and malar regions. These pains are aggravated by driving in cold air or even by inhaling cold air, and the head must be well wrapped when out of doors. Congestive headaches also are mentioned, eased by pressure and by warmth. Scalp and hair tend to be dry, possibly with eruptions on the scalp of scabby or scaly type, and associated alopecia especially on the temples and eyebrows.

Eyes

Lancinating pains may be felt in the eyes. Dimness of vision can be a frequent occurrence, especially after coitus. There is often a complaint of troublesome muscae volitantes before the eyes. Swelling of the medial angle of the upper lid is characteristic, and other puffy swelling as mentioned above.

Ears

Asthenia may be accompanied by disturbances of hearing, by tinnitus, by cracking in the ears. A curious sensation as if 'cold air was blowing into the ear' may be noticed.

Respiratory System

The nose may be swollen and very red, and nostrils uncomfortably dry. The nasal passages tend to be blocked with foetid mucus and crusts, associated with thick, fluent yellow discharge. The nose becomes stuffed up in a warm room and this gives relief, whereas out of doors, although the nose is less obstructed, headache recurs. Epistaxis may occur about 9 a.m. or when washing the face. There is a great tendency to constantly take fresh 'colds', and these often involve the larynx with loss of voice. Enlargement of tonsils may occur, possibly associated with swelling and induration of the parotid glands. Sore throats are characterized by sticking pains or a sensation as if a fish bone were lodged in the throat. There is much hawking of mucus from post-nasal discharge. Stinging pains are felt on swallowing and there is a persistent feeling of 'a lump in the throat'.

The lower air passages are liable to become involved with a resulting incessant dry, violent, racking cough, worse from 3 am to 5 am, and associated with bag-like swelling above the upper eyelid, more marked when coughing. The chest feels cold. Cough may be paroxysmal with much wheezing, gagging and vomiting. Sputum is scanty, sticky and apt to be swallowed; or little grey balls of inspissated phlegm are shot from the mouth during a fit of coughing. There are stitching pains in the chest, increased by movement but occurring also when at rest. These pains are mainly located in the lower one third of the right lung and spread to the back. Chronic catarrhal conditions of the chest may follow an attack of measles or pneumonia, associated with a productive cough and copious, offensive, tenacious, lumpy sputum, yellow or yellowish-green in colour and often blood-streaked. The sputum may have a pungent taste as of ripe cheese. Dyspnoea is noticed when going upstairs or uphill, but not when walking on the level. The remedy is indicated in asthma when there is aggravation between 3 a.m. and 5 a.m., causing the sufferer to sit up and lean forward with head on knees for relief. The attacks are usually associated with cardiac weakness.

Alimentary System
Toothache results from exposure to a cold wind or draught. Pyorrhoea alveolaris may accompany the general debility with loosened teeth and a foul taste in mouth. The tongue may become covered with small painful vesicles, or a painful pimple may be present on the tip of the tongue. The swallowing of food may be rendered difficult by excessive dryness in the pharynx and may be associated with a pricking sensation. Atonic dyspepsia occurs, accompanied by a sinking feeling that is not relieved but rather increased by eating, both at the time and after the meal. After taking food there is a sensation of coldness and leaden weight in the stomach, or the organ feels 'full of water'. There is a good deal of heartburn and at times pyrosis. These symptoms are made worse by cold drinks, but relieved temporarily by belching and also by warmth. Pain may be felt in the stomach on stooping.

Severe bloating is common, associated with belching and the passage of offensive flatus. The bloating comes on soon after meals, even if only a small quantity has been consumed; everything swallowed seems to be turned into gas. Recurrent attacks of flatulent colic cause very severe pains of a cutting nature and are associated with a desire for warmth, hot water bottles, hot drinks and bending double for relief. The remedy may be called for in liver disorders, associated with fullness and pain in the right hypochrondrium, in the right side of the chest, extending to the right shoulder-blade, gastrointestinal disturbance and periodic bilious attacks. Constipation is usual with large hard stools, followed by burning in the rectum and anus. But chronic diarrhoea may occur, possibly alternating with constipation, especially in asthenic, pallid, broken-down subjects. Piles are liable to be very large, constantly prolapsed, to burn like fire and bleed profusely. They are extremely painful, exquisitely tender to touch, and cannot be properly replaced. They may cause insomnia, and may give rise to the sensation of 'a hot poker pushed up the rectum'. Contrary to the usual modality, some relief is obtained by sitting in cold water. Coughing and urination make matters worse.

Cardiovascular System
Cardiac asthenia is prominent with weak, irregular or intermittent pulse, tendency to palpitations, especially when hungry, and constrictive pain in the region of the heart. The symptoms are worse when eating, when recumbent and at night. Pulsations may be felt all over the body, even without actual palpitations. The enfeebled circulation encourages oedema in various sites, and dyspnoea may become extreme on least effort. The heart may feel as if 'suspended by a thread'. Endo- and pericarditis, associated with the typical pains and exhaustion, may call for the remedy.

Urinary System
The bladder takes part in the general hypotonus. Frequency of urination occurs with delay in starting the act and feeble stream. Dysuria occurs with burning, both during the passage of urine and after. The urine may be loaded with urates.

Genital System
The menstrual period is apt to be preceded by increased chilliness and colicky pains. Constipation is likely during the period. Low back pain is specially troublesome during pregnancy. The remedy should be considered in relation to threatened abortion, amenorrhoea and persistent uterine haemorrhage despite curettage and other treatments. Coitus is followed by excessive exhaustion associated with dimness of vision.

Nervous System
Hypersensitivity is evidenced in this sphere by the onset of tingling and numbness in response to the least degree of pressure in any site. Also twitchings and tremors may occur, or even actual convulsions, but without loss of consciousness.

Locomotor System
The prominent feature here is marked muscular weakness. The legs may suddenly give way, the back gives out and forces the sufferer to lie down; on attempting to walk, the back feels as if 'it would break'. Pains are frequent in the back extending both up and down, but especially affecting the sacral region with the tendency to spread through the hips to the thighs. The pains are worse when walking, and before the onset of the menstrual period. Relief is felt when lying down and by firm pressure on a fairly hard object in the small of the back. (This last modality is shared also by Cimicifuga, Natrum Mur. and Sepia.) Accompanying

stiffness is eased by movement. Pain may be felt in the spine when eating. An itching sensation may be noticed in the bones. A triad of cold sweats, great weakness and low back pain is said to point with precision to Kali Carb.

MODALITIES

Aggravation results from exposure to cold air, from the least draught, and from weather changes. Also from taking soup or coffee; from least touch or pressure and from lying on the painful part of the affected side. Chronologically the worst time is from 3 a.m. to 5 a.m.; headache tends to be worst at 9 a.m.; a hungry faintness comes on about 10 a.m.; there is often a stubborn chilliness at noon.

The symptoms tend to be ameliorated in warm moist weather, as is the case with Causticum, Hepar Sulph. and Nux Vomica. Relief is obtained by leaning forward, and during the daytime.

CLINICAL NOTES

This is a rather tricky remedy, said to be very dangerous in asthenic gouty subjects if given higher than 30c. It is of special value in the older age groups.

It should be considered in asthenic and anaemic states following severe or protracted illness, or deriving from childbirth or abortion.

Kreosotum

SOURCE

The source of this remedy is a mixture of phenols obtained from beechwood tar. It is an almost colourless or yellowish oily fluid with a penetrating odour and a burning taste.

PHARMACOLOGY

Affinity with mucous membranes leads to profuse offensive secretions, coagulation of protein, necrosis and sloughing; the skin is similarly affected. Action on the central nervous system induces profound depression and collapse; on the blood, results in disorganization and cell destruction; on the kidneys, produces acute irritation associated with dark green urine or anuria.

PROVING

Kreosotum was first proved by Dr Wahle of Rome, and published in the *Archiv*.

APPEARANCE

Physical features are a yellowish pallor, a sickly semi-cachectic appearance, with blue rings round the eyes. Reddish blotches may be seen on the face; lips are apt to be dry and bleeding; corners of the mouth ulcerated.

Children look old, wrinkled and marasmic, or may appear lean, ill-developed and tall for their age.

There is marked foetor of breath; discharges have a foul odour.

PSYCHOLOGY

The mental state is described as nervous, excitable, never satisfied and tearful over trifles. Restlessness is marked; wants to be constantly on the move. Is very irritable if in pain. Any emotional upset is accompanied by pulsations all over the body. Memory is impaired.

PHYSIOLOGY

Very chilly with cold legs and feet; but the face may be hot.

Appetite is keen with desire for meat, or there may be a deep and persistent disgust with food, especially during convalescence from illness.

There may be a craving for alcohol, especially spirits. Thirst may be intense and burning.

Drowsiness is marked during the daytime, accompanied by frequent yawning, but at night lies awake till all hours, restless and tossing with burning and itching skin. May start awake when dropping off to sleep; may laugh while asleep. The child moans constantly or dozes with half-closed eyes. Dreams are frequent, varied, vivid and fearsome or unpleasant.

Sweating occurs mainly in the morning hours.

SYMPTOMATOLOGY

General

Pains are described as pulling, shooting, burning, fiery, accompanied by heaviness, stiffness, numbness, tingling, crawling and itching in affected parts. Fingers or other areas go pale, cold, 'dead'. The least injury bleeds profusely. There is a tendency to haemorrhages of dark blood, oozing in type, e.g. epistaxis, haemoptysis, post tonsillectomy or tooth extraction. Discharges and secretions are profuse and putrid in odour. Symptoms tend to predominate on the left side of the body.

Head

Vertigo is of the whirling type. A throbbing, bursting frontal headache is associated with drowsiness. A severe headache may occur before and during the menstrual period, like a board pressing against the forehead. Pain in the occipital region is accompanied by a sensation of weight and a feeling as if about to topple over backwards. Scalp may be tender to touch. Alopecia may occur.

Eyes

Chronic blepharitis may occur with agglutination of lids. Lachrymation is salty. Lids may be red with itching. There is discharge of hot, scalding tears, especially in early morning. Eyelids may quiver uncontrollably. Vision may seem obstructed by something floating before the eyes.

Ears

External ear inflamed, red hot, burning and itching associated with enlargement of cervical lymph nodes, pain and stiffness of neck on the affected side. Roaring or humming tinnitus with some deafness, preceding and accompanying menstruation; this is worse when lying down. Moist herpetic eruptions around the ear.

Respiratory System
Nasal discharge is very offensive. Catarrh becomes chronic in old people. Epistaxis occurs mostly in the morning; type of blood variable. Frequent sneezing, especially in the morning. Throat is dry with burning and choking sensations, worse on swallowing. Larynx painful with accompanying hoarseness. A sensation of fullness and tightness in the chest gives rise to a desire to take a deep breath, but there is a seeming inability to do so; this is worse in a warm room and better in the open air. Stabbing burning pains may be felt in the chest. Cough may be very troublesome, dry and wheezing or spasmodic with retching, especially in the morning. Winter cough in old people comes on in bouts, is worse at night; there is much green purulent sputum, possibly stained with dark blood, and foetor is marked.

Alimentary System
Dentition is painful, associated with much restlessness and screaming. Drawing, throbbing, jerking pains are felt in the teeth. Early and rapid caries occurs, teeth show black specks almost as soon as they erupt. Gums are painful, black and bleed easily. Aphthous ulcers occur in mouth. There is marked foetor and a foul taste in the mouth. The tongue is pale and flabby and feels 'cold'. The lower lip may be red, painful with cracks. Fullness is felt in the stomach, with burning immediately after a meal. Belching is frequent and violent. There is a peculiar type of vomiting; food is either returned at once or brought up unchanged, perhaps several hours after ingestion. The vomitus is acid and burning and may have a cadaveric odour. The condition is aggravated by taking cold food; warm food gives some relief. Pinching shooting pains occur around the umbilicus or in the hepatic region. Diarrhoea occurs with dark brown, undigested, putrid stools. Children strain and scream while passing a stool. Cholera infantum may call for the remedy. A curious symptom may be complaint of a sensation of ice-cold water in the stomach.

Cardiovascular System
There is a liability to palpitations, and widespread pulsations all over the body. Cardiac distress may be induced by emotional stress. Music causes tears and palpitations. Actual fainting may occur in a warm room.

Urinary System
Frequency of urination accompanied by urgency with passage of copious pale urine. Or urine may be turbid and offensive with red sediment. Burning occurs both during and after urination, when itching may be

aggravated. May be unable to pass urine except when lying. Enuresis, especially during first sleep.

Genital System

Menstruation too early and too profuse, with associated deafness and tinnitus; blood is dark and offensive; flow is intermittent, only occurring when lying down. Leucorrhoea associated with intermittent haemorrhage. Much burning in pelvis like red hot coals, with discharge of clots of foul-smelling blood. Lochia are dark, brown, offensive, acrid; almost dry up, then start again. Uterine complaints are worse after menstrual period; are accompanied by dragging pain in back or bearing down pains in genitals. Smarting and itching affect pudenda or are felt deep in vagina. Yellowish offensive vaginal discharge stains linen; worse when standing or walking; less when sitting.

Nervous System

Facial neuralgia with burning pain is worse from motion and when talking. Long-standing neuralgias. Finger tips become numb; parts go 'dead'.

Locomotor System

Pain radiates from sacral region upwards to between scapulae, also forwards causing rectal or urethral urging. The pain may also spread downwards into the thighs; it is worse at rest and relieved by movement. Gnawing, drawing pains in limbs. Hip and knee likely to be affected. Sprained stiff feeling in left thumb. Soles of feet tender, as if 'treading on balls'.

Skin

Eruptions, either pustular or urticarial. Vesicular eruptions with violent itching, worse at 5 or 7 p.m. and at night. Moist, offensive eczema of face with intense itching at night. Foul-smelling ulcers are liable to become gangrenous.

MODALITIES

Worse from cold; out of doors; from washing in cold water; when at rest, especially when lying down; from touch; from coitus; during the menstrual period; between 6 p.m. and 6 a.m.

Better from warmth; taking warm food; when moving about; from pressure.

CLINICAL NOTES

Pruritus, putridity and dark haemorrhages suggest consideration of the remedy.

Lac Caninum

SOURCE

This remedy is prepared from bitch's milk. The dog and the serpent were formerly associated in the sphere of healing, and the milk of the bitch was used medicinally in ancient times, mostly in connection with uterine troubles. It was also credited with the power to counteract poison.

PHARMACOLOGY

From available provings it would appear that the potentized substance has an affinity with the tissues of the pharynx, leading to severe types of inflammation with exudation. There is also an affinity with the nervous system, resulting on the one hand in neuralgic type pains and on the other in aberrations of thought and sensation.

PROVING

This remedy was revived by Reisig of New York, and the present drug picture was developed by Swan. Provings were conducted with the 30th potency and higher, and appear in Swan's *Materia Medica of the Nosodes and Morbific Products*, 1888, arranged by Berridge.

APPEARANCE

There are no very characteristic physical features related to the remedy. It may be considered when faced with a child who cries and screams all the time, or with an adult subject to bouts of rage and a penchant for cursing and swearing.

PSYCHOLOGY

It is in the mental and emotional sphere that the remedy presents several well-marked features. Moreover, these disturbances of the psyche tend to be severe, prolonged and distressing.

The sufferer is typically hopeless, despondent, says 'there is nothing to live for', but nevertheless carries on with the chores. There is aversion from solitude and a plethora of fears and weird imaginings – fear of snakes, fear of falling downstairs, fear of disease, fear of death with anxious distraught mien.

or other eye. The headache is aggravated by looking upward, by the use of the eyes for reading or close work, by noise or a lot of talk. Headache above the eyes brought on by the impact of cold air is relieved in a warm room. Dandruff may be excessive, and extremely sensitive sores may occur on the scalp.

Eyes

The eyes are very sensitive to cold air. Upper lids may seem heavy – can hardly keep the eyes open. Vision may be obscured as if a film were before the eyes, or, when reading, the page appears to be covered with pale spots of red, yellow, green and other colours. A pricking sensation may be felt in the eyeballs. The remedy may be called for in such conditions as acute conjunctivitis, corneal ulcer or stye on lids.

Ears

Severe pain in the right ear tends to be worse at night. The voice seems to reverberate in the ear or sounds seem far away.

Respiratory System

Coryza may present a blocked nostril on one side associated with fluent discharge from the other nostril. Chronic rhinitis may occur with profuse discharge at night, staining the pillow greenish yellow. The condition may progress to a frank ozaena. Severe inflammatory lesions of the throat are associated with extreme sensitivity of both the internal and external throat. The throat feels as if it were closing up and the mouth is held open 'lest he choke'. The whole throat feels tight or stiff. Swallowing may be almost impossible despite a great desire to do so. The throat feels dry, as if scalded. As with Hepar Sulph., Kali Bich. and Phytolacca, the pain tends to extend from the throat into the ear. Unlike the pain of Lachesis, which is relieved by taking solids, the reverse is the case in this remedy. It is worse, too, on empty swallow, but better by taking either cold or warm drinks. As with Ignatia, there is often a sensation of a 'lump stuck in the throat', relieved somewhat by swallowing, but only temporarily. The appearance of the throat is shiny, almost glazed, very red, or showing white silvery shiny patches of exudate, like china. The remedy has proved its value in diptheria, and also in relation to diphtheritic paralysis of the soft palate with regurgitation of fluids through the nose. The throat symptoms appear first on one side, probably the right, clear up on that side, then appear on the opposite side; may indeed alternate in this way back and forth from side to side. A sore throat may be a concomitant of menstruation.

Alimentary System

Cracks occur at the corners of the mouth, as well as ulcers inside the mouth with a putrid taste. The teeth are very sensitive to cold water. The tongue may be coated white; white or glazed patches may be seen on the buccal mucosa. Nausea with headache may be present on waking and continue all morning. A variety of pains and discomforts may occur in the belly, notably acute pain in the left groin, which is relieved by the passage of a stool. Frequent urge to stool associated with tenesmus on passing stool, which though soft tends to adhere to the anal verge. Constipation may occur before and after menstruation, and quite loose stools during the period.

Lymphatic and Glandular Systems

Engorgement of breasts is associated with a lumpy condition of the organ and great sensitivity to least jar or jolt, so that the breasts must be supported with the hands when going up or down stairs. The breasts tend to become painful at the menstrual period. Acute mastitis in nursing mothers and irregularities in lactation are indications for the remedy. It may also be indicated in connection with throat infections.

Urinary System

Frequency of urination may be complicated by the fact that delay in emptying the bladder when full may give rise to severe pain. Even after emptying the organ the sensation of a full bladder may persist; and likewise the desire to pass water. Polyuria and nocturia may both occur.

Genital System

A variety of ovarian and uterine pains are described, with a tendency to spread across the lower abdomen or down into the thigh. Vulval itching or hypersensitivity may cause distress. Uterine haemorrhage may occur, the blood being bright in colour, stringy and tending to flow in gushes. Dysmenorrhoea may be of a membranous type, associated with pain in the left groin or a bursting sensation in the pelvis. A curious symptom is the escape of gas per vaginam.

Locomotor System

Intense unbearable aching in the spine extends from the base of the skull to the coccyx, and the whole spine is very sensitive to touch and pressure. The pain is worse when at rest or when stooping forwards, but is relieved by leaning backwards. Pain is felt in the limbs, especially in the wrists and knees. It is sharp in nature, or as if bruised, and accompanied by stiffness and lameness. The pain is apt to shift from side to side, or fly from joint to joint. Cold gives relief.

Skin

Ulcers have a red, dry, glazed look. Hyperaesthesia is widespread. Formication may be present in neck and shoulder regions. Herpetic eruptions have been observed in the axilla, especially on the right side.

MODALITIES

There is marked aggravation from cold air; symptoms also tend to be worse at night, after sleep, from movement, from extension and from touch. An aggravation may occur on alternate days, or in the morning one day and in the evening on the following day.

Relief is experienced from warmth, when at rest, when lying down, by flexion, and in the open air.

CLINICAL NOTES

The remedy has been used with success in diphtheria, both curatively and as a prophylactic. It may also be indicated when there is a past history of diphtheria or severe throat infection. It is of proven value in drying up lactation, where this is desirable.

It is described as a deep and long-acting remedy. A single dose often suffices.

Lachesis

SOURCE

This remedy is prepared from the venom of *Lachesis muta*, the dreaded surucuccu snake of South America. The deadly brute, locally known as the bushmaster, may measure up to twelve feet in length. Its body is patterned with orange and black lozenges and may be as thick as a man's thigh. Its rainbow-coloured head is armed with fangs an inch to two inches long; these hollow teeth, like hypodermic needles, are attached at the front of the upper jaw in a hinge-like manner and fold back along the roof of the mouth when not in use. If a fang is injured it is shed and a new one grows in its place.

This reptile is the largest of the pit vipers, a family which includes the rattlesnake and the copperhead. It lives in humid forests, especially near rivers. Its young hatch from eggs, whereas all the other New World pit vipers bring forth their young fully formed. Its bite is particularly deadly, causing quick death from massive thrombosis if a vein is pierced, or death in a matter of hours from vasomotor paralysis. More delayed death may result from secondary haemorrhage, from haemoptysis or from sepsis. Anti-serum is seldom effective against its virulent poison.

Strong poison makes good medicine, when suitably potentized and appropriately prescribed. *Lachesis* venom is no exception, being a remedy of very wide usefulness.

Interestingly, there are a number of correspondences between the character and behaviour of snakes in general, and this one in particular, and the characteristics of the Lachesis 'subject'.

Unlike the general run of snakes the bushmaster is an aggressive brute, and will attack even human beings without provocation. 'Lurking in the grass, it waits patiently for someone to approach, then darts like lighting at its prey.'

The Lachesis subject has been described as 'given to fault-finding and reproach; also to cavilling and quarrelling'.

The expression of the reptile, with its thin unsmiling lips and glazed unwinking eye, is anything but attractive. Indeed, with its evil-looking forked tongue constantly flickering in and out the impression given is one of repulsion and even threat. The thin taut lips conceal the venom sacs;

the eyelids, being fused together, form a translucent covering for the cornea; and the whole flattened head conveys an air of balefulness that is not belied by the beast's behaviour. It is essentially concerned with its own appetites and ruthless in the pursuit of its prey.

The Lachesis mentality is egocentric in a marked degree, unable to laugh with those who laugh or weep with those who weep. The Lachesis subject may shed tears, but they will be of self-pity and not of sympathy with others.

The excessively active tongue is a marked feature of the snake, although this organ is not used for speech but as 'an efficient odour-detecting device'. Unable to hear their fleeing victim they 'rely on their darting tongue to literally taste their way along the fresh trail until they overtake the dying animal'.

The Lachesis subject also possesses an extremely active tongue, pouring forth a flow of words in veritable spate, and darting from subject to subject with bewildering rapidity. Our particular snake is not as silent as most of its kind, and is described by one writer as 'waiting for whatever may come along, singing cucucucucucu to itself.' This, for a snake, is quite unusual loquacity.

Complaints of a sensation of tightness or constriction are common with the Lachesis subject, especially in the region of the throat. Moreover the Lachesis fear has been described as 'a stupefied, venostatic, congested fear – a restrained fear such as is depicted in the facial expression of Laocoon and his sons in the deadly coils of the constricting serpents'. In other words, fear is felt as strangulation – the icy clutch of fear.

The snake is limbless, arms and legs being replaced by endless pairs of ribs, up to four hundred in some reptiles. It swallows its victims whole, and to this end has discarded any constriction at neck or waist, the better to facilitate the inward or downward progress of the meal. This is accomplished by a steady left-right, left-right movement of the ribs, leading off with a forward movement of the left mandible.

Notably the Lachesis subject strongly resents anything tight round neck or waist and is frequently aware of a fullness in the throat, accompanied by a constant desire to swallow. Moreover, there is relief from swallowing solids when the throat is sore, but not from swallowing liquids.

Curiously enough there is a left-sided laterality about the symptoms of the Lachesis subject and a tendency for symptoms to spread from left to right.

The movement of the snake is fascinating. It does not hop, skip or jump, but just flows through the undergrowth – 'that rivulet of pure silver' – streaming sinuously with amazing speed.

Relief from 'flow' is characteristic of Lachesis. The inward anxiety and pent-up emotion finds expression in the spate-like flow of speech. Whereas rest, inaction, warmth and sleep all diminish circulatory flow and aggravate the sufferings of the Lachesis patient in consequence, activity, cool fresh air and taking food all improve the flow of blood and afford a measure of relief. Active flow of discharges will have the same effect.

One last feature. The snake has no proper ear but is highly equipped with the sense of touch and acutely aware of any vibration. In the Lachesis subject all the senses are intensified and there is a special sensitivity to noise, the equivalent in the human to the sensitivity to vibration in the snake.

These parallels and correspondences are sufficiently numerous and striking to deserve mention, as well as being an aid to the understanding and memorizing of the materia medica picture of the remedy.

PHARMACOLOGY

The venom of *Lachesis muta* contains a full range of potent enzymes, proteolytic, cytolytic, neurotoxic and coagulant. One or more of these effects may predominate. The blood is attacked primarily, while the nervous system is at first aroused and excited.

The main affinities therefore are with the blood, causing disintegration of red cells, lowered coagulability after initial tendency to thrombosis, and impaired resistance to infection with associated liability to gangrene and necrosis. Also with the central nervous system, with ensuing delirium, coma and paralysis of vital centres. Also with the cardio-vascular system as evidenced by hypotension, cold sweats and collapse.

In the actual region of the bite the effects are extreme swelling of the part, purple or black discoloration, formation of blood blisters and terrible pain.

PROVING

Lachesis was first inadvertently proved by Constantine Hering in 1837, whilst he was attempting to extract the venom from a snake in the course of his zoological work in the upper Amazon. A graphic description of this event, taken from Hering's own account, appears in Clarke's *Dictionary of Materia Medica*, p.211. Subsequent provings were made with the 30c potency.

Lachesis

APPEARANCE

The Lachesis patient is usually either a dark, spare over-active person or a redhead with freckles.

The complexion tends to be pale, the nose bulbous and dull red, but lacking the varicosities associated with Carbo Veg. and Thuja. But the face, or indeed any affected part, may acquire a purplish and bloated or red, congested, swollen appearance and be hot to the touch.

The expression is apt to be anxious, suspicious, even furtive, and the eyes wide as if with fear.

Speech, as already mentioned, is either a torrential logorrhoeic spate, or may be slow and hesitant from obvious difficulty in pursuing a connected train of thought.

Other physical signs that may be present are a shiny tongue with a 'varnished' look, spontaneous bruising, purplish discoloration and foul-smelling discharges.

A tremulous type of delirium may be observed, accompanied by constrictive spasms and much clutching at the throat.

PSYCHOLOGY

The emotional features of the Lachesis subject are characteristic. It is suggested that they derive from 'a state of anxiety', restlessness and hypersensitivity due to the threat of an eruption of repressed emotionality and sexuality'.

Typically an unstable, unattractive, egocentric individual, full of schemes and projects, but seldom seeing anything through to completion.

Liable to be self-conscious, selfish, conceited, jealous, even suspicious without cause. There is often an urge to confess to crimes never committed, presumably from a desire for notice or notoriety resulting from self-importance.

Unbearable anguish and anxiety may assail, especially on first waking from sleep. Although wide awake and alert in the evening, during the night becomes melancholy and depressed, and is even more so after the night's sleep.

There are tendencies to apprehensive irritability, alternation of gloom and fury, taciturnity and confusion of time sense.

Great sensitivity to all stimuli, but especially to touch and noise. Whilst quite slight pressure is resented, quite firm pressure may be tolerated. Noise is intolerable, even noise at a distance. May in fact 'hear noises' or become paranoic, or show manic-depressive tendencies.

A peculiar fear is 'of someone lurking behind' (the snake lurking in the grass), which results in an unwillingness to turn the back towards anyone or to sit in the forward seats on a bus.

An odd sensation may be as if 'the bed was swaying from side to side', reminiscent of the undulatory movement of the serpent either on the ground or when preparing to strike.

Other features recorded include: 'sees the blackest side of everything', 'puts the worst possible interpretation on the most innocent facts', 'apt to lay plans to hurt people and hatch evil plots', 'in a constant hurry and flap; must do everything quickly', 'no sense of duty, insensitiveness of conscience'.

This is a somewhat staggering list, but obviously in the Lachesis subject there is a great tendency to emotional instability and over-sensitivity, which may reveal itself in various ways.

PHYSIOLOGY

The circulation is extremely labile, probably due to hypersensitivity of vasomotor control, and is subject to easy fluctuations with the combination of cold extremities and a hot head, or a sensation of waves of heat coursing through the body (the weaving and waving undulations of the serpent in motion).

In the realms of appetite there is often a desire for wine or for milk, both of which may disagree. There may be a strong dislike of bread, which can scarcely be swallowed. The appetite is frequently capricious and there is a tendency to wolf the meal with resultant bloating and belching.

Thirst may be insatiable and there is intolerance for hot fluids.

Sweats may be profuse and afford relief in fevers.

Sleep is noteworthy, being liable to disturbance by suffocative attacks and horrific dreams. The night is dreaded because of the suffering it brings. Sleep is feared, because of waking feeling worse than before going to sleep and generally confused and disorientated.

SYMPTOMATOLOGY

General

Many of the Lachesis symptoms are psychosomatic in origin. Complaints are often left-sided or, having started on the left side, tend to spread to the right side. The left is, of course, the shield side, denoting the awareness of danger and the need for protection, in this case from the threat of emotional upsurge from the unconscious into disruptive psychosomatic disturbance. In the abdomen many symptoms are on the right side, especially in the right lower quadrant, but it must be remembered in this connection that the gut in the embryo is a left-sided organ and only swings over to the right on its mesenteric pedicle at a later stage. Pains tend to be hammering, throbbing or bursting in type, due to circulatory disorder, irrespective of site. The pain is often associated with excessive exhaustion, as is also the case with Arsenicum Alb. and Phosphorus, presumably the result of a sudden severe hypoxia of the tissues. Easy bleeding is common, or periodic haemorrhage; the blood tends to be dark and non-coagulating with little black flecks floating about in it. Serious disturbances on the metabolic plane lead to irregularities of blood and tissue fluid distribution, and this in turn gives rise to independent vegetative activity of bacterial life. Hence the tendency to inflammations, congestive states, septic processes, blood decomposition, haemorrhages and purpura.

Head Region
Vertigo is apt to occur in the daytime and is aggravated by closing the eyes and when walking. It is relieved by lying down. A throbbing headache above the left eye may extend to the root of the nose; it is worse after sleep and during the morning and is relieved by warmth, by lying down and by free nasal discharges or after a nosebleed. A neuralgic type of headache occurs in the occipital region as the result of exposure to cold or to draughts; it is accompanied by great soreness to touch, even the pressure of the pillow being resented; the scalp also is so tender that the sufferer is unable to use a comb. A rush of blood to the head may give distress, especially at the menopause. Head pains, moreover, are liable to shoot downwards to the eyes, or from the zygoma to the ear, or down the nape to the shoulders. A headache is also described resulting from exposure to direct sun, associated with pallor and relieved in the open air.

Eyes
Intense photophobia is accompanied by pain, itching, stinging and sensitivity to touch. In spite of this there is a desire to rub the eyes. Clarity of vision may be affected by weakness of the ocular muscles, especially after diphtheria. Haemorrhages may occur, either subconjunctival or intraocular. The eyes may feel 'pulled backwards'. There may be a marked awareness of muscae volitantes before the eyes.

Ears

A great variety of ear noises may be complained of, especially on the left side. Also the ears feel stuffed up, a sensation of 'fullness'. Pain in the ear is often a concomitant of sore throat.

Respiratory System

Nocturnal rhinorrhoea may be troublesome, associated with much sneezing and at times a sensation of nasal blockage, especially in the morning. There is a tendency to epistaxis, which affords relief to symptoms. Throat symptoms are specially prominent. Morning hoarseness may be very persistent. Pain in the throat occurs without associated inflammation. There is a constant tickle in the throat, or a feeling as if a fishbone were lodged there. Quite common is a distressing sensation of choking, as if caused by a lump which cannot be swallowed or by a definite constriction. This is aggravated by attempting a dry swallow, or by drinking hot fluids, also by exertion, especially that of using the arms above shoulder level. Curiously the sensation is eased when swallowing solids (reminiscent of the snake which swallows its meal whole).

Another characteristic is an unusual sensitiveness of the throat, even on the surface, so that a tight collar is unbearable. Ulceration may occur in the fauces with dark purplish or greyish discoloration. The ulcer tends to be deep, spreading and haemorrhagic. The lesion tends to start on the left side and later spread to the right. Associated with the sense of constriction in throat or in the chest is a frequent desire to take a deep breath, and breathing may almost seem to be arrested on falling asleep. A sharp pain may be felt in the left chest, associated with the sensation of constriction. Asthmatic attacks may occur, relieved by the expectoration of watery sputum.

Alimentary System

The tongue is apt to be tremulous and may be deflected to the left on protrusion. There is much tenacious saliva. There may be a feeling as if 'the mucous membranes of the roof of the mouth were peeled off'. The tongue is dry and red, at times with a brown streak down the centre. Bloating is common, necessitating loosening the clothes round the waist. Intestinal pain is relieved by the passage of a stool. There may be much ineffectual urging to stool, associated with throbbing pain or a sensation of pressure, or of a plug, in the rectum. Piles tend to bleed or become strangulated and are aggravated by straining at stool. Spasm of the anal sphincter adds to the difficulty of defaecation. Stools are apt to be extremely offensive. The remedy is also associated with enlargement of the liver, which is soft, and stabbing pains may be felt in the organ.

Special mention should be made of the remedy in connection with septic conditions in the abdomen. The picture here is as follows: There is a dry brown tongue, thick difficult speech, and the tongue is tremulous and protruded with difficulty. Thirst is acute. The belly is extremely distended and drum-like and excessively tender, the least touch being resented, even the pressure of the bed-covers or of a forearm laid across the abdomen. There is a horrible sensation as if the contents of the abdomen were being twisted into a ball and something would give way and burst. With an appendix abscess or other right-sided abscess, pain tends to start in the caecal region and extend to the thigh and sacrum on the right side. With gallbladder infections the pain spreads across into the region of the stomach. The face appears dusky, the body feels hot but the extremities are cold. There is a sensation of suffocation and a craving for air. Pus, if present, is very foul; wounds tend to slough and ooze and show little, if any, sign of healing.

Cardiovascular System

Hypotension is common, accompanied by attacks of dizziness associated with pallor. Syncopal episodes are associated with cardiac pain, or accompanied by nausea and vertigo. Hard thumping palpitations are associated with the sense of tightness in the chest; these are aggravated by lying on the left side and may interfere with sleep. Hot flushes alternate with chills down the spine and are associated with surges of heat to face and head. Spasmodic feelings of oppression in the precordium are associated with a weak, rapid, possibly irregular pulse. Odd sensations are described, as if 'the heart was suspended by a thread and every fresh beat would tear it away', or as if 'the heart was several sizes too large'. States of venous stasis lead to hypoxia of tissues, thrombosis, embolism or thrombophlebitis. Blood dyscrasias such as leukaemia and agranulocytosis are also related to the remedy.

Urinary System

Frequency of urination occurs in the daytime with great variation in the amount passed. Violent pain may occur in the urethra. There may be a sensation of 'a ball rolling round inside the bladder'. Nephritis may occur with dark, albuminous urine.

Genital System

This is an important sphere for the remedy, especially in connection with menopausal disturbances such as hot flushes, floodings, melancholy and listlessness. Uterine cramps and profuse sweats may occur. A thin pale leucorrhoea may be present. Left-sided ovarian pain may be complained of. Pelvic pain occurs before the onset of menstruation, but is relieved when the flow starts.

Nervous System

Muscle spasms may be triggered off by quite light touch. Again, tremors and weaknesses may produce a picture of pseudo-paresis. The remedy may be called for in relation to petit mal or grand mal, especially when the seizures occur in sleep. It may be of value in left-sided sciatica.

Locomotor System

Pains in the neck muscles force the sufferer to hold the head erect. Low back pain is accompanied by a feeling as if the back was 'dislocated', and the pain is associated with great weakness, fatigue and trembling. Severe pain in the region of the coccyx is made worse on rising from the sitting posture.

Skin

Erythematous eruptions tend to become dark bluish in colour. Ulcers are extremely sensitive with foul discharge and bluish discoloration of the surrounding skin. There is a tendency to gangrenous necrosis and pain may be severe. Warmth gives some relief. Wounds are very sensitive, bleed profusely and persistently, the blood being dark and non-coagulating. Haemolytic icterus may be present.

MODALITIES

There is susceptibility to either extreme of temperature, but especially to heat. The subject feels oppressed in a hot room and must have air; may even faint in a hot bath.

Aggravation is caused by hot sun, hot winds, going from a cold to a warmer climate, from change to warmer weather in the spring, in cloudy weather, before a thunderstorm, from getting wet and if exposed to draughts. One is reminded of the snake which seeks to retire to a nice, cool, dark, dry hold and avoid the winter.

Other aggravating factors are touch, constriction, lying on the left side, the onset of night, and waking from sleep. This harks back to the horror of the struggle to escape from the old skin as the new-born snake comes awake after its long night of hibernation. There is an aggravation before the menstrual period with relief when the flow starts. Puberty and the menopause are also times of aggravation.

Incidentally, emotional stress may precipitate an aggravation in association with circulatory disturbance, as evidenced by icy cold extremities, feeble pulse, rush of blood to the head, profuse sweats and air hunger.

Factors which tend to afford relief are open air, cold drinks, free discharges, eating (but not to repletion) and active movement.

CLINICAL NOTES

The remedy is of special value in relation to throat affections and menopausal disorders. It has been used for the effects of alcoholism. The presence of the typical characteristics will point to its use in a great variety of indispositions.

The remedy is followed well by Iodum, Kali Bich., Lycopodium and Nitric Acid. An aggravation can be countered by Belladonna.

Latrodectus Mactans

SOURCE

The source of this remedy is the black widow spider, so called because the female of the species is in the habit of eating the much smaller male soon after fertilization has taken place. It fetters its prey, which may be many times its own size and weight, in a very strong mantle of silk strands, then approaches and injects its venom through the chelicerae or fangs, a pair of claws in the region of the mouth. In a few minutes the struggles of the victim cease.

The full-grown female has a rather obese black body about half an inch long, and eight one-inch sprangling legs. The red or orange hour-glass marking on the ventral aspect of the black belly is peculiar to the species.

Because of the spider's unobtrusive habits and its preference for dim and remote haunts it escapes much public notice, though it may sometimes turn up in a bunch of imported bananas. It is very common in the southern half of the USA.

The venom, drop for drop, is probably the most virulent poison secreted by any living organism. It is fifteen times as potent as the venom of the prairie rattler; the only reason the black widow has fewer victims to her credit is that she has at her disposal only 1/200th of the amount of poison carried by her rival. However, if the testimony of her human victims is to be trusted, her bite can produce an all-time high in pain.

PHARMACOLOGY

The effects of the venom suggest a mainly neurotropic action. These are best exemplified by records of symptoms described by those who have been bitten.

One John Bradbury, a husky 21-year-old student at the University of Georgia, on turning over in bed one morning felt a sharp prick in the small of his back. Sleepily he groped for what he supposed was a pin, but found nothing and stretched out for a final snooze. 'Just then she let me have it again', explained the victim, 'that waked me up all right.'

He jumped out of bed, threw back the covers and saw the spider. Recognising his assailant he lost no time in getting to the local hospital.

Latrodectus Mactans

About half an hour after the bite he recalled: 'I started to hurt, and I mean hurt. Pains shot all over me. It was in the stomach that they hurt most. I couldn't breath; I couldn't talk; I couldn't relax.' For two days the victim had a bad time of it, and for a month or more a muscle would suddenly without warning tighten up and quiver like a bowl of jelly for two or three minutes. Nothing he could do would stop it.

Dr A. W. Blair, a member of the faculty of the University of Alabama, volunteered to act as a guinea pig and was bitten three times on the hand by a large and healthy specimen of the spider.

In fifteen minutes things began to feel unpleasant locally. In an hour, pains of a nature and violence quite outside Dr Blair's previous experience shot across his neck, chest and stomach. His breathing became laboured and gasping, his heart action slow and weak. He could speak only with difficulty; his abdomen was as hard as a board. He turned ashy grey. A cold sweat broke out on his body. He could not straighten up. For three days he was a very sick man.

The main features of this case were severe spasms and rigidity of muscles, giving rise to a sensation of constriction – 'the spider fetters its prey'. Later great restlessness supervened; he was sleepless, perspiring freely; complained of muscular pains and feeling chilly; and became so upset mentally that he was afraid, if firm control was not exercised, he would go insane. Finally, generalized pruritus and desquamation of the hands and feet were noted.

Research at Rockefeller University, New York, has shed light on the way the black widow spider paralyses its victim (1970). There is interference to the passage of the nerve impulse at the neuromuscular junction where normal response depends on the release of acetylcholine. In experiments with frogs, physiologists at R.U. have shown that the effect of the spider venom is to trigger all the packets of acetylcholine in the nerve ending into releasing their contents prematurely. This means that until a fresh supply of acetylcholine can be synthesized, transmission of the nerve impulse is in abeyance. The disappearance of the acetylcholine packets from the nerve ending has been observed under the electron microscope. This is, of course, only a partial explanation of the biochemical effects of the venom.

PROVING

Latrodectus Mactans was introduced into the materia medica by Jones and Tafel in 1889 in the *Homoeopathic Recorder*.

303

Latrodectus Mactans

APPEARANCE

The sufferer may appear shocked, with an expression of grave anxiety. A characteristic gait is described, namely bent forward with the hands held against the abdomen, and movement of the legs is achieved slowly and with difficulty. Speech may be difficult.

PSYCHOLOGY

There is extreme anxiety, possibly amounting to fear of imminent death – the not unnatural result of difficulty in breathing. Unrestrained and causeless crying may occur.

PHYSIOLOGY

Chilliness is a prominent feature. Extremities may be icy cold.

Appetite is ravenous or absent. There is great thirst for cold water; must be constantly drinking.

Extreme restlessness interferes with sleep.

Perspiration is profuse.

SYMPTOMATOLOGY

General
Pains are cramping, constricting and very severe. There is accompanying prostration, but the sufferer is so restless he cannot stay still. The pains and spasms come and go in waves. Muscles are sore to the touch.

Respiratory System
Dyspnoea is a prominent symptom, almost to the degree of apnoea. This is, of course, the result of muscle spasm. Respiration is laboured with an uncontrollable expiratory grunt.

Alimentary System
The board-like condition of the abdominal wall may suggest an emergency laparotomy. Distension is drum-like and is only slightly relieved by the passage of flatus. Nausea and vomiting of brownish matter may be present. Rectal atony is marked. Stools when passed may be black.

Cardiovascular System

The remedy is often indicated in relation to severe angina. Violent precordial pain extends to the left axilla and down the left arm and forearm to the tips of the fingers. There is accompanying numbness and near paralysis of the affected limb. The pulse is rapid, up to 130 per minute, weak and may be almost impalpable.

Urinary System

Retention of urine may occur from paralysis of the bladder; the condition is relieved by warm applications and by sitting in a hot bath.

Genital System

Menstruation tends to be suppressed, scanty, delayed.

Locomotor System

Spastic paresis occurs with increased reflexes; there is difficulty in raising the lower limbs because of spasm of the hip extensor muscles. There is tenderness of the calf muscles and paraesthesias in hands and feet. The ankles may be swollen. Shooting cramping pains occur in the lumbar region with a feeling as if the back was broken.

Skin

There is a general hypersensitivity of the skin. The soles of the feet may burn as if on fire.

MODALITIES

Attempts at exercise aggravate the situation. Other aggravating factors are damp weather; weather changes; before a thunderstorm; night time; taking alcohol.

Some relief may be obtained by a hot bath.

CLINICAL NOTES

Although the main indication for the use of the remedy is the anginal picture, it may be called for in other conditions presenting symptoms as above.

Ledum Palustre

SOURCE

Ledum palustre is a small shrub resembling the tea plant. It is also known as wild rosemary, Labrador tea or marsh tea. Historically the plant was formerly used quite extensively in parts of northern Europe, as a popular remedy against whooping cough and bilious attacks, certain skin diseases, diarrhoea and dysentery. The Swedes used a decoction of the plant to wash their oxen and swine to kill lice. In Lapland, branches were placed among the grain to keep away mice. An infusion of the leaves was formerly used by hunters in Canada as a substitute for tea.

The plant is a member of the Ericaceae, a very ancient family; fossil forms have been found in layers of the preglacial period. The plant favours cold northern climates and is found growing in marshy places and peat bogs.

The plant grows to a height of one to three feet. Its stems are shrubby, much branched and slender; they are soft in the upper portions, where they are covered by a down of rust-coloured hairs. Lower down, the stems are woody and hard.

The leaves are alternate with very short petioles and either spreading horizontally or reflexed downwards close to the stem. They are narrow, lanceolate with entire margins; on the upper aspect they are dark green; underneath they are covered with soft downy hairs, which with the rolled-in margins serve to conserve warmth. The plant is thought to derive its name from the Greek *ledos*, a woollen garment.

The flowers are numerous, in dense, terminal corymbs; the blossoms are small, white in colour and on quite long stalks; the calyx is insignificant; the five petals are spreading, ovate, concave; the seeds are plentiful, flat, strap-like and rough to the touch.

The whole plant, especially when bruised, has a strong, oppressive, aromatic odour, somewhat like hops. The taste is bitter. The mother tincture is prepared from the whole freshly-gathered plant or from the dried twigs.

Ledum Palustre

PHARMACOLOGY

The flowers contain an antiseptic camphor-like oil, ledol, which is responsible for the distinctive odour.

The plant as a whole shows an affinity with muscles, fasciae, connective tissue and the vasomotor system, tending to induce capillary stasis, inflammation, coldness of surface and inadequate nutrition of skin.

PROVING

Ledum was proved by Hahnemann, who published the results in *Materia Medica Pura*, Vol.IV.

APPEARANCE

The subject is usually of full-blooded plethoric build, portly, robust and red of visage, possibly with large pupils.

A hot head is associated with coldness of body, or there is a purple tint with throbbing pulsation all over.

Affected parts appear bloated, mottled, swollen, and are markedly cold. Purpuric spots or petechiae may be evident.

Violent shivering or shuddering may be present.

PSYCHOLOGY

Subject is apt to be cross, morose, discontented with everybody, 'everything is disagreeable', a similar mental state to that of alcoholics beteween bouts. Sobs with a peculiar double inspiratory sighing.

PHYSIOLOGY

Coldness is a prominent feature, yet finds heat of the bed intolerable; wants cold for relief. Sometimes feet and hands are hot, especially in the evening.

Thirst may be violent, for cold water.

Nights are disturbed; is chilly and sweaty in bed, but throws off covers or actually gets out of bed in search of coolness. Much restless tossing at night; uneasy dreams; feels drowsy in daytime.

Ledum Palustre

SYMPTOMATOLOGY

General

Tendency to hard, tense swellings with tearing pains, or to dropsical swellings. Special predilection for involvement of left eye or right ear. Pains are described as tearing, pulling or stabbing, shift rapidly from site to site and spread from below upwards. Abscesses and septic conditions are accompanied by great tenderness. Ecchymoses may occur, or haemorrhages of dark, almost black, frothy blood. There may be a bruised, beaten sensation of the whole body.

Head

Vertigo is troublesome, and head tends to bend backwards. Definite aversion from having the head covered. Possibly a feeling as if intoxicated. Headaches various, mostly of pressive type, and accompanied by a desire to put the head outside the window to cool off.

Eyes

Eyes ache. Extravasation of blood in eyelids, beneath the conjunctiva or into the chambers of the eye. Cataract may occur in association with gout. Flickerings are seen before the eyes, or a halo appears to surround objects looked at. Pupils appear dilated. Sensation of 'sand in the eye' or a feeling as if the eyeball would be forced out of the orbit.

Respiratory System

Burning sensation in nose. Violent cough, resembling pertussis, associated with haemoptysis of bright red foamy blood. A mouldy taste in the mouth when coughing. Epistaxis may also be present. Haemoptysis may alternate with acute rheumatism or with pain in hip joint. Dyspnoea occurs, associated with a sensation of constriction in chest, worse when walking. Bronchitis and emphysema in the elderly. Tickling in larynx causes spasmodic cough.

Alimentary System

Sudden flow of saliva into the mouth associated with bad breath and a musty taste. Shooting pains may occur on swallowing. Thirst may be excessive or absent. Queasy nausea may be troublesome and accompanied by sweating when walking out of doors. Complains of cutting pains in abdomen or stitches in loins. Painful bleeding piles. Anal fissure.

Delusions or hallucinations abound – 'sees spiders or snakes'; imagines all sorts of horrid sights and fears he will see them in reality.

Curiously enough is not afraid in the dark; 'sees things' only in the light, and is apt to look under tables, bed, chairs.

Is extremely forgetful, absent-minded and irresolute, apt to make purchases and walk away without them. Mistakes are made in writing; concentration is difficult and there is a tendency to suddenly lose the train of thought – a symptom shared with Nux Moschata.

A peculiar sense of unreality may be present, or a delusion that 'she is a loathsome mass of disease' or 'infested with snakes'. Another odd symptom is undue sensitivity of the surface of the body, so that no contact can be tolerated between one part of the body and another, even the fingers are held widely apart.

As is the case with Lachesis, there may be complaint of a floating sensation, as if 'walking on air' or, when lying down, seems 'not to be in contact with the bed'. Moreover, as with Lachesis, there is hyper-sensitivity to touch and even the pressure of the bed-covers is resented.

There may be a distressing feeling as if 'the heart would stop beating and respiration would be arrested'.

PHYSIOLOGY

Appetite is unusually ravenous, canine hunger – as hungry after a meal as before it. There is distaste for sweet things and desire for pepper and for milk. There may also be intolerance of milk. Thirst is considerable.

Sleep is apt to be uneasy and restless, with inability to get comfortable in any position. May finally fall asleep in the prone posture; may dream of snakes or of urinating.

Sweats may be profuse and leave a brown stain on the linen.

SYMPTOMATOLOGY

General

Symptoms often alternate and show irregularity. Unlike the left-sided Lachesis, this tends to be a right-sided remedy, or the symptoms may shuttle from right to left and back again. This rather unusual charac-teristic is a strong indication for employing Lac Caninum. An extreme degree of restlessness is accompanied by undue prostration.

Head Region

Headache is severe, frontal, unilateral or alternating from side to side, or it may start in the occipital region and extend forwards to settle over one

Urinary System

Frequency of micturition associated with interrupted flow and burning in urethra after the act. Large amount of red sand in urine, especially when feeling unusually energetic. Copious, clear, colourless urine of low specific gravity associated with symptoms of gout.

Genital System

Menses are early, profuse with bright red blood associated with coldness all over the body, but nevertheless relief from cold air.

Locomotor System

Rheumatic symptoms start in the feet and then progress regularly from below upwards. Rheumatism affecting joints which are swollen and hot to touch, but not red. Pains are worse from heat of bed, also in evening and first half of night; better for coolness. Pains may involve opposite sides of body, e.g. left shoulder and right hip. Pains affect the periosteum of phalanges, worse by least pressure. Acute pain in great toe, relieved by cold. Joints are very stiff, can only be moved after bathing with cold water; desire to put feet in ice-cold water. Muscular rheumatism, especially of right shoulder, worse on movement. Low back pain and stiffness, especially after sitting for a while in one position. Chronic rheumatism of small joints with periarticular pain, affecting especially fingers, toes and jaw, possibly accompanied by painful hard nodules in feet and hands. Hands tremble on grasping objects. Knees tremble when sitting, also when attempting to walk. Soles of feet sensitive and painful as if bruised. Soreness of feet and heels, especially after exposure to damp, worse on walking; feet feel stiff and rigid in morning. Intolerable pain from sprain of foot or ankle.

Skin

Red pimples may be present on forehead and cheeks, which sting when touched. Crusty eruptions occur round nostrils and mouth. Papular, pustular or eczematous eruptions on covered parts, worse from warmth of bed and better in cool air. Bluish or violet-coloured swellings. Phagedenic ulcers. Whitlow or other septic conditions, especially if resulting from a prick or punctured wound, and pain is relieved by cold. Gnawing pruritus on dorsum of foot – must scratch till raw; worse at night from heat of bed. Indolent spreading ulcers, surrounded by mottled skin. Phlegmonous erysipelas of face or injured part. Prolonged discolouration after injuries, associated with numbness.

Ledum Palustre
MODALITIES

Aggravation results from heat of bed, by being overclad, by movement when walking, by taking alcohol and at night.

Relief is obtained from cool air, a cold bath, by bathing the feet in cold water, by cold applications, while at rest.

CLINICAL NOTES

Of frequent indication in respiratory and rheumatic troubles. To quote Hahnemann, the remedy 'is suitable for the most part only in chronic maladies in which there is a predominance of coldness and deficiency of animal heat.'

Kent claims that the remedy counteracts the effects of whisky and takes away the desire for it.

Is said to have a prophylactic value in relation to tetanus.

Can be given in erythromelalgia.

Helpful in wounds in succession to Arnica, especially where there is delay in the absorption of extravasated blood.

An important remedy in injuries caused by sharp pointed instruments and for stings and bites, especially when these are followed by great sensitivity to touch and relief from cold.

Complementary remedies are Sulphur and Tuberculinum.

Lilium Tigrinum

SOURCE

This colourful plant, the tiger lily, is found growing wild in hilly country in China and Japan. The deep orange blossoms are spotted (not striped!) with blotches of inky black. The mother tincture is prepared from the stalk, leaves and flowers of the fresh plant.

PHARMACOLOGY

There is affinity with the pelvic organs, tending to relaxation of ligaments and uterine displacements; also with the nervous system, producing a variety of mental and emotional disturbances.

PROVING

Lilium Tigrinum was proved by Dr E.W. Payne, of Maine, USA, and published in the *Transactions of the American Institute of Homoeopathy*, 1867.

APPEARANCE

The patient appears listless and inert, yet cannot sit still. There may be a wild look in the eyes. The subject is often portly and plethoric.

PSYCHOLOGY

A variety of complaints are met with in this sphere.

Inability to think; cannot read a book; has an indescribable crazy feeling. Feels hurried for no known reason; must keep walking and walking, faster and faster; has a feverish desire to undertake tasks but is unable to carry them to completion.

Is averse from solitude; hypercritical; snappy and disposed to curse, strike, think obscene thoughts; sexual excitement may be extreme.

Depression is profound, but sympathy or interference is resented; is apt to 'weep like a tap'.

Fears obtrude; fear of entering into a conversation lest makes stupid mistakes in speech; fear of incurable disease; fear of being alone; fear of becoming insane.

PHYSIOLOGY

There is aversion to heat and preference for a cold room and cool weather.

Appetite may be ravenous, perhaps with a craving for meat. There may however be aversion to bread, coffee and also to cigar smoking. Thirst may be excessive, with a desire to frequent drinks of large quantities.

Sleep may be disturbed by ebullitions of heat; palms and soles burn at night. Is often sleepless the first part of the night.

Sweats are cold, with severe symptoms.

SYMPTOMATOLOGY

General

All symptoms are acute and intense. Pains are variously described as wandering, flying about, shooting, alternatively constricting and relaxing, or opening and shutting. Pain may be felt in small spots. Mental symptoms may alternate with physical distress. Symptoms tends to be left-sided.

Head

Headache with a sensation of fullness and outward pressure is apt to develop in a hot or crowded room or hall. It is relieved by walking in the open air.

Eyes

There may be a feeling of heat in the eyes with a desire to press the eyelids together. Photophobia and lachrymation may be marked. Vision is dim. Twitching may occur in eyelids.

Respiratory System

The throat may be sore and dry. There may be loss of control over the voice. There is a tendency to frequent sighing and a desire to take a deep breath. This is associated with a sense of tightness or constriction in the chest, relieved by change of position. Sharp pains may penetrate the right lung; these are aggravated in the open air. Pains may be felt in or below the left breast, extending laterally and to the scapula; these are worse when lying down and by lying on the left side.

Alimentary System

Pain may shoot from the teeth into the left ear. Tongue may be coated yellowish-white in patches. Saliva is abundant. A peculiar bloody, foul taste may be noticed in the mouth, relieved by taking food. Hiccough and belching may be prominent. Nausea is made worse by tobacco smoke; it is accompanied by inability to vomit, by pain in the back and by fullness in the belly. A hollow, empty sensation may be felt in the abdomen, with a feeling as if the abdominal contents were being dragged downwards; this causes a desire to support the belly with the hands. There is much bloating with distension, rumbling and passage of flatus. This is made worse by the least intake of food. A sensation as if diarrhoea was imminent passes off after urinating. Clutching pains across the lower belly are relieved by gentle rubbing with a warm hand. There may be a constant urge to stool, associated with pressure in the rectum as by a heavy weight or ball. Morning diarrhoea is accompanied by griping pains and burning in rectum and anus. The stools are loose, dark, offensive and very urgent; patient is driven from bed. Stools may be frankly dysenteric. Prolapsed piles are common.

Cardiovascular System

This is an important sphere of action of the remedy, but the cardiac symptoms are usually associated with uterine conditions. Pain is felt in the heart region, as if the organ were forcibly clutched, the grip then being gradually relaxed; this is often worse at night, but lying on the left side affords some relief. The pain may be accompanied by pain and numbness in the right upper extremity. There is irregularity in the heart action and a tendency to faint in a warm room. Pulse rate is increased by the least exertion.

Urinary System

Tenesmus in the bladder both by day and at night causes a constant desire to urinate. Smarting is felt in the urethra both during and after the act.

Genital System

Menstruation is early, and the flow is only when moving about and in the daytime; it contains dark clots and is offensive in odour. Uterine displacement or actual prolapse occurs. This is accompanied by terrific downward and outward pressure or bearing-down sensation in the pelvis, involving also the bladder and rectum. It is worse when standing and moving about, and not relieved even when lying down; in an attempt to get relief the perineum has to be supported by the hand or by wearing a T-bandage. The downward dragging sensation may be described as starting from the shoulders or breasts, or from the epigastrium. There may be a yellow excoriating vaginal discharge which stains linen brown. Libido is increased. Vaginismus may be present. Pruritus vulvae may be intense. Ovarian pain on either side tends to extend to the medial aspect of the thigh. On the left side it may be associated with pain in the left breast.

Locomotor System
Soreness is felt in the nape, the shoulders and the spine. Sacral pain is noticed when standing. Contrary to the prevailing bearing-down, there may be a sensation as if the tip of the coccyx was pulled up. Tearing pains or cramps occur in the limbs, associated with tremulousness. Burning sensation may be present in the soles and palms; difficulty may be noticed in walking on uneven ground. The legs are apt to ache; has to keep moving them in search of ease.

Skin
Burning pruritus occurs on the upper chest and arms, or in other sites. Tingling and formication may also be described.

MODALITIES

Aggravating factors are heat, a warm room, a crowded place, church, theatre, lying on right side, rest, inaction. Is worse on rising in the morning and from 5 p.m. to 8 p.m. Consolation and kindly speech also aggravate the situation.

Is better if fully occupied, in cool air, when walking, when lying on the left side and from pressure.

CLINICAL NOTES

The uterine symptoms afford the chief indication for the use of the remedy, often in association with nervous or cardiac disturbances. Complementary remedies are Lachesis, Lycopodium, Sepia.

Lycopodium Clavatum

Many of the plants employed as remedies in homoeopathy may be described as strong poisons, menacing in their very appearance and nature, violent in their manner of growth and in their toxicity, but each of them in its individual characteristics separate and distinct.

Such, for instance, are *Aconitum*, *Belladonna* and *Nux vomica*. One can well imagine that these plants, with their obvious propensity for poisoning living cells and tissues, and thus creating disorder and disharmony within the body, may be transmuted into valued remedies, able to cure the symptoms they cause in accord with the homoeopathic principle – 'The Wounder Heals'.

It is, however, surprising that an apparently inert and innocuous little plant like the club moss can produce one of the most powerful therapeutic agents in the whole materia medica. Such nevertheless is the case.

SOURCE

Lycopodium clavatum, wolf's claws, is also known as club moss, lamb's tail, fox tail, names suggested by its appearance. The classification of the plant is somewhat indeterminate; it is said to lie between the mosses and the ferns. One of the characteristics of the Lycopodium subject is extreme diffidence – being in two minds, like the plant itself which cannot decided whether to be a fern or a moss.

The plant is described by C.P. Johnson, 1861, thus: 'This plant is found abundantly on heaths and mountain pastures, throwing out long straggling stems, thickly coated with hair-pointed leaves, and extending often to the length of many yards, rooting at intervals by means of long fibres. The fructification is in erect scaly spikes growing in pairs on the extremities of stalks.'

The prickly character of the plant and its persevering manner of growth are also suggestive of other Lycopodium features, namely a capacity for biting sarcasm and unkind speech and a proclivity for pig-headed, overconscientious application to a given task or pursuit.

From the creeping, prostrate branches arise aerial stems, often forked at the summit, with slender bristle-tipped bracts. These stems bear the fruit, sporophylls, which when mature contain spores which can be shaken out and sieved to provide a mobile powder of light yellow colour and devoid of odour and taste. It floats on water, and when boiled with it, sinks. It burns with a quick flash when thrown into a flame.

This seemingly inert powder, utilized as a dusting powder to prevent excoriation of the skin in babies, and in the process of pill-rolling, to prevent the pills from sticking to one another, nevertheless possesses this surprising capacity to explode when sufficiently heated. The Lycopodium subject, although to outward appearance a fairly mild and plodding type of person, can nevertheless 'blow up' under provocation, and frequently does.

The spores contain about 50 per cent of fixed oil, chiefly lycopodium-oleic acid, also sugar, phytosterin, traces of alumina, phosphoric acid and silica. Regarded as medicinally inert in the natural state, these spores become a powerful and deeply-acting remedy with a wide range of application when potentized.

PHARMACOLOGY

We are told, 'Lycopodium acts profoundly on the entire organism'. This seems a somewhat sweeping statement, but the tissue affinities of the potentized drug are certainly extensive. An effect on the endocrine glands notably the gonads, is evidenced by physical weakness, hypotonia and circulatory stasis, a combination which tends to the development of an inferiority complex in the psychological sphere.

Affinities with mucous membranes, respiratory, alimentary, and genito-urinary systems, and with the skin lead to degenerative changes, impaired function and progressive ill-health. Ultimate changes include necrosis, abscess formation, ulcerations and extreme emaciation. All this is presumably secondary to inadequacy in the circulation, with resulting oxygen deprivation in the tissues involved.

PROVING

Lycopodium was proved by Hahnemann, and the result published in the first edition of the *Chronic Diseases*.

APPEARANCE

This remedy is related to a very definite type of psychosomatic make-up. Quite a plethora of physical features are mentioned as being characteristic of Lycopodium subjects.

They tend to have a sallow complexion, often with flushed cheeks and a rather red nose; perhaps a yellowish spot in the temporal region and multiple pigmented plaques and moles, especially in the region of the upper chest and dorsum.

They appear lean, even emaciated, about the face, neck and chest, but are quite well-covered in the lower part of the body.

Freckles are common on the face. The brow tends to be wrinkled, with a marked vertical frown above the root of the nose.

Spasmodic contraction of the facial muscles can be observed in a steady alternating rhythm, and the face tends to twitch at every jar or bang. A notable feature is a curious quivering of the alae nasi, and these movements do not synchronize with respiration.

Poor muscular development is evidenced by such signs as toneless stance, head-nodding, side to side movements of head, clumsy awkward movements of limbs, even staggering gait. There is also a tendency to quite definite muscle tremor after extra exertion, or when upset emotionally.

Speech may be stammering, with delay in finding the right word, or it may become vehement and violent when heated in argument. There is a tendency to whistle softly when not talking, and to do so unconsciously.

The head hair is plentiful, but body hair is scanty and the belly smooth. Early greying of the hair may occur. A peculiar physical sign that may be present is marked coldness of one foot while the opposite member is warm or hot.

PSYCHOLOGY

In this sphere, too, the Lycopodium subject presents a wealth of characteristic features. Noticeably conscientious and orderly, he cannot bear to be corrected or found fault with or opposed, and becomes frantic if chivvied. He is a poor arguer.

He is intellectually active, must be occupied, finds relief in action, movement and active exercise, especially out of doors. He is extremely self-conscious, shuns crowds, parties, children en masse, but is also averse to complete solitude and likes to have someone around.

He is apprehensive before an ordeal, from diffidence and lack of self-confidence, but rises to the occasion when it arrives. Apt to worry about the future and may seem parsimonious as a result.

He is fearful of the dark, of ghosts, of failure, of strangers, shrinks from appearing in public, and hates being watched when at work. He is also averse to the effort of undertaking anything new.

Temper is a problem. The child flies into tantrums or goes berserk if

317

provoked or ticked off. Quick to take umbrage at any slight, insult or rebuff, the Lycopodium subject tends to dwell on injuries, real or imagined, to harbour resentment and exaggerate trifles. When sick he becomes domineering, imperious and impatient.

There is the ever-present liability to sudden explosions of wrath. The silent, sallow, rather sombre individual suddenly erupts into brilliant talk or blazing wrath, neither of which are sustained for long.

There is also a tendency to want to get on with the job and get it finished. In a hurry he pushes past other pedestrians, runs words together when speaking, drops letters out of words or gets them jumbled when writing or typing.

Black moods are common, and so is satiety of life, especially on waking in the morning. Moist eyes or a 'lump in the throat' are easily produced from sentimental emotion, as when thanked for a gift, at partings, reunions, confronted with sad or touching situations.

There is great sensitivity to music, to noise, especially loud or sudden noises, and to pain. A desire for open spaces is associated with an aversion to being shut in and confined or restricted. There is also intolerance of tight clothing, especially round the neck, and of being approached or touched.

A noticeable attribute is lack of aptitude for finance and commerce – not good at either argument or arithmetic.

Mental weariness may ensue with confusion of thought, indecisiveness, forgetfulness of names, and misanthropy.

It is evident, therefore, that there is a certain inadequacy in the Lycopodium individual, especially in relation to physique and circulation. With this is associated a temperamental diffidence, a haunting fear of failure under stress, set off to some extent by hyper-conscientiousness and a penchant for meticulous attention to detail.

PHYSIOLOGY

A definitely chilly individual, hates the cold and feels paralysed thereby in both mind and muscle, but also tends to flag in great heat, which embarrasses the not too active circulation.

While liking to be comfortably warm, is oppressed by too much clothing or a hot stuffy atmosphere.

Appetite is apt to be capricious. Starts a meal quite hungry but feels satisfied after a few mouthfuls. Or may feel ravenously hungry almost immediately after taking quite a heavy meal. May have no desire for food, but appetite returns on starting a meal. There may be complete anorexia for solid food, only fluids being acceptable. Sometimes there is hunger at night associated with an empty sinking feeling.

In the matter of food preferences and dislikes, there is a definite fondness for sugar and sweet things and a marked preference for hot meals and hot fluids, also for savouries. There is a tendency to eat too fast. Vegetables and stodgy foods are unattractive, and there is intolerance of cabbage, peas, beans, milk, pastry, onions, oysters and reheated dishes, which tend to upset the digestion.

Sleep tends to be dream-ridden, often with nightmares entailing a feeling of being suffocated or held down. Limbs may give a sudden jerk when dropping off to sleep, possibly accompanied by a sensation of falling. Wakes from sleep cross, 'ugly' and depressed, but improves when up and about with consequent acceleration of blood flow.

May perspire on quite slight exertion – a cold clammy sweat with odour of onions. Easy nervous sweats under emotional stress. Sometimes a curious inability to sweat, which tends to clear up after taking the remedy. Severe sweats may be followed by intense thirst.

SYMPTOMATOLOGY

General

The Lycopodium subject is prone to chronic types of ill-health or to exacerbations of symptoms. These are manifestations of the widespread lack of tone in the musculature, not only of the skeletal system but even more of the plain muscle of the walls of blood vessels and the gut, leading to circulatory inefficiency.

Sudden fluctuations in the blood-flow in one site or another may produce sudden flashes of heat, sudden satiety of appetite, sudden onset of pain or discomfort with sudden cessation of same.

Symptoms tend to be right-sided, or start on the right side and then extend to the left spreading either horizontally or from above downwards. There is a tendency to physical unease, with complaint that chair or couch feels uncomfortably hard.

Head

Giddiness may be noticed in the morning, both on and after rising from bed, also at times while talking, eating or drinking. This may be accompanied by a feeling that with every movement the brain seems to oscillate inside the skull. Severe headaches occur in the temples, as if the skull was being crushed in a vice. These are made worse by heat, by the warmth of the bed, by getting hot and by lying down. They are relieved by cool air, uncovering the head, by open air and gentle movement. A

319

hunger headache, often present on waking in the morning, is relieved by taking food. This in contrast with a similar headache related to Cactus which is made worse by eating.

Eyes
Symptoms worthy of note are pain in the eyeballs, swelling of the lids with sticky discharge, styes toward the medial canthus; also sparks, flickerings before the eyes and distressing awareness of muscae volitantes. Quivering of the eyelids may be troublesome. Looking intently at revolving objects causes a sensation as if something was going round and round inside the body. Vertical hemianopia may occur, only the left half of the object being seen.

Ears
Conditions that may call for Lycopodium are otitis media with thick, yellow, offensive discharge; chronic deafness; various forms of tinnitus; sensations as if 'hot blood is rushing into the ears'; eczema of the pinna and skin behind the ear with the presence of crusts and fissures. This will be specially so if the symptoms are right-sided.

Respiratory System
There are many important indications for the use of this remedy. A tendency to take cold at the least provocation, with involvement of the frontal sinuses and obstructive nasal catarrh. The nose is blocked at night with compulsive mouth-breathing. The catarrh may become chronic, with formation of yellow or green crusts, and much thick tenacious post-nasal discharge. The nose becomes swollen and sore. Sore throat, possibly with ulceration, starts on the right side, is aggravated by swallowing cold fluids and relieved by warm drinks. There may be complaint of a sensation as if 'a ball was rising up into the throat', causing a choking feeling, or a tight feeling in the throat when swallowing, associated with a constant desire to swallow saliva. Various other odd sensations related to the throat have been noted, mostly referred to the right side, e.g. 'presence of sulphur fumes in the throat'. Lycopodium has been found of value in post-diphtheritic paralysis of the soft palate, with regurgitation of fluids through the nose. Other chest symptoms related to this remedy are a feeling as if the chest were constricted by too tight a waistcoat (in keeping with the general objection to any form of constriction); a sudden violent cough from a tickle as if there was a feather or a crumb in the larynx; a cough which causes a severe headache, is aggravated by taking a deep breath and by empty swallowing. The remedy is indicated in pneumonia which is slow to resolve, and associated with flapping alae nasi and much wrinkling of the

forehead. Other possible indications are severe dyspnoea and wheezing, made worse by walking fast or climbing a hill; stubborn bronchitis with rattling respiration; burning and soreness in the sternal area.

Alimentary System
This is a sphere in which Lycopodium comes very much into its own. In the mouth there is often a salty or putrid taste; the teeth tend to become yellow and discoloured or covered with a gummy deposit, and to be tender to the touch so that chewing is painful. The tip of the tongue may feel 'scalded and sore'. An important symptom is severe heartburn extending up to the pharynx. It is prolonged and almost intolerable, and probably associated with pyloric spasm. Pyrosis is common, with eructations which taste of food ingested, and burning pain like hot coals between the shoulder blades. These symptoms are aggravated by cold fluids but helped by heat. Food tends to be bolted too rapidly, with resulting bloating in the epigastrium which becomes distended like a drum, perhaps after a mere mouthful or two of food. Gastric distress may come on immediately after a meal, possibly with a 'whirling sensation in the stomach' or a feeling as if 'the stomach would fall down'.

Lycopodium has a special relation to the colon, with much flatulent rumbling, irregular spasm giving rise to peristaltic tumour, incarceration of flatus causing a feeling of something pressing outward in the right inguinal region. There may be an actual right inguinal hernia present. The clothing has to be loosened for relief, and leaning forward gives some temporary comfort, as does also the passage of flatus. The flatus passed is non-odorous. The remedy is often indicated when the liver is affected with local tenderness in the right hypochondrium and, possibly, evident jaundice. Also when there are recurrent bilious attacks or actual bile duct spasm. Lycopodium shares with Crocus, Pulsatilla and Thuja the rather common complaint of 'something alive moving about in the belly'. It shares with Belladonna sensations of clutching – 'oesophagus being clutched and twisted', 'a hand in the abdomen clutching the guts'. A further indication for the remedy is constipation resulting from the abuse of purgatives associated with anal spasm, a sensation of incomplete evacuation after passage of stool, which is at first lumpy then changing to soft and narrow. The diameter of the stool varies according to the degree of spasm in the anal sphincter muscles. There may be an absence of any desire for stool for days, followed by much ineffectual urging, a symptom shared with Nux Vomica. Other rectal symptoms are pressure and tearing pain in the rectum, piles which tend to prolaps, bleed and become very painful, and pruritus ani.

Cardiovascular System

The circulatory atonia associated with the remedy results in a tendency to get short of breath and distressed on exertion. Irregular alterations in blood flow may cause a sudden rush of blood to one site or another, or the reverse, with the result that fingers or toes 'go dead'. The remedy is mentioned in connection with aneurysm, varicose veins, varices of external genitalia, naevus, and anasarca of the lower half of the body.

Urinary System

There are a number of symptoms associated with the remedy. Aching pain in the loins before urination, relieved by emptying the bladder. A tendency to shiver at the close of urination. Much frequency with the passage of large quantities of pale urine. At other times, highly concentrated urine is passed containing a sediment of 'brick dust' or 'red sand' appearance. There may be delay in starting the act of urination, with a slow stream. Nocturia is common, the bladder having to be emptied several times during the night. The remedy may be called for in renal lithiasis with colic, especially if right-sided, also possibly in connection with chronic nephritis with anasarca.

Genital System

In the genital system in the male, Lycopodium has proved of value in relation to psychogenic impotence, and also in pruritus affecting scrotum and groins. In women, irregularities of menstruation, severe menorrhagia with clots, metrorrhagia with passage of dark blood and large clots may require the remedy. Also mentioned are great depression with irritability before the menstrual period, which is relieved when the period starts, as is the case with Lachesis. A curious sensation may be complained of as if 'gas was discharged per vaginam'.

Locomotor System

A number of symptoms are recorded as being related to Lycopodium. A tearing pain in the right side of the neck extending downwards to shoulder, arm and fingers. Drawing and tearing pains in the lower limbs. Restlessness in the limbs at night, interfering with sleep. Severe back pain, aggravated by any movement and relieved by the passage of large quantities of urine and by heat. Knees feel as if they would 'give out', a symptom shared with Ruta. Soreness and swelling of joints, especially small joints, associated with nodular deformity, and relief of pain by gentle movement.

Lycopodium Clavatum

Skin

The following conditions are mentioned. Chronic indolent ulcers which are painful, stinging, burning, and smarting, aggravated by heat and soothed by cool applications. Urticaria in weals or nodules which itch and burn and are aggravated in a warm room or by warmth of bed. Eczema behind the ears with tendency to spread to the scalp and exude a sanious, watery discharge. Eruptions of various types which itch violently. Intertrigo of persistent nature. Dryness of the skin, especially of the palms.

MODALITIES

Generally symptoms are aggravated by impact of cold air, by taking cold food or drink, in a stuffy hot atmosphere. Physically they are made worse be touch, pressure, the weight of clothes or bedcovers, by overexertion and when lying on the right side. Aggravation also results if emotionally hurried, harried or worried, also if idle or unoccupied. Chronologically, the worst times are on first waking in the morning and from 4 to 8 p.m.

Conversely, relief is afforded by reasonable warmth, by taking hot food or fluids, by loosening the garments, by uncovering, and in the open air. Active movement and active occupation also help.

CLINICAL NOTES

A main guide to the use of the remedy will be such characteristics as physical mediocrity associated with intellectual alertness, emotional diffidence and hyper-conscientiousness, circulatory inadequacy, tendency to liver complaints and flatulent dyspepsia. The higher potencies, especially the 200c, are apt to cause quite severe aggravation. In chronic disease it may be wise to start treatment with another anti-psoric remedy, e.g. the sequence Sulphur→ Calcarea Carb.→ Lycopodium.

Magnesia Phosphorica

SOURCE

The phosphate of magnesium occurs in hexagonal crystals, which are sparingly soluble in water and sweetish to the taste. This salt is present in various body tissues. It is also found in the grain of cereals.

PHARMACOLOGY

There is affinity with both nervous and muscular tissues, inducing neuralgic pains and muscle spasm; a later effect is to produce anaesthesia and paralysis. The anaesthetic effect can be countered by Calcium.

PROVING

Magnesium Phosphate is one of the twelve Tissue Salts introduced by Schuessler. It has not received a satisfactory proving, and the present drug picture is composed of observations recorded from clinical practice.

APPEARANCE

The remedy is especially suitable for thin, emaciated subjects of dark complexion.

There is a lean, thin, nervous look, possibly with staring eyes. The individual appears tired, exhausted, almost unable to sit up. May be found talking to herself or sitting motionless in stony silence.

May be found doubled up with pain or groaning and pacing to and fro.

PSYCHOLOGY

The subject appears listless, languid and averse to mental effort (not given to fits of rage as with Colocynth).

Is forgetful, unable to think clearly; much inclined to tearful lamentation. There may be a tendency to stammer.

PHYSIOLOGY

A very chilly subject, complains of cold, especially up and down the spine. Shows a great dread of uncovering.

There is craving for sugar and aversion to coffee. Curiously enough there may be thirst for very cold drinks.

Drowsiness is a feature, especially if making an attempt to study. Severe spasmodic yawning may occur, as if to dislocate the jaw.

SYMPTOMATOLOGY

General

Pains are violent, shoot like lighting, cramping, boring, maddening and prostrating. They may be so severe as to cause retching. Pains are apt to change location and may be felt anywhere in the body. They both come and go with sudden abruptness. It is interesting that although there is such a variety of pains, burning pains are not met with, as is so markedly the case with Arsenicum Alb. In both remedies, however, there is relief from heat. The neuralgic pains increase in severity until the victim becomes almost frantic, and may recur every night. Pain may be accompanied by or alternate with a sensation of constriction. Extreme exhaustion is also a frequent concomitant symptom. Pain may be induced by overexertion or too prolonged use of particular muscles, and be accompanied by occupational cramp. Symptoms tend to be right-sided and often show periodicity.

Head

Headache is usually severe and associated with a red face and much throbbing. One type starts in the occiput and spreads over the whole head; it is worse on the right side, from 10 to 11 a.m. and from 4 to 5 p.m.; it is relieved by warm wraps. Neuralgic headache occurs in young people, increased by intensive study. Severe facial neuralgia of trigeminal distribution is often on the right side; it is aggravated by cold, by the least touch, by pressure, at 2 p.m. and at night; local application of heat may give some relief. Headaches are usually relieved by warmth, by firm pressure and in the dark, but sometimes the impact of cold air is preferred. The head may feel as if full of fluid or as if portions of the brain were swishing about. There may be a sensation of a cap on the head.

Eyes

Pain is felt in and above the right orbit from exposure to cold; it is accompanied by spasms of the facial muscles. Other eye symptoms are double vision, spasmodic squint, dimness of vision, dark spots, sparks, rainbow colours seen before the eyes, nystagmus, constriction of pupils, twitching of eyelids, ptosis.

Ears

Sharp intermittent pains occur behind the right ear, worse in cold air or from washing the face in cold water.

Respiratory System

A sore throat is associated with chilliness and constant desire to swallow, though doing so causes pain. Spasmodic contraction occurs in the throat on attempting to swallow fluids. Laryngismus stridulus is associated with tetany. A dry paroxysmal cough may be so severe as to make it difficult to lie down or to speak coherently; the subject goes red in the face, chokes and retches; the cough is worse in a warm room and better in the open air. Intercostal neuralgia occurs with sharp, intermittent pains; there is a desire to take a deep breath to relieve a feeling of constriction; the condition is worse on first entering a warm room, but better after being in the room a short while. Walking aggravates.

Alimentary System

Lips apt to be sore and cracked. Mouth is sore with red, raw-looking patches on tongue, gums and buccal surfaces. Mouth feels scalded and eating is painful. Severe toothache moves from spot to spot; it is made worse by eating and drinking and is also worse after retiring at night; heat gives some relief. Teeth are very sensitive to touch or cold air. Hiccough is troublesome both day and night, and is associated with retching. Gastric distress is aggravated by cold drinks, touch and physical exertion; drinking hot water, local warmth and taking food afford relief. Very severe flatulent colics with radiating pains cause the sufferer to bend double, press the hands into the abdomen and use massage in search of relief. Distension makes it imperative to loosen the clothing; passage of flatus does not afford relief. Infants with colic lie, crying in pain, with thighs flexed on the belly, application of a warm hand gives some relief. Dysentery or choleraic diarrhoea occurs in association with severe cramps.

Cardiovascular System
Anginal pain is recorded, accompanied by a sensation of constriction round the heart. Palpitations are associated with nervous tension.

Urinary System
Nocturnal enuresis may occur from nervous disturbance. Spasmodic retention is accompanied by tenesmus and painful urging. Cutting pain in the bladder may precede passage of urine. Frequent urge to urinate occurs when standing or walking; it may also disturb sleep at night.

Genital System
Severe dysmenorrhoea occurs, especially before the flow starts. Menstrual periods are too early, with dark blood containing stringy clots.

Neuromuscular System
Neuralgic pains occur in the limbs, worse from movement and at night. Right-sided sciatica is associated with sharp pains, aggravated by the least touch, the slightest draught and on getting undressed; is better if warmly clad. Stiffness and rigidity affect the limbs. The remedy to be considered in paralysis agitans, chorea and tabes dorsalis. Tremors and twitching may occur all over the body. Cramps and tonic spasms may follow over-use of certain muscles. Convulsions in children or adults are followed by extreme sensitivity to touch, wind, noise or any exciting stimulus.

MODALITIES

Aggravation results from cold air, cold wind, contact with cold water, a cold draught – in fact from cold in any form; from touch; from movement; at night.

Relief is obtained from warmth, by applied heat, from pressure, rubbing or bending double; when resting.

CLINICAL NOTES

The remedy is of great value as a pain-reliever, in contrast to narcotics which merely dull pain. It is especially related to excruciating pain accompanied by extreme exhaustion. It has given good results in all potencies; is said to act more promptly if given in hot water.

327

Medorrhinum

SOURCE

Medorrhinum is a nosode prepared by the homoeopathic potentization of the purulent discharge from an untreated case of gonorrhoea.

Microscopically, such a specimen would show a large number of polymorphonuclear leucocytes, epithelial cells, and Gram negative diplococci of *Neisseria gonorrhoeae*. The nosode is thus complex, including human tissue and bacteria. and is not just a potency of gonococcal toxin (which in fact also exists, under the name of Gonotoxinum).

Gonorrhoea is a sexually transmitted disease involving chiefly the mucous membranes of the genito-urinary tract, rectum and cervix, and occasionally of the eye, with possible haematogenic spread to serous and synovial membranes.

In the male, the onset consists of an acute purulent anterior urethritis with dysuria. Following spread to the posterior urethra, frequency and urgency appear, and there may be involvement of the seminal vesicles, Cowper's glands and the urethral follicles. Vasitis, epididymitis, sterility and urethral stricture can result. In the female, primary infection of the urethra, the cervix, or Skene's or Bartholin's glands is usual, and in many cases rectal infection follows. Symptoms and signs of acute infection may be severe, but frequently they are absent, and asymptomatic female carriers can be responsible for the spread of the disease.

Local complications include acute Bartholin's abscess, endocervicitis, endometritis and salpingitis, leading to pelvic peritonitis and sterility. The symptoms of pelvic inflammatory disease closely resemble those of acute appendicitis, with fever, nausea, vomiting and pain.

Arthritis is a common complication of gonococcal infection and may be associated with conjunctivitis, iritis, iridocyclitis, and occasionally keratoderma blenorrhagica. Rarer complications include gonococcal myositis, serosynovitis, pleuritis, meningitis.

Gonorrhoea may be associated with Reiter's Syndrome, which is characterised by urethritis, conjunctivitis and polyarthritis, but gonococcal bacteria are not found, and the condition is resistant to antibiotic therapy.

Medorrhinum

PROVING

The first proving of Medorrhinum was published by Swan in his *Materia Medica of Nosodes* in 1888, and subsequent provings are listed by H.C. Allen.

APPEARANCE

The general impression is of a weak, undersized, prematurely-aged person, with pallid, moist, unhealthy skin and a permanently worried expression. Children are anaemic, with large heads, sweaty faces, swollen glands and respiratory catarrh. The adenoid facies is common, as are warts, moles, papillomata, polyps and other soft-tissue tumours.

PSYCHOLOGY

Medorrhinum people are worried and hurried; time passes too slowly for them.

They are full of shame and blush easily; children are especially sensitive to reprimand.

They are sensitive, start at the slightest sound, and weep easily.

They feel exhausted in the morning but come alive in the evening, when they are ready to go out on the town.

Memory is poor for recent events, proper names and figures; in writing, letters or words may be omitted.

The time sense may be disturbed, and they have difficulty in sustaining a conversation.

Visual and auditory hallucinations may occur.

PHYSIOLOGY

The Medorrhinum subject is chilly and very sensitive to barometric changes. He is better by the seaside, but worse in mountain regions.

There is canine hunger even immediately after eating, and great thirst, with a desire for beer and spirits – in fact a craving for all stimulants, tobacco, coffee and drugs, and also for sweets, ice cream, acid fruits and bitters.

A keynote of this remedy is that the subject sleeps in the genupectoral position. He is very tired in the morning, but wakes up at bedtime and could then stay up all night.

SYMPTOMATOLOGY

General

The general picture is of:

a) Debility and anxious depression.

b) Fluid retention (hydrogen constitution).

c) Mucous discharges from the respiratory and urogenital tracts.

d) Soft-tissue tumours and swollen glands.

Head

Frontal headache, with the sensation of a band round the head. Neuralgia which comes and goes quickly, worse in the morning, and better in damp weather or by the sea.

Eyes

The eyelids are stuck together in the morning, and there is a feeling as of sand under the eyelids. The eyelashes fall out. There is induration of the edge of the upper eyelid. The eyeballs are painful and feel as if pushed outwards. Brown or black patches appear in the field of vision. Objects appear double, or else reduced in size.

Ears

There may be loss of hearing, or even total deafness. Auditory hallucinations – thinks he hears voices. Pain in the Eustachian tubes, extending to the ears. Itching of the external auditory meatus.

Respiratory System

Nose. The sense of smell is deficient or absent. The nose is blocked, with dry nasal mucosa; or copious white, yellowish or bloodstained nasal discharge; or watery coryza with frontal pain, worse at 10 a.m. The tip of the nose itches; there is sensitivity to inspired air. Epistaxis is common.

Throat. The pharynx is full of thick mucus coming down from the post-nasal area. Spasm of the glottis and dryness of the throat causes a cough at bedtime.

Chest. There is a dry painful cough, worse at night, better from lying on the stomach, worse in a warm room. Asthmatic dyspnoea in children is relieved by lying on the stomach with the tongue protruded. Difficult expectoration of viscous secretions containing small white lumps. All respiratory troubles are better at the seaside.

Alimentary System
The teeth are yellowish, brittle and carious. The mouth is dry and burning, with offensive breath and a taste of copper. The tongue is coated at the base, with aphthous ulcers. There is canine hunger, even immediately after eating. Thirst is intense. Nausea occurs after eating, or drinking water. There is glairy, bilious vomit. Cramp-like pains in the stomach are not relieved by eating or drinking. Anxiety is felt in the solar plexus. Pains in the liver and spleen are associated with nausea, vomiting and pale foetid stools. Constipation; it is difficult to expel stools, but this is relieved by leaning backwards. There are pricking pains in the anus, with redness and a foetid sweat smelling of fish-brine. Rectal prolapse may occur in young children.

Cardiovascular System
There is a tendency to collapse, with a need to be fanned. In spite of a cold sweat, he uncovers himself. Dyspnoea and palpitations. Cutting precordial pain is aggravated by movement, and extends to the left arm.

Urinary System
Nocturnal enuresis. The urine is dark yellow, covered with a greasy film, and has a strong stale smell of ammonia. Albuminuria is accompanied by hyaline casts in the urine. There is oedema of the feet and ankles. Inflammation of the kidneys, bladder and prostate. There is weakness of the bladder, with a feeble stream of urine.

Genital System
Men. Nocturnal emissions are followed by weakness and impotence. Pain in the testicles and spermatic cord, especially the left, associated with left sciatica; worse from the slightest draught.

Women. Dysmenorrhoea with pain in the sacrococcygeal region and front of the thighs; better from drawing the legs up to the belly. Abundant leucorrhoea smelling of brine, with intense vulvovaginal pruritus. Warts on the labia majora and perineum. Chronic ovarian pain. Increase of sexual desire after periods, with hot flushes and sweats; chronic metritis; the breasts are as cold as marble, and sensitive to touch.

Endocrine System
Pituitary dysfunction is indicated by impotence, amenorrhoea and asthenia. Disorders of basal metabolism and sleep. Hypogonadism.

Locomotor System

Neuralgic type pains which come and go quickly, and are worse in cold damp weather and before a storm. Acute and chronic rheumatic pains; acute rheumatism is worse from movement; chronic rheumatism is better from movement. Burning pain of the vertebral column, hands and feet. Pain in the shoulders and small joints of the hand. Deformity of the finger joints, with stiffness. Pain in the lumbar region, lumbo-sacral joints, hips and thighs. Left sciatica. Sharp pains in the heels and soles of the feet. Restlessness and burning pains of the feet, which are better from fresh air and cold sweating of the soles. Constant movement of the feet and legs, which cannot keep still.

Skin, Hair and Nails

The skin is cold, damp and shiny, with copious cold sweat and a stale odour. Sweats at the least effort. Cold in localised spots: the tip of the nose, the nipples, the palms of the hands and soles of the feet. Yellow marks on the back of the hands. General irritation, worse from thinking about it. Recurrent labial herpes. Cutaneous and mucous growths: pedunculated warts, which may be flat-topped, peaked, seborrhoeic or soft; polyps of the nose, the uterus, the vagina or the perinanal region. Intensely irritating herpetic eruptions of the scalp. Dry hair. Dandruff. Brittle deformed nails with transverse ridges.

MODALITIES

Aggravation: from thinking about the complaint, from touch, in the mountains, from draughts, during the day, from dry cold weather, on Saturdays and Sundays.

Amelioration: by the seaside, in damp weather, from lying on the belly, during the night.

Laterality: weakly left-sided.

CLINICAL NOTES

Medorrhinum is closely related to the sycotic remedies, especially Thuja, Natrum Sulph. and Argentum Nit. It is often given as a single dose in cases where such remedies, though apparently indicated, do not complete the cure.

Mercurius

SOURCE

Mercurius Solubilis, also known as Mercurius Oxydulatus Niger from its black colour, was the ammonium nitrate salt of mercury introduced by Hahnemann into medicine in 1788. It was also used by him in provings. However, the preparation of the salt 'required much care and labour'. In accordance with the precept 'That which can be done simply should not be done extravagantly', Hahnemann therefore recommended triturations of metallic mercury, Mercurius Vivus, as being of equivalent value therapeutically. The two preparations, therefore, may be considered as one from the materia medica angle.

Mercury was not used medicinally before the fifteenth century. The employment of mercury, which in its poisoning effects can produce symptoms similar to those of syphilis, as a cure for the pox was an early example of inadvertent homoeopathy.

PHARMACOLOGY

Mercury is a general poison having affinity with a wide range of tissues, notably mucous membranes, bones, salivary glands, lymph nodes, liver, kidneys, nervous system, blood and skin. Inflammatory lesions are produced, tending to degenerative changes, especially necrosis of tissues.

It is recorded that the symptoms of mercury poisoning range through erethism, stomatitis, sialorrhoea, tremors, skin rashes to albuminuria and the nephrotic syndrome. Dysphonia, dysarthria, ataxia and severe constriction of visual fields have also been described.

PROVING

Hahnemann's proving of Mercury appears in the last edition of the first volume of his *Materia Medica Pura*.

APPEARANCE

The Mercurius subject has usually a sickly, even cachectic, appearance. The face shows yellowish pallor or a lead-coloured earthy look, with dull lustreless eyes. A bloated look may be noticed, especially round the eyes, which are encircled by a bluish red discolouration. The face may be covered with perspiration, but the lips are dry, rough and blackish. They may show pustules, scabs or small ulcers. Rhagades are common at the corners of the mouth.

A pale, swollen, flabby tongue shows the imprint of the teeth; it is usually quite moist, but fairly thickly coated. Foetor oris is pronounced and the whole body odour is offensive.

General tremors may be evident, and the hands so shaky as to make writing impossible.

Speech may be hurried and rapid, but is perhaps more often slow with long pauses before answering questions.

PSYCHOLOGY

The subject is restless, agitated, anguished – just cannot stay still for one minute. There is often excessive fear from quite trivial causes. Mental turmoil and torment is most pronounced at night, associated with a desire to flee, to escape, and a feeling 'as if he had committed a crime'.

The mind is weak and tremulous; memory and will-power are impaired – is apt to forget names of people, of streets, of places etc. At times feels hurried and does things in great haste. The mental state may be one of extreme indifference, of homesickness, of suicidal or even murderous intent.

PHYSIOLOGY

The Mercurius patient is essentially a chilly person, especially when out of doors and in the evening. Flashes of heat in the face may coincide with shuddering and icy-cold extremities. Heat and cold sensations may alternate or intermingle. A peculiar creeping chilliness precedes the onset of coryza, fevers and malaise from other causes, and is rendered more noticeable by uncovering, even slightly.

Hunger may be constant and insatiable, but there is an aversion to meat, fat and butter. There is intolerance of sweets.

Thirst is intense and excessive, despite the presence of a moist tongue. It is a burning thirst for cold drinks, especially for milk or beer.

Excessive drowsiness makes keeping awake difficult in the daytime, but insomnia of various types and degrees disturbs sleep at night. Vivid, often terrifying, dreams cause frequent waking which may be accompanied by palpitations or sweats. Sweats are profuse, offensive, of sickly or nauseous odour, and stain linen yellow. They afford no relief, however.

SYMPTOMATOLOGY

General

A feature of Mercurius is very easy exhaustion after quite slight exertion. There is a tendency to emaciation and paretic weakness, associated with a liability to fainting attacks or sudden myocardial failure. Blood dyscrasias occur, resulting in profound anaemia which renders the subject liable to ready suppuration, characterized by sanious pus or necrotic ulceration. Oedema of face, hands and lower extremities may develop.

Head

Vertigo associated with stumbling or swaying is especially noticed on rising from bed or from sitting. Headache is severe; the whole head is tender to the touch, feels compressed as if in a vice, or it may feel as if growing larger or being pressed on from above. Boring pains occur in the head, notably in the left temple or occiput. Headache is worse at night and on waking, but better when up and moving around. Hair tends to fall out. The scalp is extremely itchy. Skull bones necrose.

Eyes

Various inflammatory eye conditions are described which are aggravated by the heat of a fire or a stove, and also worse at night. Photophobia is very severe, and vision is dimmed, with a mist before the eyes or seeing black specks floating around. Severe neuralgic pain may be felt in the eye, associated with a sensation of cold all round the orbit.

Ears

Otitis media is accompanied by lancinating pain and a purulent, offensive, excoriating discharge. The pain is especially severe at night. Tinnitus of roaring type may occur.

Respiratory Sytem

Frequent sneezing may occur without actual coryza. The bridge of the nose may be swollen. Actual caries of nasal bones may be present, or necrotic ulcers inside the nose. The associated discharge is acrid, often yellowish green in colour, and the nostrils are raw and sore. There is a liability to epistaxis with blood which coagulates easily, perhaps causing a clot to dangle from the nostril. The throat feels very dry and swallowing is painful, but owing to excessive salivation frequent swallowing is unavoidable. Ulcerative tonsillitis occurs. Cough is worse at night, and suffocative paroxysms occur with an inclination to vomit. There is a good deal of mucopurulent sputum. The cough is aggravated when lying on the right side. Stitching pains occur in the chest, especially in the pectoral regions. Involvement of the right lower lobe is accompanied by sharp pains shooting through to the back. Haemoptysis may occur.

Alimentary System
A foul mouth is associated with much soapy, slimy or stringy saliva. The tongue is moist, flabby and indented at the edges by contact with the teeth. It may be swollen. Greyish ulcers may be present on the buccal aspect of the cheeks, on tongue, gums and palate. An unpleasant taste is noticed in the mouth, metallic, salty or like rotten eggs. Teeth are apt to ache, especially at night, and the pain is aggravated by taking either hot or cold fluids; it is eased somewhat by rubbing the contiguous cheek. Teeth may feel 'too long', become loose and be discoloured, turning black. Gums become swollen, recede and bleed very easily. Involvement of the liver results in biliousness, jaundice, ascites and inability to lie on the right side. Pyrosis, violent vomiting, extreme epigastric tenderness and other forms of gastric distress are described, generally made worse on bending forwards. Pinching pains occur in the belly. Hiccough is frequent. Excoriating watery diarrhoea may occur, especially toward evening, with bright yellow, green or dark brown stools; and great exhaustion follows the passage of the stool. Actual dysentery may be present with slimy, blood-stained stools, severe tenesmus and the 'never get done' sensation. The stools are foetid in odour. In very severe attacks Mercurius Corr. is of signal value.

Lymphatic and Glandular Systems
Involvement of lymph nodes is common, especially in the cervical and inguinal regions, with a strong tendency to suppuration and abscess formation. Painful swelling of the salivary glands also occurs.

Urinary System
Frequency and urgency of urination may be present both day and night, only small quantities of urine being passed, and with the accompaniment of much burning both during and after the act. The urine excoriates. Nephritis with generalized anasarca may be present.

Genital System
The testicles may become swollen and indurated, associated with a feeling of coldness in the parts. Priapism may be painful and persistent.

Chancre, bubo, balanitis, greenish urethral discharge are associated with the remedy. Ovarian pains may occur of a stinging and burning nature. Lactation has been observed in non-pregnant women during the menstrual period. Leucorrhoea is greenish and is more marked in the evening, during the night and when urinating. It tends to be accompanied by severe pruritus which is relieved by cold bathing. Ulcers occur on the cervix and vulva.

Nervous System
Neuromuscular incoordination is a frequent feature. Tremors are prominent, causing difficulty in grasping small objects. The tremors may be so violent as to throw the patient down, or they may take the form of constant choreic movements associated with difficulty in articulation and indistinct speech. The tremulousness is aggravated by exposure to the least draught, by even slight exertion and by emotional stress.

Locomotor System
Burning and drawing pains occur in the nape and back, accompanied by rigidity. Sacral pain tends to spread to the thighs. Caries of the spine may be present with stitching pains in the thighs, worse on walking. Severe pain is felt in the bones, especially at night when warm in bed. Cramplike pains occur in the hands with stiffness suggestive of tetany. A bruised weariness in the lower limbs causes restless unease of limbs which makes it impossible to keep still or stay put, even in bed. Joints become painful, puffy, pale and tender, and the pain is worse both from the heat of the bed and also from uncovering.

Skin
Eruptions occur of many varieties, but are inevitably aggravated by extremes of temperature and at night. Ulcers tend to spread rapidly, are serpiginous in outline, have a yellow sloughing base and a foul foetid discharge. Excoriations occur in contact areas. Fissures may be present in hands and feet. Severe pruritus is common in various sites, worse in the evening and at night.

MODALITIES

There is aggravation from either extreme of temperature, in a warm room or a warm bed; also from change in weather, especially to humid or rainy weather, and from the least draught. Perhaps the most important modality is severe aggravation at night, but the sufferer is also worse in the evening, when lying on the right side, from touch and pressure, from eating and from sweating. The autumn is a bad time.

Some relief is obtained when at rest, and the subject feels better at high altitudes.

CLINICAL NOTES

The remedy is indicated in syphilitic lesions. It is often of value in cachectic conditions due to malignant disease or tuberculosis.

Low potencies tend to hasten suppuration; high may abort.

Mercurius and Silicea are inimical if either is given in sequence to the other before the action of the first dose is completed. Mercurius is seldom indicated if the tongue is dry.

Mezereum

SOURCE

This remedy is prepared from *Daphne mezereon*, one of the Thyme-laceae, and closely related to spurge laurel. Quelch describes the plant thus: 'A shrub about four or five feet high, which is found wild in the woods of the southern counties. Its leaves which are smooth and lanceolate do not appear until after the flowers, which are purplish in colour and appear in February and March. They grow in groups of three or four and have rather a powerful fragrance.'

The stems are covered with a light brown bark, which is silky on the inner surface. The young branches are covered with dense white hairs. The fresh bark has an unpleasant odour; the taste is sweetish at first but soon becomes acrid and intensely burning to mouth and throat. The berries are bright red, fleshy, ovoid, bluntly pointed, about three-quarters of an inch long; they appear close to the stem in July.

The whole plant is a dangerous irritant. The vesicant principle is an acrid amorphous resin, mezerein; other constituents are a bitter crystalline glucoside, daphnin, a fixed oil, malic acid, sugars, starch. In large doses the plant causes vomiting and acute catharsis; the berries have proved fatal to children.

The mother tincture is prepared from fresh bark collected just before the flowers appear in February.

PHARMACOLOGY

The plant manifests an irritant affinity with bones, nerves, mucous membranes and skin, inducing such effects as very severe pain, acute swelling, vomiting and purging, erythema and blister formation.

PROVING

The proving of Mezereum appears in the second edition of Hahnemann's *Chronic Diseases*.

APPEARANCE

Possible features are a grey earthy pallor, light coloured hair, brown rings round eyes, blue nails. There may be red, inflamed-looking patches on the cheeks. The child scratches its face constantly till it becomes covered with blood.

In pain the sufferer lies perfectly still and only responds to questions with a 'Yes' or 'No'.

Frequent shuddering or trembling may be noticed, or constant stretching and yawning.

Discharges are coloured green.

Finds it hard work to talk.

PSYCHOLOGY

The patient is irritable over trifles, irresolute, averse to everything, despondent, takes no pleasure in anything.

May be apprehensive, complaining of a queer feeling in the stomach; wants to 'run away'.

While speaking may lose the thread; is unable to recollect or take things in; becomes oblivious to surroundings.

PHYSIOLOGY

Is a chilly subject with cold hands and feet; feels chilly even in a hot room.

There is a constant desire for food, not from actual hunger but because gastric discomfort is eased by eating or by drinking milk. There may be a craving for fat ham. During the day is irresistibly drowsy; sleep at night is interrupted by dreams and is unrefreshing; nightmare may wake at 2 a.m. to 3 a.m.

SYMPTOMATOLOGY

General

Symptoms are characterized by violence: violent pains, violent itching; violent hunger; violent burnings in mouth and stomach; violent inclination to cough; violently acute fever. Pains are associated with chilliness and sensitivity; they shoot upward, seeming to draw the patient up from the bed. Sudden alarming oedema may occur, e.g. of the face, lips and tongue. The swelling may be accompanied by vesication and, later, shedding of skin or mucosa. The patient may complain of sensations of constriction, contraction, stiffness in limbs, chest, neck and throat. Symptoms spread from above downward, from within outward, from right to left.

Head

Vertigo is associated with a tendency to fall to one side, and sparks before the eyes. Headache is described as 'splitting', 'as if the top of the head had gone', 'as if scalp was bruised'; it is relieved by stooping or by wrapping the head warmly. The vertex and occiput are tender to touch. Violent neuralgic headache extends to the eye, with profuse lachrymation; it is unilateral and radiates downward, involving teeth and jaws. The malar bone is tender and there is a cold feeling in the eye, or a sensation as if 'cold air was blowing on the eye'. The pain is made worse by eating, from the least touch; worse also at night. Curiously the pain may be eased by proximity to the fire but not by any other form of heat. The pain may even extend to the shoulder region. Periostitis of the lower jaw may occur with swelling and burning pain. There may be a boggy tumefaction of the scalp, which is covered by thick leathery crusts; under the crusts thick white pus collects, glueing and matting the hair. The head may be lousy with much itching and burning.

Eyes

Sharp, pricking pains cause a desire to rub the eyes, which are red, injected and extremely dry. Eyes may feel 'too large' or 'as if drawn back into the orbit'. Eyelids twitch, especially the left upper lid; twitching of the muscles of the right cheek may also be noticed.

Ears

Deafness and tinnitus are associated with great sensitivity of the external auditory canal to the impact of air, and a sensation as if 'air was blowing into the meatus' or 'distending it'. There is a desire to bore the finger into the ear. Itching may occur behind the ear with an oozing eruption. Deafness may follow suppression of eruptions on the scalp by ointments.

Respiratory System

Burning pain may be felt in nasal bones. Sneezing may be troublesome with yellow discharge, possibly blood-streaked, and excoriation of nasal mucosa. Sensation of smell may be impaired and nose feels dry inside. Hoarseness is accompanied by burning and dryness in the throat. A dry hacking cough with a desire to take a deep breath is worse in the evening and first part of the night. Syphilitic ulceration in pharynx and larynx, with dryness and burning relieved by drawing in cold air, may call for the remedy. The chest may be painful on inspiration with a feeling of constriction and some dyspnoea.

Alimentary System

Intense burning in mouth, pharynx, oesophagus and stomach is relieved to some extent by inhaling cold air. Teeth feel blunt and elongated. Toothache is worse on biting and at night; is also eased by breathing in cold air. The tongue is coated only on one side. Belching accompanies the burning. Nausea occurs with vomiting of bitter fluid. Burning in the epigastrium is aggravated by pressure but eased by drinking milk. Peptic ulcer occurs with uneasiness, rawness or burning in stomach, relieved temporarily by eating; food seems to stay indefinitely in stomach. Colicky pains are felt in the umbilical region with burning and diarrhoea of sour, watery, undigested stools. Flatulent colic is associated with shivering. Constipation is associated with stools of stony hardness which seem to split the anus when passed, with resulting exhaustion. There may be a tormenting rectal urge; also protruding piles associated with anal spasm. Coldness and shuddering may occur before and after passage of stool.

Urinary System

Burning in anterior urethra is felt at the close of urination. Several drops of blood may be passed at the end of micturition. Red flakes float on surface of urine.

Genital System

Testicles enlarged and tender on pressure. Increased libido. Menses too frequent; profuse discharge. Leucorrhoea like white of egg; discharge excoriates.

Locomotor System

Pain and stiffness in nape of neck, worse in cold, wet weather, also from heat of bed and by movement. Rheumatic pains in back and limbs, worse in hot weather. Pain in long bones, especially tibia; pains are burning and violent, often located on left side. Pains in bones of feet, worse when walking.

Skin

Herpes zoster accompanied by intense itching and burning; may be followed by severe and intractable neuralgia in affected area. Skin subject to constant irritation, tinglings, itchings, formication, bitings, changing from site to site as result of scratching. Parts become cold after scratching. As soon as warms up in bed or becoming heated in a warm room the itching starts. Pruritus in the aged. Vesicular eruptions behind the ears, on nose, at elbow or knee, become moist. Eczema on dorsum of hands and wrists. Psoriasis of palms. When eruptions are in full bloom patient feels well, but if suppressed, catarrhal, nervous and rheumatic affections ensue. Varicose ulcers are bluish-red in colour and very sensitive to light. Chronic ulcers exude a purulent discharge and become covered by yellowish-white crusts and surrounded by vesicles which itch and burn and have a brick-red areola.

MODALITIES

There is aggravation in cold air, from damp, from change of weather, from warm food, in a hot stuffy atmosphere, when hot in bed; also from touch, during the menstrual period, in the evening and at night.

Some relief is obtained in the open.

CLINICAL NOTES

Neuralgias, long bone pains and skin symptoms provide the main indications for the use of the remedy.

Muriaticum Acidum

SOURCE

Hydrochloric acid is a colourless gas with a pungent suffocating odour; it is produced by action of sulphuric acid on sodium chloride. It is freely soluble in water.

PHARMACOLOGY

The pure acid is actively destructive to tissues with which it comes in contact. It causes irritation of alimentary and respiratory mucosa and tends to produce a grave degree of debility and discharges of a putrid nature.

PROVING

Hahnemann's first proving of Hydrochloric Acid appears in the fifth volume of his *Materia Medica Pura*.

APPEARANCE

Cheeks are shiny and coloured red or livid. The expression is one of restlessness and the subject is constantly changing posture. Pimples and freckles are common on the face.

On attempting to walk, staggers about, owing to weakness of thigh muscles. Or may present a picture of extreme prostration, vacant staring look in eyes, lids half closed, dropped jaw, slides down in the bed, legs drawn up, extremities cold, moaning or muttering delirium.

Tongue is dry, shrunken, narrow, pointed and either paralytic or rattles in dry parched mouth. Lips are dry, sore, cracked.

Skin is hot and dry; so burning hot in fever that the bedclothes are pushed off.

The breath and body odour are offensive. Discharges are thin, excoriating and foul-smelling.

PSYCHOLOGY

The subject is reserved, silent, sad and unwilling to talk. Tends to be restless, irritable, peevish, fretful, possibly with loud moaning.

PHYSIOLOGY

Complains of extreme chilliness with or without actual shivering.

May have a ravenous appetite or on the other hand cannot bear the thought or sight of food, especially meat.

May have a constant desire for fluids but is not thirsty in fever.

Feels drowsy but is unable to get off to sleep; if he does fall asleep, wakes frequently. Tosses and turns constantly.

There may be actual shivering accompanied by much yawning and desire to stretch limbs.

SYMPTOMATOLOGY

General

Symptoms may be accompanied by burning sensations and are associated with extreme prostration and muscular weakness. There is a tendency to ulcer formation.

Head

A whirling type of vertigo is aggravated by movement and by lying on the right side. A stupefying headache is relieved when walking slowly in cold air. The hair feels as if standing on end. The occipital region feels as heavy as lead. The brain may feel bruised or torn.

Eyes

There may be complaint of dim vision or optical illusions. Hemianopia may occur.

Ears

Pinching or tearing pain is felt in an ear. The sound of people talking is unbearable.

Respiratory System

Sneezing is frequent. Epistaxis common. Throat symptoms are severe, e.g. swelling of uvula, formation of ulcers and false membrane. Pharynx is oedematous, dark coloured and raw. Chokes on attempting to swallow. Respiration is rapid, weak and rattling. Stitching or boring pains are felt in chest.

Alimentary System

Herpes labialis is common. Mouth is very dry with a bad taste, tongue like leather and feels heavy, shrivelled and paralytic. Aphthous ulcers occur with foetor oris. There is queasy nausea, worse on sitting up. A curious empty sensation in oesophagus and stomach, possibly associated with dysphagia. Violent pinching and squeezing may be felt below left costal margin and in the umbilical region. Stools are dark, thin and offensive in odour. Stool is apt to be passed involuntarily when urinating or when passing flatus. Haemorrhage occurs from anus of dark fluid blood. Haemorrhoids are excessively sensitive to least touch; are specially troublesome during pregnancy, when they are bluish, hot, burn when touched and cause stitching pains. Anal pruritus and prolapse occur while passing urine.

Cardiovascular System

Heart action is weak and pulse rapid, with a tendency to intermit at every third beat. Cirrhosis of the liver may occur, associated with dropsy.

Urinary System

Bladder musculature is weak; there is delay in starting act of urination, and straining causes prolapse of anal mucosa. Or there may be frequency of urge and the passage of copious dark clear urine.

Genital System

In male, there is loss of libido and impotence. In female, menses are early and associated with anal pain. The genitalia are unduly sensitive to the least contact.

Locomotor System

There is paralytic weakness in limbs, especially the thighs, accompanied by tearing, cramping, lancinating pains and unsteady gait. Cramp-like pain occurs in the thumb muscles, better for movement. Similar pain affects the left thigh, especially when resting in sitting position. The back aches when sitting, and relief may sometimes be obtained by standing or when walking. Pain is felt in the Achilles tendon.

Skin

Voluptuous itching is felt in palm of hand. Papular or vesicular eruptions occur, accompanied by intense itching. Boils are associated with shooting pain when touched. Painful putrid ulcers with bluish margins are associated with burning at edges. Scurfy eczema occurs on the dorsal aspect of the hands. Itching and pricking may occur on the dorsum of the left foot.

MODALITIES

Is worse in damp humid weather, from contact with cold water, taking cold drinks, from least knock or jar, when at rest, and after sleep.

Obtains relief from warmth, by moving about, and when lying on the left side.

CLINICAL NOTES

The remedy is indicated in low states supervening in the course of illnesses such as diphtheria, scarlet fever, typhoid fever, septicaemia; also especially in lesions affecting mouth or anus. May be needed after recovery from the above to restore strength. Complementary remedies are Phosphoric Acid and Carbo Veg.

Natrum Muriaticum

SOURCE

The source of this powerful remedy is sodium chloride, common salt. It is noteworthy that two such active, even aggressive, elements as sodium and chlorine become relatively harmless, almost indifferent, when their atoms are bound together in a molecule of salt.

Sodium chloride is an indifferent electrolyte; in the body it is the least disturbing to the cell colloids. However, in contact with water the atoms become once more bearers of electric charges, and their active energy increases in direct proportion to the degree of dilution and subdivision. The lower three potencies should be prepared by trituration.

In nature the oceans are the main reservoir of sodium chloride; solid deposits in the earth's crust are rare.

PHARMACOLOGY

In the body, sodium chloride provides the mainstay for the regulation of the flow of water and salts by means of osmotic pressure. It belongs almost exclusively to the extracellular fluids, in striking contrast to the potassium salts which are in the main intracellular and with which the sodium chloride maintains balance.

In the body fluids the concentration of sodium chloride exceeds that of other necessary salts by a factor of 40 to 100, and it constitutes about 0.9% of those fluids. There is a stock of approximately 1½lb of this salt in the human body, the skin providing the main depot for storage. The subcutaneous tissues can apparently serve either for storage or for liberation of the salt according to the demands of the blood and other tissues. Excretion of the salt is mainly through the kidneys, but the skin also participates in this by the process of perspiration.

Maintenance of osmotic fluid balance is held to be the function of the sodium ions which remain outside the cells. Chlorine ions can penetrate into the cells and are thought to be responsible for the action of the salt in increasing oxidative metabolism. A consequence of this is, of course, emaciation, which may be associated with elevation of body temperature – salt fever.

The halogen element is also probably instrumental in causing seborrhoeic changes in the skin and a tendency to eczematous eruptions at the margin of the hair.

In general sodium chloride stimulates appetite and steps up the flow of saliva and gastric juices – Natrum Mur. subjects are usually inordinately hungry and also extremely thirsty – but excessive salt intake inhibits the secretion of hydrochloric acid in the stomach.

In the absence or diminished secretion of suprarenal corticosteroids, the body fluids become greatly depleted of sodium chloride. The condition known as Addison's disease develops with its concomitants fatigue, lethargy, irritability and progressive asthenia – a picture met with in the course of Natrum Mur. provings.

Despite its apparent harmlessness, common salt, sodium chloride, and solutions of pure salt can cause many toxic symptoms, and chlorine is considered to be the poisonous principle. Investigators have tested the effects of excessive salt intake on themselves. They became more or less seriously ill. The skin responded with inflammation, urticaria, wart-formation, becoming dry and cracked and at the same time tending to perspire freely. There was loss of hair, and nerve pains, headache, eye-pains and attacks of vertigo developed. Mucous membranes became inflamed with resulting gastro-intestinal catarrh and mucilaginous diar-rhoea. Gingivitis and gouty pains were also noted.

Connective tissue overloaded with salt undergoes a change. An excess of sodium chloride upsets the balance between the chlorides of sodium, potassium, calcium and magnesium, and demineralization ensues.

It is of particular import to note that fluctuations and variations in sodium chloride metabolism and electrolytic balance may result in alternating extremes of symptom picture.

Thus, hair may be dry or greasy, growing luxuriantly or falling rapidly; eyes may be dry or watery, sunken or bulging; the features may appear puffy or hollow and scrawny; the face may be ruddy or show distinct pallor.

The explanation for this paradoxical duality of effects lies in the fact that the remedy is two agents in one. The bipolar nature of the symptoms in different individuals, or in the same individual at different times, will result from the preponderance of effect of either the sodium or the chlorine element.

Again, the electrolytic balance may be disturbed in either of two opposite directions:
a) Over-elimination, with increased salt loss through the kidneys and skin. This leads to dehydration, weight loss and asthenic states.

b) Sodium retention as the result of diminished renal excretion. This results in waterlogged tissues, anasarca and weight gain.

It has to be realized, therefore, that the Natrum Mur. patient may exhibit puzzingly paradoxical symptoms, both physical and psychological.

PROVING

Natrum Mur. has a pathogenesis in the first edition of Hahnemann's *Chronic Diseases.*

APPEARANCE

With the foregoing in mind, it is not surprising that the appearance of the Natrum Mur. subject may vary. Often the countenance presents a pale, puffy, rather waxy look, probably due to sodium chloride stagnation in the skin. Or the face is greyish, dry-looking and wrinkled, as the result of sodium chloride depletion.

The skin has a greasy, shiny, pimply, seborrhoeic look, and may even break out in a greasy sweat during a meal. Or, again, the skin may be fine, thin, almost translucent, with prominent distended veins. White patches are common on the nails.

The whole patient appears weak, wan, wasted, demineralized, with cold clammy hands and perhaps ragged-looking hang-nails. As with Lycopodium there is a thin, scrawny appearance about the neck but lower down, below the waist, the subject is usually well-covered. But, once more, the opposite picture may present, with obesity or oedema from salt and water retention.

The lips tend to be dry, often with a crack in the centre, especially of the upper lip. The upper lip may be swollen, and herpes labialis is often observed.

The eyes may look watery with much redness of the conjunctiva.

The manner is often languid, and speech is not forthcoming. Much questioning may be required to elicit symptoms, which are divulged with reluctance. The whole patient seems almost aggressively on guard against any exposure of the ego, either mental or physical. Sympathy may result in a burst of weeping or in a display of anger in the effort of trying to hold back the tears.

PSYCHOLOGY

Children are often slow in learning to talk.

There is a tendency to oscillate emotionally from one extreme to the other. Either the subject is very depressed, terrified and miserable, or else over-excited, very bright and gaily laughing. All the senses are over-acute. Responses may be paradoxical. The mere idea of one type of emotion arouses its opposite: laughs when should be solemn; is the death's head at a feast; tears mingle with laughter.

Or an emotion may become intensified in its own direction. Thus excessive impulsion may lead to extravagant behaviour, even criminal actions.

The extreme sensitivity results in a strong aversion to fuss, sympathy and attempts at consolation. There is a desire to be alone, to be left alone and not interfered with or admonished.

Attempts at pleasantries are not appreciated, but neither is neglect or total lack of attention. A difficult, decidely independent and definitely unpredictable individual, inclined to take up new enthusiasms and later on to drop them.

There is a liability to harbour resentment over old insults and disappointments, with constant rumination; tends to dwell on every little injury, real or imagined; may shed tears in private; suffers silent grief over unrequited love or disappointed affection.

Sensitivity to noise is a prominent feature, especially to sudden noises or those of a scratchy, squeaky or rasping nature. Sensitivity also to music, which may please or irritate.

Fear may be obtrusive, even panic, felt especially in closed spaces, such as tube trains, caves or phone boxes. Another fear is that of robbers or interlopers, driving the individual to look under the bed, in the wardrobe and so on, to 'make sure'.

The possibility of underlying emotional stress, even remote emotional shock, must always be borne in mind.

PHYSIOLOGY

The subjects of this remedy are usually chilly and often complain of patchy coldness, perhaps on the vertex or round the heart, or from the knees downwards, or as if 'a cold wind was blowing through the head'. They do, however, thoroughly enjoy cold, sunny, frosty weather.

The appetite is often ravenous, but despite 'eating like a horse' the individual remains thin and does not put on weight. On the other hand, appetite may be entirely lacking with an aversion especially to fat, meat and bread. There is a desire for salt, possibly excessive, also for fish, milk and bitter things. Intolerance may be present in relation to bread, fat, rich food, eggs, starches and honey.

Thirst is liable to be unquenchable, especially for tea.

Sleep is apt to be disturbed by the relentless recurrence of unpleasant thoughts, and this despite unconquerable drowsiness during the course of the evening, especially after a heavy meal.

Sweats usually occur in the second half of the night.

SYMPTOMATOLOGY

General

Symptoms tend to be excessive in nature, rather than mild. Periodicity also is a frequent feature, with recurrence at the same hour each day, or perhaps every weekend. Again, symptoms may show much inconsistency, at one time perhaps suggesting hyperthyroidism, at another corresponding with hypocortinism. Or at times showing great dryness of mucous membranes and at other times much catarrh and excess of normal secretions. A condition of anaemia associated with depletion of body fluids is accompanied by very easy exhaustion from quite trifling cause and by a distressing sensation of throbbing all over. Tiredness is frequent and especially noticed in the morning.

Head

These symptoms are important. Giddiness is associated with a tendency to fall forwards or to the left, and is relieved by lying down. Headaches are various and severe. They are apt to be induced by railway travel with accompanying nausea and vomiting. They often result from delay in the usual meal time. The headache is often frontal or else unilateral, of migraine type with associated pallor, nausea and vomiting. It tends to be worse from sunrise to noon, but may last till sunset, or continue for two or three days. The pain may be described as throbbing or 'beating like little hammers', perhaps accompanied by a bursting feeling and made worse by every movement of the eyes. Some relief is afforded by lying down, by vomiting, as a result of sweating, and sometimes after sleep. Tingling and numbness of lips, tongue and nose may precede the headache, and it is often associated with dryness of the tongue and terrific thirst. The headache may be brought on by thunder, or by eye strain or by emotional stress. It is often associated with spots or fiery zigzags in front of the eyes, or even temporary loss of vision. Periodic recurrence is common.

Eyes

Vision tends to 'give out' while reading or sewing; the letters or stitches run together. The eyeballs may feel 'too large'. Spasmodic closure of the lids occurs, and the lids feel stiff on attempting to move them. There is a sensation of 'grit in the eye', and the eyes are apt to water profusely in the wind.

Ears
This remedy shares with Elaps and Nitric Acid the complaint of 'crackling in the ears' when chewing.

Respiratory System
There is a great tendency to recurrent colds. These often start with excessive sneezing accompanied by a profuse flow of clear watery discharge, much lachrymation and loss of taste and smell. The free discharge tends to give place to nasal blockage. Chronic nasal and nasopharyngeal catarrh may ensue, with thick mucoid discharge like white of egg. This is usually worse in the morning, giving rise to much hawking of mucus. There may be a complaint of hoarseness and a very persistent tickle in the throat or in the trachea, causing a cough, often accompanied by headache. The throat may feel 'plugged' and food seems to be 'swallowed over a lump'. The lungs may feel 'too tight'.

Alimentary System
The gums tend to be unhealthy. Lips and mouth are either excessively dry or, possibly, there may be copious salivation. Herpetic eruptions are common around the mouth; aphthous ulcers may occur on the tongue and the buccal aspect of the cheeks. The lips are apt to become swollen at frequent intervals. Food lacks taste. Dyspeptic symptoms occur, accompanied by a weak sinking sensation in the stomach. An important modality here is amelioration from tightening the clothes in spite of accompanying flatulence. This is contrary to the usual inclination to loosen the clothes associated with the flatulence of Lycopodium or Nux Vomica. There may also be complaint of a 'lump in the stomach' after meals, which seem to take a long time to digest. The remedy may be called for in acute gastric upset characterized by attacks of vomiting. The vomiting is arduous and productive of white slimy mucus, possibly streaked with blood. An actual gastric ulcer may be present; if so, it is usually situated at the cardiac end or on the lesser curvature. With these gastric symptoms the tongue may present a 'mapped' appearance, coated with clear areas as if the coating had been stripped off in patches. Or the tongue appears red and shiny with small flecks of frothy saliva along the edges. Chronic watery diarrhoea may occur, aggravated by moving about and by eating starchy food. It may be associated with a horrid dragging

sensation in the belly as if everything was sagging downwards. The condition may be a chronic colitis and associated with enlargement of the liver. Constipation, if present, is associated with dry stools, passed only with great effort. Naturally enough under these circumstances there is a liability to anal fissure with accompanying bleeding, burning and soreness.

Cardiovascular System

The remedy may be called for when there is a feeling of cardiac distress associated with fluttering sensation and faintness. This is worse in a warm room and when lying on the left side. Relief is obtained in the open air. Or there may be a complaint of very violent palpitations which shake the whole body. Pulsations and flushes extend to the chest and head, while the legs remain cold. An intermittent pulse may be noticed, every third beat being missed.

Urinary System

A feature of this remedy is the inability to urinate in the presence of other people, owing to nervous spasm of the sphincter urinae. Cutting pain may be felt in the urethra after passing water. Involuntary loss of urine may occur when walking, or coughing, or sneezing. This is associated with a general slackness and atonia of the pelvic organs. Polyuria or diabetes insipidus may call for this remedy.

Genital System

Menstrual disorders are frequently met with in the Natrum Mur. subject, and in this sphere also manifest opposite polarities. The periods may be too early and too profuse, or on the other hand may be delayed, with only scanty flow. There is often an associated low back pain, which is relieved by sitting or lying down with a firm pillow or other support in the hollow of the back. Uterine prolapse may occur with considerable distress, which is worse on rising in the morning, and may compel the sufferer to sit down and cross one thigh over the other for support.

Locomotor System

Tremor may result from over-use in writing or other activity, or may be induced by emotional stress. Backache is common and the back 'feels broken'. The feet feel heavy as if 'full of lead'. There may be a sensation as of 'water trickling into a joint'. Atrophic changes lead to local weakness of muscles. Sclerotic changes may produce conditions such as Dupuytren's contracture.

Skin

Disorders of salt metabolism are liable to cause quite a variety of skin affections. Eczematous eruptions are specially common behind the ears and at the hair margins. These are often accompanied by a glutinous exudate which mats the hair. Herpetic eruptions frequently affect the region of the mouth, and may also occur on arms and thighs or in flexures. Urticarial lesions may occur showing large red blotches which itch, burn and smart. They are liable to be present in proximity to joints and are aggravated by taking exercise. The skin of the fingers may be dry with a tendency to form cracks. Other degenerative lesions may occur such as brown or black pigmented warts, palmar warts, atrophic spots on nose, face, ears and orbits. Dandruff, alopecia, acne, boils, pustular eruptions may also call for consideration of the remedy, especially if the lesions are symmetrical.

MODALITIES

Aggravation is caused by extremes of temperature, by hot sun or radiant heat from a hot stove, also by a warm, stuffy atmosphere. Aggravation may be marked at the seaside, but here again the reverse may be the case. Physical exertion may aggravate. There is aversion to walking and also touch or pressure and the recumbent posture. Over-excitement or emotional or mental stress make things worse, and the patient is usually worse after sleep. There is peak aggravation at 11 a.m. Symptoms are worse during and towards the end of the menstrual period.

The patient feels better in the open air, on bright sunny days, when fasting, after a sweat, by washing in cold water, and as the result of gentle exercise which does not over-heat.

CLINICAL NOTES

Low potencies are said to be ineffectual. On the other hand, the higher potencies administered to the hard-pressed over-tense city dweller are liable to give rise to aggravation. In this case it is better to start with medium potencies and proceed to higher, if repetition is called for.

In any case it is wiser not to administer the remedy during an acute exacerbation, for instance of severe headache, but to give it in between attacks. Bryonia is the acute of Natrum Mur.

The remedy is frequently of great value if there is a history of malarial infection, or even of much dosing with quinine. It is indicated also in acute malaria.

Natrum Sulphuricum

SOURCE

This remedy is a preparation of sodium sulphate – Glauber's salts – which occurs in large, colourless, transparent, prismatic crystals. The crystals are deliquescent, melting in warm air in their own water of crystallization. The salt constitutes the chief ingredient of many mineral spa waters.

PHARMACOLOGY

Sodium is one of the big four – potassium, sodium, magnesium and calcium – on the relations of which depends the maintenance of optimal electrolyte balance in the body fluids. The sulphate is not so readily absorbed as the chloride, but its involvement in electrolytic imbalance may lead to waterlogging of the tissues and catarrhal states.

The claim that this salt stimulates intestinal and biliary secretions has not been substantiated. Its action on the bowel in inducing purgation is due to retention of the water content of the ingesta as the result of retarded absorption. There may be an additional increase of fluid content in the bowel as the result of withdrawal of water from the blood, owing to increase in osmotic pressure. The net effect is to cause distension of the bowel with fluid and consequent increased rate of downward propulsion with hyperactive peristalsis.

The ensuing dehydration and associated malnutrition tend to produce physical debility and mental depression.

PROVING

Natrum Sulph. was first proved by Schieler and Nenning, and published in Hering's *Materia Medica*.

APPEARANCE

A sallow, pimply complexion of earthy hue is described.

There is an air of depression, accompanied by definite disinclination to indulge in conversation.

There is obvious weakness, perhaps associated with trembling or twitching in the limbs.

The tongue shows a dirty yellow coating towards the root. Discharges are green or yellow in colour.

Despite the debility there is a restless urge to keep constantly changing position or moving about.

Audible rumbling in the belly may be noticed.

PSYCHOLOGY

The subject is restless, discontented, tired of life; may have to use restraint to keep from committing suicide.

There is aversion to meeting people and to talk. The individual is sensitive and suspicious, and apt to harbour feelings of hate and vengefulness. There is fear of people, of crowds, of evil.

There is great sensitivity to noise; music may be intolerable, even inducing tears. Depression is worse in the morning; it may take the shape of despair of recovery.

Is always worse when the weather turns wet; change of scene or circumstances gives some relief.

PHYSIOLOGY

The characteristic feature about Natrum Sulph. subjects is a marked susceptibility to every change from dry to wet weather. They cannot tolerate sea air, and are unable to digest plants which grow near water. They feel best on dry days.

Appetite is usually poor, perhaps with a repugnance to food. There may be an acquired aversion to bread.

Food intolerances include vegetables, fruit, pastry, cold dishes, cold drinks, anything grown near water.

Thirst varies; there may be considerable thirst for cold, iced water, despite the fact that it disagrees. A dry mouth may be associated with lack of thirst.

Drowsiness is usual during the daytime. At night there is a liability to start awake in fear shortly after dropping off to sleep.

Sweating is unaccompanied by thirst.

SYMPTOMATOLOGY

General

Pains are tearing, shooting, boring or jerking in character; they are often accompanied by a sense of oppression in the chest, which is worse in the

357

evening or at night. Oedematous states occur, possibly associated with yellow, watery or mucoid discharges. Marked weariness of the body forces the subject to lie down. Symptoms of ague are accompanied by bilious vomiting, induced and aggravated by damp. Periodicity of symptoms is common, e.g. violent colic recurring at 2 a.m., asthma attacks coming on at 4 a.m. to 5 a.m., onset of diarrhoea at 9 a.m. Recovery after an illness tends to be slow. Symptoms are predominantly left-sided.

Head

An attack of giddiness at 6 p.m. may be accompanied by acid vomiting. A sensation of heat may be noticed on top of the head. Another sensation described is as if the brain were loose inside the skull. Severe headache of the bursting or splitting variety is aggravated by mental effort, by use of the arms, when walking, by coughing, by vomiting, and during the menstrual period. Some relief is obtained by lying down in the quiet and by firm pressure of the hand. The scalp is unduly sensitive and a creeping sensation may be felt in it. A boring sensation occurs in the facial bones. Violent pains in the head and in the nape may follow a head injury, or may be related to injury incurred at a remote date in the past. Periodic headaches occur in association with stomach or liver complaints, and are accompanied by bilious vomiting. The remedy may be called for in relation to cerebrospinal meningitis associated with lateral decubitus.

Eyes

Pain may be experienced in the eyes when reading by artificial light. Eye complaints may be accompanied by thick, green discharges, agglutination of the lids in the morning, and an extreme degree of photophobia. Eyes burn and eyeballs seem to radiate heat; there may be a crawling sensation in the eyes; the lids feel as heavy as lead. All eye symptoms are worse near the fire, but rubbing affords some relief. Scintillations may be noticed before the eyes on blowing the nose.

Ears

A sensation of forceful outward pressure may be felt in the ears. Sudden violent stitches occur in the ears. A sensation of boring may be felt behind the ears. Chirping sounds in the ears occur in the evening. There may be noises as of bells tinkling in the distance. The remedy may be called for in purulent otitis media.

Respiratory System

Nasal catarrh is associated with profuse, thick, green, tenacious, offensive, blood-streaked discharge. The nostrils become obstructed with thick mucus at night. There may be much itching of the alae nasi. Boring pain is felt at the root of the nose. This is likely to be associated with sinus involvement. Post-nasal discharge is associated with much hawking of salty mucus in the morning. A choking feeling may be noticed in the throat when walking, perhaps in association with thyroid enlargement. A loose cough is accompanied by soreness and pain in the left side of the chest, much greenish, mucopurulent sputum and noisy râles. The cough is painful and may cause the sufferer to spring up in bed and hold on to the chest with both hands, a symptom shared with Drosera. The cough is worse in damp weather, when lying down, and at 3 to 4 a.m. It is somewhat better when sitting up, and may be paroxysmal. There is often an all-gone feeling in the chest, associated with a frequent desire to take a deep breath; this is especially so in damp evening air. Asthmatic attacks occur with every change to wet weather or at the seaside, and are apt to be associated with bronchial catarrh.

Alimentary System

Tongue feels burning, and may be thickly coated with greenish brown fur. Extremely sensitive blisters occur on tongue or palate; the soreness is relieved by taking cold food or fluids. Much slimy or sticky salty mucus is present in the mouth. Gums become ulcerated and burn. Toothache is aggravated by warmth or by taking hot drinks; it is relieved by inhaling cold air, by holding cold water in the mouth, and by smoking tobacco. Nausea occurs in the morning, associated with hiccough; it is not relieved by vomiting. Stomach upsets are associated with a tendency to regurgitation of food ingested; quantities of thick, viscid, slimy mucus are hawked up. There is persistent nausea with vomiting of green bile. Much bloating of the belly occurs with great aversion to anything tight around the waist; both belching and passage of flatus afford relief. Borborygmus is marked. A dragging sensation is felt in the right hypochondrium when lying on the left side. Pain and soreness is located in the right iliac fossa, associated with colic. The liver may be enlarged, painful, with stabbing pains, and hurts if touched or jarred, as when walking. The remedy may be called for in relation to the presence of gallstones. Acute diarrhoea occurs after the early cup of tea, with stools like a jet from a hose, watery, spluttery, yellow and burning. Chronic diarrhoea also occurs, with a stool at the same time each day, usually soon after rising in the morning (compare the early morning diarrhoea of

Sulphur, which drives from bed). The stools are thick, watery, gushing and spluttery, accompanied by the passage of enormous quantities of flatus, and may be associated with pain in the region of the descending colon. The stools may on occasion be passed involuntarily.

Lymphatic and Glandular Systems
Lymphadenitis shows a tendency to suppurative lesions.

Urinary System
Chronic urethritis is associated with thick, greenish-yellow painless discharge. The remedy may be called for in relation to post-exanthematous nephritis, glycosuria, polyuria, phosphaturia, nocturnal frequency, burning and cutting sensation both during and after urination. It is of value in relation to enlargement of the prostate. The urine may show a white sandy deposit, a copious jelly-like sediment, or a brick red or yellowish deposit. There may be excess of uric acid in the urine; much urging to urinate with cutting pain at the meatus and a sticking pain in the groin.

Genital System
Menses tend to be scanty, late and associated with colic and constipation. The flow is only in the morning, is acrid, contains clots and excoriates the thighs.

Nervous System
The remedy is indicated in Jacksonian epilepsy following a head injury. Tremors of hands may occur on waking or when writing.

Locomotor System
Limbs tend to feel bruised and weary. There are sudden onsets of heaviness of the arms, tearings or shootings in the hands and fingers, trembling and weakness of hands with inability to hold anything at all weighty, tinglings in finger tips. Sharp pains occur in the hips on stooping or when rising from sitting, and at night. Tearing pains, heat and pulling sensations are felt in the legs, especially in the calf muscles and the Achilles tendon. Lancinating pains occur in the heels. There is much unease or actual pain in the feet; possibly violent itching of and between the toes, especially on removing shoes and stockings at night. Is apt to constantly move the feet in search of relief. The limbs are often extremely restless in bed. Pain and stiffness may affect the temporo-mandibular joint, also the muscles of the neck. Pains spreading from

nape to occiput may be so violent as to extort cries; the pains are made worse by movement, but relieved by massage. Stabbing pains occur between the shoulder blades. Fingers may become swollen and stiff. Sharp pains, burning or numbness may affect the toes; these are relieved by rubbing. The soles of the feet are apt to burn at night.

Skin
Vesicles or pimples may occur on face or chin and burn when touched. An itching eczematous eruption may occur on the face, with watery oozing. A generalized pruritus is aggravated on taking off the clothes. The remedy is indicated in paronychia, which may tend to be recurrent. Other conditions calling for its use are chronic sinuses, with undermined edges; psoriasis of palms; raw, sore palms which exude a watery discharge; gonorrhoeal warts; intertrigo; red wart-like excrescences all over the body. A sensation is described as of 'blood trickling down the legs'.

MODALITIES

The outstanding modality is aggravation from damp in any form, cold wet weather, even warm weather if humidity is high, seaside, damp dwellings, proximity to water. Is worse when lying on the left side, and often has to turn on to back; worse for contact, tight clothing, when at rest, in early morning, in the spring.

There is relief in warm dry weather, from firm pressure, from change of posture (for a short while), in open air.

CLINICAL NOTES

Causal factors which may point to the possible use of the remedy are emotional strain from nursing relations for a prolonged period; the onset of humid weather; a head injury with or without loss of consciousness, which may have occurred some years before the present illness.

Complementary remedies are Arsenicum Alb. and Thuja.

Nitricum Acidum

SOURCE
This remedy is prepared from nitric acid, *aqua fortis*, an extremely corrosive acid which on contact stains the tissues yellow.

PHARMACOLOGY
The acid possesses a destructive, ulcerating affinity with skin and mucous membranes, especially at the mucocutaneous junctions, resulting in cracks, rhagades and fissures.

PROVING
Nitric Acid was first proved by Hahnemann in the 30th potency, and published in the second edition of his *Chronic Diseases*.

APPEARANCE
The face appears pale, pinched, bluish or sallow in complexion, with dark rings round the orbits. The eyes are lack-lustre in expression and the pupils are large. The visage is deeply lined. The subject is likely to be emaciated with obvious weakness manifested by a constant desire to sit or lie down. The limbs show tremors or twitching of muscles. In fevers the pulse is apt to be intermittent.

Discharges are offensive, thin, excoriating and possibly of a dirty yellowish-green colour.

PSYCHOLOGY
Is depressed and anxious, especially in the evening. Worries about disease; fears death; feels tired of life.

Easily startled; the least thing annoys; intolerant of sympathy. Is hypersensitive to noise, pain, touch, any jolt or jar.

May be obstinate, taciturn, or exhibit vindictiveness.

Memory is poor; thoughts vanish when attempting to concentrate.

PHYSIOLOGY
Feels chilly and shivery, even near the fire; has cold hands and feet; feels chilly on getting into bed.

Craves both fat and salt; has also a fondness for herrings and may show perversions of appetite with a desire for chalk, lime, earth and so on. Bread may disagree.

Thirst may be unexpectedly absent in fevers.

Tends to be drowsy during the day. At night may wake about 2 a.m. and stay awake; may get out of bed to pace the floor; sometimes starts suddenly awake in fear. Is apt to wake with a headache and pain in the nape of the neck.

Profuse sweats occur on hands and feet, especially at night in the latter half; the sweats are very exhausting and malodorous.

SYMPTOMATOLOGY

General

A prominent feature is extreme weakness, exhaustion, even cachexia; this is accompanied by sweating, soreness in bones and shortness of breath. Peculiar sharp, splinter-like pains accompany lesions, and both come and go with suddenness. These peculiar pains are touched off by contact, by movement, when swallowing, when passing a stool, or from contact of dressings with the surface of an ulcer. Haemorrhages are apt to occur from any mucous surface and are usually of bright blood. Complaints may derive from loss of sleep or night-watching.

Head

Darting pains occur in the forehead, radiating to jaws and ears. Head is very sensitive; pressure of hat is resented; combing the hair is painful. Head feels as if constricted by a tight band or as if compressed from side to side as by a vice. Moist, burning, offensive, haemorrhagic eruptions occur on the scalp. Alopecia may be prominent, the hair coming out in handfuls.

Eyes

Eyes smart, feel hot and full of grit; water profusely. There may be double vision. There is difficulty in opening the eyes in the morning. The remedy may be called for in ophthalmia neonatorum, or with syphilitic iritis.

Ears

Ears crack when chewing. Deafness is less severe when riding in a car or in a train. Ears feel stopped up; are very sensitive to the noise of traffic. Otitis media is accompanied by discharge of foetid ichorous pus.

Respiratory System

There is a great liability to constant colds; no sooner is one recovered from than another follows. Contact with the least draught brings on a bout of sneezing. The nasal discharge is acrid, yellow, offensive and watery at night. The nasal catarrh is often accompanied by swelling of the upper lip and violent itching inside the nose. Ozaena may be present with discharge of green crusts. Ulcerative tonsillitis may occur, possibly associated with a membranous exudate and bad breath. There is a sensation as if a fishbone were stuck in the throat. Painless aphonia may occur. A dry tickle in the larynx gives rise to a paroxysmal cough, which is aggravated by laughing or crying and also when lying down at night; it is worse in a warm room. A dry barking cough may be accompanied by haemoptysis of dark blood and clots. There may be sputum which is sticky and glue-like, containing greenish white plugs, or offensive, sanious, purulent and of a dirty green colour. A burning sensation may be noticed in the chest; the chest may feel as if bound by an iron band. The muscles of the chest feel sore and bruised.

Alimentary System

Blisters and vesicles are present on and around the lips. The corners of the mouth are apt to be cracked, ulcerated and crusted. Stomatitis occurs with the presence of aphthae, ptyalism and swollen spongy gums.

Foetor oris is present. The mandibular joints crack when chewing. Food seems to stick in the throat; splinter-like pains are felt when swallowing, extending to the ears. Nausea and sweating may follow a meal. The liver may be painful, possibly in association with jaundice. There is a constant ineffectual urge to stool, and faeces when passed are not hard. Stools may be green, slimy and offensive. The passage of the stool may be accompanied by pain as if the rectum would be torn asunder; the pain persists after the stool is passed, continuing perhaps for some hours. This is so even with a soft stool. Diarrhoea tends to be chronic and accompanied by great weakness. Piles are extremely sore and liable to bleed and prolapse with every stool. Anal fissure is associated with constant oozing of foetid moisture, much burning at stool, and after the stool smarting as if cut with a knife.

Cardiovascular System

There is very easy palpitation; also a tendency to intermittent pulse.

Lymphatic and Glandular Systems

Involvement of lymph nodes is common, especially in the cervical and axillary regions. Lumps occur in the breasts; the nipples show fissures which are accompanied by much tenderness and by splinter-like pains.

Urinary System

Frequency occurs, with scalding on urination. The urine is apt to be dark brown, scanty and strong-smelling, like horse's urine. The urine feels cold as passed.

Genital System

Libido is increased in both sexes, but not to the intense degree met with in Cantharis. In men urethritis may become chronic. Balanitis may be present or paraphimosis with inflammation. There is loss of pubic hair. In women, pruritus vulvae may be severe, aggravated by cold. There is easy haemorrhage from the uterus. Menstrual periods are early and profuse; the flow is dark and thick; the period is accompanied by extensive malaise. The parts become fissured and bleed easily; warts and condylomata may occur. Extremely sensitive urethral caruncle may be present.

Locomotor System

Joints crack on movement. Soreness or boring pains are felt in bones, especially skull and tibia; these are worse with every change in the weather. Exostoses may be present.

Skin

Jagged bleeding warts and condylomata occur. Ulcers are of rapidly spreading type, deep, punched out with irregular borders and offensive discharge; the base is filled with exuberant granulations which bleed at the least contact. The ulcers are associated with sticking or burning pains, aggravated by contact with cold water. Coppery eruptions may occur.

MODALITIES

There is aggravation from cold, wind, thunder, change of temperature or weather; also from washing or bathing; from sweating; while walking; in the evening after midnight, on waking from sleep.

There is some relief on lying down; feels better when driving smoothly in a car.

CLINICAL NOTES

The leading indication for the use of this remedy is a lesion at one or other mucocutaneous junction, especially if associated with the typical splinter-like pains. It was formerly found to be of value in the treatment of syphilis, notably secondary lesions. It should be considered in typhoid fever complicated by haemorrhage and with an intermittent pulse.

Complementary remedies are Arsenicum Alb. and Caladium.

Nux Vomica

SOURCE

This remedy is obtained from the well-known *Strychnos nux vomica* or poison nut plant. It is a tree of the Loganiaceae family, found growing in the East Indies, the Malay archipelago and northern Australia. It has a crooked trunk and irregular, somewhat ataxic-looking branches, with a smooth ash-coloured bark. The leaves are large, four inches long and three inches broad, ovate, short-stalked, shiny and smooth on both aspects. The flowers are small, funnel-shaped, greeny white, in small terminal cymes. They bloom in the cold season and have a disagreeable odour. The fruit is an orange yellow globular berry, about the size of a large apple, having a hard rind, and filled with a soft, white, jelly-like pulp containing five seeds. These are disc-shaped, up to three-quarters of an inch in diameter, and covered with a soft woolly substance. They have been dubbed Quaker's buttons, though anything less Quaker-like than the typical Nux Vomica subject would be difficult to imagine.

The dried seeds are used in preparing the mother tincture. They are exceedingly bitter and contain, among other alkaloids, brucine and strychnine. Other constituents are a glucoside, loganin, caffeotannic acid, fatty matter and a trace of copper.

PHARMACOLOGY

The tissue affinities of the drug are largely associated with the action of the alkaloid strychnine, which has a marked effect on the nervous system. Its poisonous symptoms are only too well known as the result of its use as a homicidal poison and in connection with destruction of animal pests. They are vividly described by Schenk – 'Strychnine can lead to an atrocious death. Doses of 10 to 20 milligram lead to dyspnoea and unbearable feelings of anxiety (this is a marked symptom in the early stage of tetanus). Twitching and spasms gradually develop and lead to violent tetanic seizures in which the head is often bent right to the buttocks, so that the spine may be broken, as in insulin shock.

'Breathing may cease for intervals of one to two minutes at a time; in this event the seizures may also stop, only to recommence at the least excitation – a loud noise or a gentle touch – until death from exhaustion finally supervenes. No death could be worse than this and no man is likely to endure greater agonies.

'Despite the virulence of the poison, strychnine habituation may develop. Preparations of the drug may be taken medicinally for many years, until one day the patient is suddenly struck dead by convulsions.'

Strychnine is poisonous to almost all common animals and birds, but cats are remarkably tolerant to the poison and snails are unaffected by it.

The action of the poison on the motor elements of the pons and spinal cord results in exaggerated motor responses to sensory stimuli; probably by lowering the threshold for impulse transmission through inhibition of the activity of choline-esterase, the enzyme which normally controls the flow of acetylcholine. The latter is responsible for the transmission of nerve impulses at synapses and myoneural junctions.

A further effect involving the sensory elements of the nervous system induces enhanced sensitivity to all stimuli, with abnormal acuteness of all senses, especially that of touch.

The excessive excitability of the nervous system, while resulting initially in muscle spasm, leads at a later stage to exhaustion and paralysis. This is an instance of the phenomenon of dual effect: two opposite reactions being brought about by one and the same drug, which at different stages, or meeting varying degrees of tissue susceptibility, can swing the balance of function in either of two opposite directions towards hyper-activity or towards hypo-activity.

Pharmacologically, therefore, the drug suggests tension, increased tone of muscles, increased response to irritation. It is noteworthy that mental tension is accompanied by and associated with muscle tension – the one can scarcely be present without the other. Moreover, the increased muscle tonus affects not only the skeletal muscles, leading to clenched jaws and jerky limbs, but also involves the plain muscle in the walls of blood-vessels and gut. This is of great import, as the consequent disturbance of steady adequate blood-flow to every cell in the body, with resulting impairment of oxygen supply and inadequate removal of waste products, can be responsible for a wide range of physical disorders and distress.

PROVING

Nux Vomica was proved by Hahnemann, and he describes its pathogenesis in the third editon of the first volume of *Materia Medica Pura*.

Nux Vomica

APPEARANCE

In general the Nux Vomica patient is spare, lean, active, 'on his mark', appearing hearty and full of life.

The complexion is usually sallow, possibly with a red flush super-imposed, a dusky flush, not bright red.

The visage is lined and there may be a dark shadow under the eyes. Movements are brisk and jerky. Talks, eats, walks, does everything, rapidly.

Another type is mentioned – a slow, studious, wary-looking indivi-dual, who looks as if he sat up all night reading; slouching gait, prominent belly and appears thoroughly miserable.

With fever the sufferer appears to be boiling hot, with a very red countenance, but nevertheless feels extremely chilly and desires plenty of covering. When exhausted, the limbs may show tremors.

PSYCHOLOGY

A tense, over-anxious individual; full of zeal but often irresolute and jittery. Is very apt to feel frustrated by his limitations, with resulting discontentedness.

He may be scheming, even malicious. Is disposed to pick a quarrel, highly irritable and must have an outlet. Liable, therefore, to sudden outbursts of peevish rage, and takes it out on the furniture, or his family or associates. He feels better after a good blow-up.

The Nux Vomica patient is over-sensitive to touch, pain, noise, odours, music, food, even medicines; he finds things or people intolerable and gets very sorry for himself, but curiously is not usually very worried over his health.

He is fussy over order and accuracy, quite tidy, tends to overdo things and gets unduly exasperated over trifles. If startled may turn round and curse the offender. He resents consolation and cannot stand contradic-tion. Gets impatient with others but shows a lack of perseverance in himself.

There is a peculiar fear of knives, the sight of a handy weapon begetting an impulse to kill. Is liable to a sudden unaccountable urge to do some violent act.

As one author puts it – 'Nux Vomica is a drug for the highly civilized races, for town dwellers and those who under the stress of life develop both physical and mental symptoms. They are often sedentary brain workers, more inclined to the waste of nervous tissue than of muscular; persons who get through their work largely on stimulants.'

PHYSIOLOGY

The Nux Vomica subject feels the cold terribly, is permanently chilly, hugs the fire, cannot get warm even in bed. Is averse to the least draught or exposure; even if the body is burning hot, still cannot make any movement or uncover the smallest area without feeling chilly. Nevertheless he does object to being in a stuffy airless atmosphere.

He feels extra tense before a thunderstorm and simply hates the wind, even the sound of it.

Appetite is most unreliable; tends to be that of the gourmet rather than the gourmand. There may be complete anorexia with a loathing towards all food, or a ravenous hunger, especially just before a nervous crisis.

There is a desire for fat, tasty foods, alcohol, beer, condiments. Meat and milk tend to disagree, as also coffee, which causes a sleepless night. Cold food is not appreciated; even talking about cold food may cause a pain in the belly.

Feels better by taking food, but only in a small amount. If eats more gets a feeling of fullness and weight in the stomach, accompanied by the inclination to yawn.

Owing to the hypersensitivity of all senses, sleep tends to be light and cat-nappy, much disturbed by frightful or horrific dreams, from which the subject wakes feeling anxious and apprehensive. There is a tendency to awake in the small hours feeling pretty good, then, after lying awake for a spell, to drop off again and wake later feeling tired and headachy.

Drowsiness is common after lunch and also in the evening, with a heavy feeling in the eyes. May sleep on the back with one or other arm placed under the head. Often sleeps with the mouth open and is apt to dribble saliva. Seems to require a lot of sleep.

Perspiration is not a marked feature. Profuse sweats may occur in the morning, but not involving the face.

SYMPTOMATOLOGY

General

In general, complaints calling for Nux Vomica may be induced by prolonged mental or emotional strain or, on the other hand, by over-indulgence in food or drink, especially if associated with lack of sufficient exercise. Nux Vomica pains are variously described as shooting, tearing, jerking, stitching, but are characteristically insupportable, driving the sufferer frantic, as is the case with the pain of Chamomilla and Coffea. Limbs and joints feel bruised, constricted, numb, heavy, even paralysed.

These symptoms are worse when lying still in bed and are relieved to some extent by getting up. The sudden onset of extreme weakness or exhaustion may force the sufferer to sit or lie down. A somewhat similar type of exhaustion is met with under Arsenicum Alb. and Phosphorus. As regards laterality, abdominal symptoms tend to be right-sided and chest symptoms left-sided.

Head

A plethora of symptoms are described. One type of vertigo comes on while in bed and persists in the open air. Momentary blackouts may occur, especially when standing or walking. Malaise is brought on by exposure of the head to cold air or cold draughts. The 'hangover' type of headache is described under this remedy, occipital in site or over one or other eye; it is accompanied by nausea and a loathing of food, tobacco, coffee; it is aggravated on attempting to get up in the morning and from any exertion; some relief is obtained by warmth, quiet, holding the head in a firm grip or pressing it against something hard. The head feels muzzy and confused. The remedy is also related to a facial neuralgia associated with watery discharge from the eye and nostril on the affected side.

Eyes

Eye symptoms which may call for the remedy are various – severe photophobia in the morning; gushing of water from the eye when the lids are forced apart; burning, smarting and itching, especially at the inner canthus, with some relief by rubbing; much lachrymation; discharge of purulent secretion, especially from the canthi; complaints of sparks or greyish spots before the eyes. Toxic amaurosis from abuse of tobacco or alcohol may call for Nux Vomica.

Ears

Itching in the middle ear and in the pharyngo-tympanic canal causes frequent swallowing in search of relief. Pains as of sharp blows may be felt in the ear, worse in bed and first thing in the morning. Noises seem exaggerated, even the speaker's own voice sounds too loud.

Respiratory System

The remedy is of great use in coryzal troubles which are worse indoors and better in the open air. The nose is alternately dry and blocked or pouring profusely with a watery discharge from one or both nostrils. Fluid coryza by day gives place to complete obstruction at night, especially on the side next to the pillow. There is much distressing sneezing, with hot face and raw throat. The sense of smell is very acute, so much so that a very strong odour may cause fainting. Odd smells may be detected without adequate source. Sore throat is accompanied by shootings and stitches which are worse when not swallowing, and the throat feels raw and scarified. Complaint is made of a sensation of tightness across the chest, aggravated by walking or going uphill.

Under the remedy is described a dry cough due to a tiresome tickle; it is worse from midnight to dawn, and is accompanied by a bursting headache; a drink of warm fluid gives some relief to the cough, but the act of drinking induces fresh chilliness.

Alimentary System

A tension symptom sometimes met with is a form of dysphagia, when the food seems to stick some way down the oesophagus, causing discomfort, and then regurgitates without any actual pain. In the mouth the gums become swollen and sore, with loosening of the teeth. Actual toothache may be brought on by a chill, and is aggravated by cold air, cold fluids, and worse immediately after a meal; warmth gives relief. The tongue is apt to be coated in the posterior half, and there is an unpleasant, even putrid, taste in the mouth.

There is a tendency in Nux Vomica subjects to sudden flushing during a meal, especially if taking a favourite dish; the sufferer becomes hot and sweaty, and after the meal is unconscionably heavy and drowsy. Again, if taking a meal accompanied by plenty of alcohol and in a hot atmosphere, there may be a sudden onset of acute gastric distension, faintness, dusky colour in face, and the necessity to loosen the clothes round the waist. In this condition a dose of Nux Vomica gives very rapid relief. If worried or chivvied, indigestion is apt to ensue, atonic in type, but accompanied by pyloric spasm with resultant sensation of weight or stone in the epigastrium, queasiness after food or in the morning, nausea with much ineffectual retching and gagging, and vomiting of food as soon as swallowed. The vomiting is difficult and distressing but does afford relief. Pain in the region of the stomach may occur 1 to 1½ hours after food, either a dull ache or violent and cramping; it is accompanied by a sense of constriction round the waist, and the clothes have to be loosened; the pain is apt to spread to the chest and also to the back between the shoulderblades or down the back to the anus. Heartburn, pyrosis, waterbrash occur, associated with gagging and retching, and ultimately actual vomiting which gives relief. Flatulent distension accompanied by colic is aggravated by eating or drinking.

Liver complaints, possibly accompanied by jaundice, may be brought on by anger. In febrile states there is a tendency to jaundice with enlargement of the liver and a feeling of distension in the epigastrium. Cutting or pinching pains occur in the belly, resulting from spasticity and irregular peristalsis; these pains are relieved by sitting or lying down. Biliary duct spasm with its severe pain increased by movement and pressure, but somewhat relieved by heat, calls for Nux Vomica. By contrast the pain of Colocynthis is better for pressure. Rectal symptoms are a constant ineffectual urge to stool, scanty mucoid stools associated with a feeling of incomplete evacuation, spasm of anal sphincters, and proctalgia. Morning diarrhoea may occur with slimy sanious stools; the passage of the stool is very difficult. The stool may be watery with hard lumps covered by mucus. The passage of the stool affords temporary relief. Diarrhoea may alternate with constipation. Piles are aggravated by mental exertion and resulting rectal congestion; they cause pressive pain in the rectum after meals, pain too after stool and accompanying constipation. Bleeding piles are associated with hypersecretion of rectal mucus. Pruritus recti and ani may also be troublesome.

Cardiovascular System
The vasospasm or other circulatory irregularities associated with mental tension may give rise to palpitations. This is especially noticed when lying down or in the morning, and is associated with nausea, inclination to vomit and a feeling of weight or blows in the chest. The condition is aggravated after taking a meal, by drinking coffee and from mental stress.

Urinary System
Tension here may be manifested in renal colic, especially liable to affect the right side. Other symptoms are: much ineffectual urging to pass water, even to the degree of strangury; burning in bladder at night; itching or burning in urethra when passing urine; nocturia; polyuria. Retention of urine may occur from spasm of the sphincter, or sometimes from an opposite state of atony of the bladder wall.

Genital System
Menstrual irregularities are accompanied by chilliness and tendency to fainting. The remedy may be called for in pregnancy when morning nausea is associated with headache and insomnia.

Locomotor System
Muscle spasm is, of course, a prolific source of pains, often dubbed 'rheumatic'. Nux Vomica may be called for in relation to various aches,

pains, stitches, bruised sensations from nape to sacrum. A feature of the Nux low back pain is inability to turn over in bed without sitting up. Other symptoms mentioned in this sphere are sudden weakness, pseudo-paralysis in arms or legs, occurring in the morning; also paraesthesia and numbness in the hands, which feel cold and clammy, or in feet and toes. Twitchings and quiverings may be noticed in the thighs. Tottering unsteady gait may result from weakness. Complaints of tensive pain in calves, cramps in bed, heaviness in the limbs, dragging the feet, are mentioned also.

MODALITIES

There is aggravation in cold dry weather, in windy weather, also before the rain, but relief when the rain starts. Stimulants, spices, narcotics all aggravate, and there is a liability to feel worse immediately after a meal. Touch causes irritation. Disturbed or insufficient sleep aggravates, as also mental overexertion. The worst time is about 3 a.m. to 4 a.m. or after waking in the morning.

The Nux Vomica subject feels better in wet weather, gets relief by lying down and when at rest, and after adequate unbroken sleep. Firm pressure ameliorates, and the close of the day is a better time than the morning.

CLINICAL NOTES

Nux Vomica is a remedy of wide application with well-marked indications, especially along constitutional lines. Coffee is said to be inimical when taking the remedy, as also are Acetic Acid and Zincum Met. in sequence. Complementary remedies are Sepia and Sulphur.

The best time to give the remedy is some hours before bedtime, not first thing in the morning or immediately after meals. These are both aggravation periods.

The treatment of a much-medicated patient, so frequent a type nowadays, may well be started with Nux Vomica in high potency.

Opium

SOURCE

Opium, Da Yen – Big Smoke – in Chinese, name of enchantment and enchainment; source of untold wealth to individuals and rings in control of the illegal trade in the drug, whether in the form of the crude product or its derivatives, morphine and heroin. The story of opium is full of drama and tragedy, linked with war, murder, forced labour, adventure and vice.

In association with medicine the drug has been employed down the centuries to induce sleep, allay pain and banish care, but its therapeutic benefits are tragically offset by the horrors and miseries of addiction. As Gerrard remarked, 'It mitigateth all kindes of paines, but it leaveth behinde it oftentimes a mischiefe worse than the disease itselfe, and that hard to be cured, as a dead palsie and such like.'

Crude opium is obtained from the poppy, *Papaver somniferum*, which is cultivated mainly in India, China, Persia and Asia Minor. The name derives from the Greek – *opos* juice – and the drug consists of the hardened, dried juice or latex of the plant. A few days after the flower has fallen, horizontal incisions are made in the unripe seed capsules towards sunset. A white milky latex exudes and soon hardens on the outer surface of the capsule into a brownish mass. This is scraped off the following day and, when sufficient quantity has been collected, the pulpy mass is kneaded by hand to a uniform consistency and then shaped into balls or cakes.

The crude substance has a characteristic and unmistakable pungent odour and a very bitter taste. It owes its powerful narcotic effects to the presence of a large number of alkaloids, of which morphine, codeine, apomophrine and papaverine are among the most important.

From the lobed silvery blue-green foliage the annual herb rises rapidly and energetically with its flower stem which reaches up to one and a half yards in height. At first the top of the stem bends over, unable to hold up the somewhat bulky flower bud, but it becomes erect again before the bud bursts into bloom. The flower is particularly beautiful, clear lavender or white, with a heavy stain of rich purple at the base of each of the four petals, which form a deep cup open towards the sun. A field of flowering

374

poppies provides a breathtaking spectacle, breathtaking in more senses than one with its overpowering heavy narcotic scent.

PHARMACOLOGY

The predominant affinity of opium is with the central nervous system. Following an initial stimulant effect accompanied by increased capacity for effort, of short-lived duration, the narcotic action sets in.

This is evidenced by a dulling of perception and awareness of sensation, with resulting relief of pain and induction of a state of euphoria characterized by aberration of time sense – the past is now; the present is some other time, as in dreams. There is a special action on the respiratory centre, which is depressed, giving rise to progressive interference with respiration accompanied by cyanosis, stertor and sopor, from which the subject can be roused at first. But increasing narcosis leads to paresis, coma and death.

Irritation effects cause contraction of the pupils to an extreme, pin-point, degree. Tetanic convulsions have been recorded but are rare. Other effects may be nausea and vomiting (especially in sensitive subjects), inhibition of glandular secretion, increased tone of sphincters associated with diminished peristalsis and loss of rectal sensitivity. These latter effects tend to result in an extremely severe type of constipation.

PROVINGS

There is a pathogenesis of Opium in the first volume of Hahnemann's *Materia Medica Pura*.

APPEARANCE

The typical Opium picture is one of stupor, contracted insensitive pupils, face mottled and purple in colour, with stertorous breathing, the paretic cheeks puffing in and out. Eyes look red with half-closed lids.

But a state of excitement may be present, with twitchings or tremors and staring eyes.

Paralysis is progressive with sagging of the lower jaw. There is marked insensibility to stimulation. The pulse is full and slow. Delirium is accompanied by incessant muttering. Infants appear marasmic and stuporous. Adults have a sallow, wrinkled countenance and show marked emaciation.

375

PSYCHOLOGY

The Opium subject shows mental obtuseness and moral turpitude. The condition may be one of hypersensitivity, peevishness and phantasy, or a picture of unnatural placidity, desiring nothing.

There are perversions of time and space sense. Phobias may obtrude and give rise to suicidal gloom. On the other hand the patient, though almost moribund, may assert that he 'feels fine' and may resent any interference. Again, the sufferer is apt to think that he is 'away from home' when actually in his own bed – a symptom also met with under Bryonia.

There may be acute awareness of distant noises, also of quite small, near sounds.

Following a severe shock or fright the sensation of fear persists, even for years. The drug is often indicated under such circumstances, but also when the symptoms ensuing on the original shock persist although the actual fear is forgotten.

PHYSIOLOGY

The Opium subject in bed feels too hot, wants to push off the covers or move about in search of a cool spot.

Appetite tends to be poor, possibly with actual repugnance for food. Thirst is apt to be violent.

Sleep is either heavy with stertorous breathing, or light, the subject lying awake for long periods with all senses hyperacute. Quite distant noises, not normally noticed, obtrude into consciousness and increase wakefulness. Dreams are euphoric, fantastic, nightmarish, phantasmagoric. Sweat tends to be copious and hot.

SYMPTOMATOLOGY

General
Symptoms are marked by painlessness when complaint of pain might be expected, e.g. in peptic ulcer; also by placidity, when owing to fever and malaise a condition of restlessness would be more likely. Extreme drowsiness accompanies all symptoms; and grave prostration may supervene, associated with loss of sphincter control of both bladder and rectum. Subsultus tendinum may be present.

Opium

Head

Vertigo is noticed on sitting up, compelling the sufferer to lie down again. Old people feel light-headed. Various unpleasant sensations are related to the head; it feels empty, or heavy, or confused and stupid with heat in eyes and a desire to close them.

Respiratory System

Breathing is noisy, stertorous, rattling. During sleep, spasms of suffocation may occur, as also on attempting to cough. Haemoptysis is associated with a hot chest and cold limbs.

Alimentary System

Extreme dryness of throat may be accompanied by spasms which cause dysphagia. The tongue is paretic, making both speech and swallowing difficult. Nausea tends to be persistent and accompanied by sweating and prostration. Vomiting is associated with colic and tympanites. The picture may be one of paralytic ileus with constant belching which affords no relief. Intestinal hypotonus results in an inveterate type of constipation with total absence of any urge to stool. An enema produces masses of black scybala. At times diarrhoea may occur as a sequel to fright, and probably involuntary. Or perhaps bouts of diarrhoea alternate with constipation. Cholera infantum accompanied by stupor. This picture may also suggest Ferrum Phos.

Cardiovascular System

Following severe trauma or an operation a state of shock is accompanied by ashy pallor, impalpable pulse, cold sweat and appearance of collapse.

Nervous System

Twitching, possibly convulsions, are aggravated in a warm room or by immersion in a hot bath. In infants an attack of convulsions may occur on the approach of strangers.

Urinary System

Retention of urine may occur from insensibility or atony of bladder, especially after a fright or post-partum.

Genital System

Disturbances of libido in either sex. Impotence in male.

Skin

Indolent ulcers occur, characterized by painlessness.

MODALITIES

Aggravation from heat, during and after sleep, from stimulants and while sweating. Fear and anxiety also make things worse.

There is relief from cold and when walking about, also possibly from black coffee.

CLINICAL NOTES

Indications for the use of Opium may be present in typhoid fever, also with cerebral haemorrhage. It may be called for in delirium tremens, especially when hallucinations are prominent, accompanied by an expression of fright or terror.

The 1M potency is recommended in acute fright. The remedy also is indicated when a fright, either recent or remote, is the causal factor in illness.

In desperate illness the 10M has proved effective, a dose given every four hours.

In poor reactors not responding to the apparently indicated remedy Opium may prove of value, as may be the case also with Lycopodium or Sulphur.

Low potencies are recommended in constipation of the type described above. Chamomilla or Nux Vomica may be of service in relation to opium addiction.

Phosphoricum Acidum

SOURCE

The substance potentized and investigated by Hahnemann was prepared in the following manner. 'One pound of bones calcined white and broken into small pieces placed in a porcelain jar, covered by one pound of the strongest sulphuric acid. The mixture to be stirred with a glass rod several times during twenty-four hours, then well mixed and diluted with two pounds of good brandy, and the whole tied up in a linen bag and pressed out between two smooth boards loaded with weights. What remains in the bag may be again diluted with two pounds of brandy, and the expressed fluid added to the first quantity. The whole is to be allowed to stand for two days, so that the cloudiness may settle down. The clear fluid is now to be decanted off, evaporated in a porcelain dish over the fire, and melted at a red heat. The melted phosphoric acid should be as clear as crystal, and while still warm it is to be broken into small fragments and preserved in a well corked bottle, because when exposed to air it soon completely deliquesces into a thickish fluid as clear as water.'

This process produces metaphosphoric acid, HPO_3, and present-day potencies are prepared from the commercially pure variety.

PHARMACOLOGY

The main tissue affinity of this acid is with the nervous system, evidenced by its effect of inducing both mental depression and muscular weakness of progressive type.

PROVING

The original proving of Phosphoric Acid is in the fifth volume of Hahnemann's *Materia Medica Pura*.

APPEARANCE

The subject in need of this remedy is often a child or adolescent who appears weedy, overgrown and overwrought. The adult too has a hopeless, haggard, worn-out look.

379

The face is pale, pinched, with blue rings around the eyes. The pupils may be unequal and the eyes have a glassy look.

The hair tends to be prematurely grey and sparse.

There is a disinclination to answer questions; replies in monosyllables and with obvious reluctance – too much bother to talk or to reply at length.

PSYCHOLOGY

Psychological asthenia precedes the physical weakness and is a prominent symptom.

The subject is listless, apathetic, sullen, indifferent and thoroughly 'browned off'. May be stupefied with grief; in a state of settled despair; worn down by adverse circumstances; unable to cope.

The mind is confused, and any effort to concentrate brings on a dizzy feeling. There is great sensitivity, notably to music and also to odours. The subject is easily startled. May complain of various odd sensations such as widespread formication; may be afflicted with homesickness.

The condition may be brought on by emotional shock or continued stress; it may also be induced by excess, sexual or other.

PHYSIOLOGY

Chilliness is prominent. The subject feels cold even in a warm room. The extremities are constantly cold. Moreover, chills and heat are apt to alternate owing to a labile state of the circulation. Appetite is poor or absent. There may be a distaste for bread, which seems bitter, the unpleasant taste remaining in the mouth for a long time after eating. There may be an aversion to coffee. Intolerance is noted for acid foods, fresh fruit, cold drinks and rich food.

Thirst may be insatiable, especially in some cases for milk or beer.

Drowsiness in fever may simulate stupor, but the sufferer can be roused to full consciousness for the moment. Agitation and dry heat may cause wakefulness at night. Jerking, moaning, talking, involuntary biting of tongue may occur in sleep. May dream of death, with fear on waking. Sleep, however, is refreshing, even quite a short nap.

Cold sweats occur on arms and hands and along the spine.

SYMPTOMATOLOGY
General
Emotional stress, grief, care, sorrow, chagrin, homesickness, disappointed love, if prolonged or persisted in, result in a dual state of

mental apathy and physical exhaustion. This can be compared with Staphysagria, in the picture of which remedy resentment, envy and wounded pride – the injured feeling – predominate; also with Ignatia with its picture of emotional instability, unpredictability and lack of poise. Symptoms are often accompanied by a sensation of pressure or constriction, whether local or general.

Head
Giddiness is noticed, especially when standing or walking. Accompanying sensations may be as if one would fall forwards, or as if the feet were rising and rising till one was standing on one's head or, when lying down, as if one's body were floating off the bed. The head feels empty or muzzy. Actual headache may occur, often occipital and severe, accompanied by a sensation as if there was great pressure crushing the vertex, or as if the temples were being squeezed together. The sufferer is compelled to lie down, and the pain is aggravated by the least shock, movement or noise.

Eyes
Styes are liable to occur, especially on the upper lids. The eyes feel pushed backwards into the skull. The lids are heavy and swollen.

Ears
Tinnitus of varying type occurs and impairment of hearing is also common. There may be drawing pain in the external ear or in the external auditory canal.

Respiratory System
Severe itching has been recorded at the tip of the nose. There is a tendency to 'catch cold' easily and the 'cold' goes to the chest. Sore throat is accompanied by severe hoarseness, and the soreness is aggravated by swallowing which causes shooting pain. Pinching pains occur in the chest, especially on expiration, or an oppressive tight feeling may interfere with respiration. Talking causes a 'weak feeling' in the chest. A 'stomach cough' is associated with tickle, as from a feather or dust, and is felt along the whole length of the trachea. The cough tends to be worse in the morning and again in the evening, also on first lying down at night, and is aggravated by contact with cold air. Yellowish, salty sputum is brought up in the morning.

Alimentary System
Aberrations of taste are common. Burning pain occurs in the lower lip.
Dryness of tongue and palate are noticed. Gums tend to bleed easily.
After a meal, distension, discomfort and a sensation of weight in the
stomach occur in about half an hour, possibly followed by nausea and
vomiting some hours later. Warm food and fluids give relief. This is in
contrast to Phosphorus, which shows preference for cold, even ice-cold
fluids. Extremely violent pinching and squeezing pains are felt in the
belly, especially around the umbilicus; these pains are aggravated by
bending the body either forwards or backwards. There is much
accompanying gurgling and rumbling, as well as the passage of large
quantities of flatus. Painless diarrhroea occurs with white or yellow,
profuse, watery stools containing undigested food particles. Rather
unexpectedly the patient feels better after the passage of these fluid
stools. This is in marked contrast to the Calc. Carb. picture of 'only
comfortable when constipated'. Phosphoric Acid may be indicated when
the 'typhoid state' supervenes in grave illness and both bowel and
bladder are emptied involuntarily.

Cardiovascular System
Heart muscles and circulation are involved in the general asthenia. There
may be complaints of palpitation and irregularity of pulse. A tendency to
passive haemorrhages or purpura has been noted.

Genital System
Seminal emissions may be unduly frequent, associated with impairment
of function. There may be herpetic or papillomatous lesions of the
external genitalia. Menstrual periods tend to be too early and too
copious. The period may be followed by a yellowish vaginal discharge,
associated with pruritus.

Urinary System
Passes copious, pale, watery urine which quickly forms a thick cloud of
phosphates on standing. Frequency may occur, also nocturnal enuresis.

Locomotor System
A bruised sensation is noticed in hips, thighs, arms, and nape of neck.
There may be tearing or squeezing pains in both upper and lower
extremities. Legs feel weak when walking; stumbles easily or makes mis-
steps. Children complain of 'growing pains'. A burning sensation may
occur in the spine, which is worse at night, and aching in the sacral

region. Involvement of periosteum causes a feeling as if the bones were being scraped with a knife.

Skin

Eruptions of red pimples occur on face, neck, chest and back. Also itching or pricking sensations in various sites.

MODALITIES

There is aggravation from the least draught, from exposure to wind or snowy atmosphere; also from any exertion, mental or physical, from touch, when lying on the left side. Noise, bad smells, music all have an adverse effect, and there is aggravation in the evening and during the night.

Warmth, walking and sleep afford relief.

CLINICAL NOTES

The remedy is often effective in low potencies, 3x or 6c. It acts well either before or in sequence to Cinchona.

Phosphorus

SOURCE

Phosphorus was first discovered and manufactured from urine in 1669. The homoeopathic preparations were made from phosphorus obtained from bone ash. This was the yellow toxic variety which may also be obtained from the mineral apatite (a phosphorus-calcium compound), from animal bones and from basic slag, a by-product of steel-making. Potencies are prepared from a saturated solution of the yellow phosphorus in alcohol.

Phosphorus is an element essential to life, whether animal or vegetable. Its presence, for instance, is necessary for the transfer of energy within plant cells through chemical reactions. The first substance in which carbon, newly absorbed from the atmosphere, has been shown to be present in a plant also includes phosphorus.

The physical properties of phosphorus are noteworthy. By reason of its combustibility in air at normal temperatures, it has to be stored under water or in alcohol. When exposed to the air it oxidizes and rises into the atmosphere in the form of vapour apparently to disappear. In this way the element exemplifies the force of 'levity', in contrast to the force of 'gravity', which pulls earthward, tending to the condensation of vapour into liquid or solid forms of ever-increasing density.

The tropical plant Spanish moss, *Tillandsia usneoides*, grows and flourishes without taking from its support any material whatsoever for the building up of its substance. It grows on the dry bark of forest trees and has been found growing even on telegraph wires. It has been found to possess the ability to absorb, materialize and utilize phosphorus from the surrounding atmosphere, despite the fact that no phosphorus can be detected in the atmosphere. It is obviously therefore present in a highly ethereal or dematerialized state.

This is of significance in revealing the intrinsic nature of phosphorus to be non-materialistic, a trend upward, a reaching out in art and imagination to the realm of the invisible and imponderable, a realm that is nevertheless real and imperishable.

The Phosphorus subject is essentially an artistic, imaginative, creative, even clairvoyant type.

PHARMACOLOGY

Yellow phosphorus is highly poisonous, whether absorbed accidentally in industrial contact or administered with homicidal or suicidal intent. Easily-obtained rat-paste may contain from 1% to 4% of the poison. Several phosphate compounds employed as insecticides are also very dangerous, being powerful inhibitors of cholesterinase and possessing toxic properties similar to those of nicotine, two or three minims of which in pure form are sufficient to cause death.

The symptoms of acute poisoning are not immediate. Several hours after ingestion a burning sensation is noticed in the throat and oesophagus; nausea follows with eructations tasting like garlic, and then vomiting of typical vomitus – dark in colour containing blood, smelling like garlic and luminous in the dark; later there is diarrhoea with darkish luminous stools. If death is delayed, intermissions of these symptoms occur with super-added jaundice, enlargement of liver, purpura and epistaxis. Oliguria ensues with the presence of bile, albumin, casts and occasional red blood cells in the urine, associated with much nervous restlessness, and finally death from uraemia.

The tissue affinities of Phosphorus are thus widespread; with mucous membranes, causing inflammation, ulceration and consequent haemorrhage; with the liver, leading to hyperaemia and enlargement, rapid disappearance of glycogen and fatty changes; with lungs and kidneys, resulting in pneumonitis or nephritis; with pancreas, heart, blood-vessels and the blood itself, tending to fatty degenerative changes and anaemia; with the central nervous system, inducing over-excitability and hypersensitivity; with bones causing central osteolysis and cortical osteosclerosis.

Research with radioactive isotopes has traced phosphorus in the body to both red and white blood cells, the latter retaining the element a very long time, also to bone marrow, lymph nodes, spleen and liver. Leukaemic and neoplastic tissues also show a selective affinity with radiophosphorus.

It is obvious, therefore, that Phosphorus in potency is likely to be a remedy of very wide usefulness in a variety of conditions of disordered cell and tissue metabolism.

PROVING

A pathogenesis of Phosphorus was published by Hahnemann in the first edition of the *Chronic Diseases*.

APPEARANCE

There are a number of characteristic features by which it is possible to recognize the Phosphorus subject

The complexion is variously described as pink and white, or possibly in anaemic subjects of a sickly pallor with a somewhat waxy look. One author speaks of long silky eyelashes and easy graceful manners. There is a tendency to flush easily, especially if embarrassed or excited.

The hair tends to be fine, often blonde or red, but the subject may be a bright-eyed brunette. Tufty baldness may be present, with a tendency to dandruff and inclination to scratch the scalp constantly.

In build the Phosphorus subject is tall and slender, with rather weak musculature resulting in a tendency to stand with a stoop and stagger in gait. Actual trembling may be noticed in the limbs from slight cause. Constant fidgets and inability to sit still are prominent features. In a child the eyes follow every movement of the doctor and nurse.

In sickness there may be a puffy appearance of hands, feet and eyelids, with blue rings round the eyes.

Speech is characteristic. Either questions are replied to rapidly and with quick eager understanding, or answers are slow and somewhat hesitant owing to a desire for accuracy in detail.

PSYCHOLOGY

The Phosphorus subject is intelligent, cooperative, overactive, affectionate, attractive, artistic, given to enthusiasms which, however, tend to wane, owing to exhaustion.

Spasmodic brilliance is followed by exhaustion both physical and emotional, often associated with a tendency to tears and either apathy or irritability.

There may in fact be outbursts of sudden rage, followed by remorse and prostration.

A noteworthy point is that the child not only wants affection but returns it, and is soothed by being stroked and cuddled. The Pulsatilla child wants affection but is not so responsive.

The Phosphorus subject is excessively sensitive to all external impressions and stimuli – light, colour, odour (may even faint from contact with strong smelling flowers), music, touch, confined space. The effect of such stimulation is exhaustion. Is full of fears – fear of the dark, of disease, of thunder, of solitude, of spiders, of study (owing to mental exhaustion), of 'what the doctor is going to do'. The fear is felt in the epigastrium.

Phosphorus

There is a craving for company, attention and affection, and also a desire to show sympathy with other people and a tendency to become anxious on their behalf.

One other point, the Phosphorus subject is capable of ecstasy, clairvoyance, even delusions, or on the other hand may relapse into lethargy, forgetfulness, even stupor.

PHYSIOLOGY

Normally chilly, the Phosphorus subject may complain of inward burnings or a feeling of sudden heat as if submerged in hot water. The circulation is obviously labile and liable to sudden alterations. He may thus at times suffer from intense cold in feet and legs.

Phosphorus has several noteworthy features in relation to appetite and food and drink. There is easy hunger and a liability to a faint empty sensation if meals are delayed; the mid-morning 'sinking feeling' is also common. Ravenous hunger may be felt quite soon after a meal, and there is a desire for snacks, even at night.

There is craving for salt, condiments, spicy dishes, cold milk and ice-cream. Dislikes are often quite marked, for such things as milk puddings, sweets, tea, coffee, boiled milk, meat, beer, fish. In other words there is a tendency to be faddy about foods. There may be actual intolerance for sweets or for tea.

A violent burning thirst may be present for ice-cold drinks which, however, are likely to be vomited as soon as they become warmed in the stomach. In pregnancy, vomiting may occur even at the sight of water.

Sleep is apt to be restless and in catnaps. On waking feels as if sleep had been inadequate. On waking from a good sound sleep, however, feels definitely refreshed. At night cannot lie on the left side; children may sleep in the knee-elbow position. Hideous dreams, talking in sleep and somnambulism are associated with this remedy.

Quite profuse sweats may occur on exertion or during the second half of the night. In children a mild, generalized, slightly sticky, faint sweat may be noticed.

SYMPTOMATOLOGY

General

The Phosphorus picture may often be met with in young people who have grown rather too rapidly, and is manifested by tissue irritability and a lack of resistance and stability. There is often a great sense of fatigue associated with a disinclination for any kind of effort. The extremely labile circulation predisposes towards sudden exhaustion or actual syncope, as well as to sensations of burning and hot sweats on head and hands. Haemorrhages of persistent type may occur from small wounds, mucous surfaces, or from ulcers. There is a tendency to ecchymoses, petechiae or actual purpura. Bone affections may occur either as exostoses or in the form of caries. The jaws are specially liable to be involved. Phosphorus symptoms tend to be left-sided.

Head

Phosphorus is a valuable remedy in connection with vertigo which is liable to occur on rising quickly from the sitting or lying position, when stooping, turning the head quickly, after eating. It may come on out of doors and the sufferer has to clutch something for support or sit down. Headache is accompanied by burning pains, is aggravated in a warm room and by lying down. It is better sitting up, and relief is obtained by cold applications, contact with cool air and by taking some food. The face is flushed and hot. A periodic headache may also occur, of migraine type, associated with marked disorder of appetite, either ravenous hunger or extreme anorexia. Vomiting may or may not be present. A common complaint is that the skin of the forehead feels 'too tight'. A sensation of heat may spread from the head to the whole body.

Eyes

Disturbances of vision abound with this remedy. Eyes give out when reading; eyes water in a wind; eyes burn violently; objects appear red or blue or as if seen through a grey or green mist. Lesions of the retina or optic nerve may call for the remedy, also twitching of the eyelids.

Ears

The ears may feel 'muffled'. There is deafness especially for the human voice, and the patient's own voice seems to echo in the head, a symptom shared with Causticum. Ears may itch, burn and throb.

Respiratory System

Nasal catarrh may be very persistent with blood-streaked mucoid discharge; the nose becomes red, shiny and sore to the touch. It often feels unpleasantly dry inside the nostrils. The nose is apt to feel blocked and there is a tendency to the formation of polyps associated with easy bleeding. Actual caries of nasal bones may occur, leading to foetor and greenish-yellow discharge. The remedy shares with Lycopodium a curious tendency to unconscious fan-like movements of the alae nasi. Colds start in the head and tend to attack the throat and involve the chest. The throat is very sensitive to touch and to cold air, and feels dry or velvety. Hoarseness or actual aphonia are common, and frequently there is a constant desire to 'clear the throat'.

Phosphorus has a hard dry cough, from a persistent tickle, felt often quite low down behind the sternum. The cough is worse on first lying down at night, if lying on left side. It is also aggravated by strong odours and by changing from a warm to a cold atmosphere, or vice versa. Some relief is obtained by sitting propped up with the head inclined backwards, supported on pillows. Cough is accompanied by discomfort in the chest, a sense of oppression or tightness, or a weak feeling. There may be violent stitching pains in the left side of the chest, or a narrow band of pain behind the sternum. This is in contrast with Causticum, where the band of pain is broader. Suffocative attacks occur at night. Dyspnoea is noticed if walking against a wind. The tight feeling in the chest is relieved by heat. Sputum, if present, is more marked in the daytime, is tough and mucoid or yellow and purulent; it tastes sour, sweet or salty, and may contain blood.

Alimentary System
Symptoms in the mouth include excessive salivation, rapid caries of teeth, pyorrhoea alveolaris, easily-bleeding gums, a bitter or sour taste. The tongue appears red, smooth with a varnished look and 'burns'. Neuralgic pain in teeth or face is relieved by warmth. Burning pains are felt in the stomach. These are very acute and are associated with a horrible, faint, hungry sensation, which returns quite soon after a meal. The pains are made worse by heat, and relieved by cold food and drink. Hot food or fluids are vomited at once. Cold food and drink may be retained for up to half an hour but tend to be brought up when warmed. In vomiting, food is brought up in mouthfuls till the stomach is empty.

With acute gastric ulcer, persistent nausea with a sensation of fullness precedes a sudden violent vomiting of bright blood. This is liable to be followed by recurring attacks of nausea, burning pain and the vomiting of dark blood, like coffee grounds. Nausea with empty hunger is apt to occur in the early morning. Nausea with vomiting may be induced by a hot stuffy atmosphere or from putting the hands into hot water. Belching is extremely uncomfortable, as if 'something was being torn apart' at the cardia. Eructations are of food or are empty but tasting of food. Spasm at the cardia may cause actual regurgitation of food as swallowed, and there is awareness of the passage of food all the way down the oesophagus. There may be a weak, empty sensation in the stomach associated with burning between the shoulder-blades.

Vomiting of bile may occur at night. Stitches are felt below the ribs, or a tormenting pain in the region of the short ribs, especially on the left side. The liver may be enlarged from hyperaemia, with or without jaundice, and pain is made worse by lying on the right side and by pressure. Acute yellow atrophy of the organ may occur with shrinkage. Chronic enteritis may be present, associated with shooting pains, sensation of great weight or of icy coldness in the abdomen. Borborygmi are common, and often the gurgle seems to start in the stomach and run right down through the whole length of the gut. This is apt to be followed by an involuntary stool. Flatus is usually non-odorous. Phosphorus has a peculiar type of constipation, long, slim, hard stools being passed with difficulty. Lying on the left side often brings on an urge to stool. Chronic painless diarrhoea may occur, which tends to be worse in hot weather. At times there may be loose, foetid, gushing stools, even involuntary stools, with a wide open patulous anus. Stools may be preceded by colic and followed by violent tenesmus and, possibly, rectal prolapse. The anal sphincter may be weak with a tendency to leak mucus. Piles, if present, may bleed, causing a gush of bright blood with every stool.

Lymphatic and Glandular Systems
The remedy may be called for when the lymph nodes are enlarged, especially in the cervical region, with some cases of goitre, and in mastitis with abscess formation and thin sanious pus. It is also mentioned in relation to suppurative parotitis.

Cardiovascular System
As already mentioned, the extremely labile circulation leads to sudden alterations in blood flow in one or other location, causing a variety of symptoms. Violent palpitation may also occur, with pulsations, accompanied by an alarming sensation of pressure in the mid-sternal region or around the heart. This syndrome may well be precipitated by emotional stress or excitement.

Urinary System
Frequency of urination may occur with the passage of very scanty amounts; also burnings and twitching in the urethra. The urine is apt to be iridescent with a fatty film on the surface. Haematuria, nephritis, diabetes with intense thirst for cold water are also mentioned.

Genital System
In the Phosphorus subject the menstrual periods are apt to be profuse, prolonged and accompanied by depression and a tendency to tears.

Uterine haemorrhage may occur, copious in amount, with bright red blood and clots. There may be profuse excoriating vaginal discharge. The remedy may be called for in vomiting of pregnancy; also in puerperal convulsions.

Locomotor System

There are quite a few Phosphorus symptoms in this sphere. Much stiffness in limbs, noticed especially in the morning. Stiffness also in the nape and muscles of the back. The arms burn; the fingers go stiff; the tips of the fingers feel numb. Paralytic weakness is felt in arms and legs with consequent disability – 'the fingers are all thumbs'. The hip joint feels 'dislocated'. The spine is sore and tender to the touch, especially between the shoulder-blades. The back may be so painful that it feels 'broken' and renders the sufferer averse to making any movement. At night the spine feels hot while the knees and legs feel cold. Tingling, formication and burning may be felt along the spine. Actual caries may be present with girdle pains.

Skin

Yellow or brownish spots occur, especially on the chest and lower abdomen. Eruptions tend to be dry and scaly, such as psoriasis. Blood blisters may form. Ulcers tend to be necrotic, indolent, even malignant.

MODALITIES

Cold causes aggravation, especially putting the hands in cold water. There is aggravation both before and during a thunderstorm, also from getting the feet wet. Aggravation is also noticed when lying on the left side, in the twilight, in the dark, and from heights. Crowds, solitude and excitement all tend to cause aggravation.

Warmth, taking food, sound sleep and massage all afford relief.

CLINICAL NOTES

Phosphorus must be used with caution in active tuberculosis and not prescribed in potencies higher than 30c. It may be indicated in amyloidosis. It is of special value in acute gastric ulcer. It is prescribed often on the grounds of constitutional type.

It has been found of value in allaying apprehension before operations in children.

Complementary remedies are Lycopodium, Sanguinaria and Sepia. It may follow Nux Vomica with advantage. It should not be given in sequence to Causticum.

Phytolacca Decandra

SOURCE

Phytolacca decandra or *americana* is a perennial bushy plant found growing in waste damp ground in Eastern North America, North Africa and China. It enjoys a string of local names – pokeroot, pigeon berry, American nightshade, scoke, pocan, garget root, red ink plant – a list suggestive of the human interest taken in its properties.

Its smooth, purplish-green stems, up to three feet in height, bear alternate, ovate, pointed leaves and racemes of greenish-white flowers. The fruit is a dark purple berry containing lens-shaped black seeds. The berries are poisonous. The plant contains formic acid and calcium oxalate.

For homoeopathic use two distinct tinctures are prepared, one from the fresh root, dug in winter, and another from the berries.

PHARMACOLOGY

It is of interest that extracts from several parts of the plant induce blastic transformation and mitosis in human mononuclear cells in vitro. There is a suggestion that similar effects may be produced in vivo on the leucocytes of persons who 'undergo immoderate exposure to the mitogen'. From the homoeopathic point of view, the plant appears to have wide affinities tending to induce hypertrophic, indurating, or irritative changes in nervous tissue, mucous membranes of throat and alimentary tract, fibrous tissue, periosteum, bone, breasts and lymph nodes.

PROVING

The original proving of Phytolacca appeared in the second volume of the *Transactions of the American Institute of Homoeopathy*.

APPEARANCE

The face, normally pale, often becomes flushed after eating. The pupils are small. There is often a habit of biting the teeth together and at the same time retracting the lips – not necessarily in pipe-smokers. The skin is dry and may have a leaden hue.

PSYCHOLOGY

The outlook on life is gloomy, perhaps with a great fear of death and an expectation of imminent demise. A certain shamelessness and lack of delicacy may be apparent. There is a curious and irresistible compulsion to clench the teeth.

Various odd sensations have been recorded. The brain feels bruised. The eyes feel too large and full of sand. Nose feels as if tickled inside by a stiff feather. Tongue feels scalded. Throat feels choked as if by an apple core. A red-hot ball is lodged in the throat. The pharynx feels like an empty cavern; the chest feels hollow like an empty cask. The body feels bruised all over.

PHYSIOLOGY

Coldness predominates, though in fever the head and face may be hot. Internal shivers may be felt. Appetite varies; may be ravenous, even soon after eating, or may be absent. Thirst is often intense.

Yawning is frequent. Sleep is restless and pains may actually drive from bed. Wakes up feeling wretched. Pungent perspiration occurs at night.

SYMPTOMATOLOGY

General

Pains both come and go with abruptness, also shift rapidly from spot to spot. They are described as shooting or shock-like. There is a marked weakness; the patient feels tired all the time, utterly worn out, always wanting to lie down, and complains of aching all over as if bruised and battered. The laterality is right-sided.

Head

Giddiness and faintness are felt on rising from the recumbent posture. A dull frontal headache, extending to the orbits, is worse when walking about, or from any jar or jolt. It is also aggravated by vomiting and worse during wet or stormy weather.

Eyes

A dull ache in the eyeballs is aggravated by movement, in bright light, and when trying to read print. The eyes are tender with swollen lids, which become stuck in the morning; the lid margins become red, indurated and ulcerated, with the formation of crusts. Eyes smart and burn, and water profusely. Itching is felt at the medial canthus. Styes and tumours of the lids may occur.

Ears

Shooting pains are felt in the ears, especially on the right side, aggravated by swallowing.

Respiratory System

Coryza is associated with pain at the root of the nose. Itching is felt inside the nostril. One or other nostril becomes alternately blocked or discharging acrid, excoriating mucus. Or the nose may become totally stuffed up, necessitating mouth-breathing, and no relief is obtained by blowing the nose. The throat is a most important sphere of activity of this remedy. A sore throat is accompanied by rawness, roughness, stiffness of neck muscles and painful involvement of the tonsillar lymph nodes. The pain shoots into the ears, especially on swallowing. It is aggravated by taking hot drinks and is usually worse on the right side. Swallowing may in fact become impossible. The tonsils are likely to be chronically enlarged, and recurrent attacks of follicular tonsillitis commonly occur. The uvula is liable to become swollen and oedematous.

The remedy has proved of great value in diphtheria, especially when associated with severe pains all over the body, chilliness, prostration and scanty, dark, albuminous urine. The fauces show a typical dark red discoloration. The throat feels full as if choking, or on the other hand may feel empty, as if it were a hollow cavern. A raw roughness in the trachea is accompanied by a frequent desire to cough. The cough, which is dry and croupy, is worse in cold air and at night. It is eased in a warm atmosphere.

Alimentary System

Teeth may feel 'too long'. Tongue looks yellowish at the base and has a very red tip. Sharp pains are felt in the tongue, and blisters may be present at the sides. The root of the tongue is painful on swallowing. There is considerable yellowish, ropy saliva. Pain is located in the region of the pylorus. After a meal the stomach feels as if 'contracting', accompanied by a sinking hungry sensation, pain, nausea and vomiting. The remedy may be called for in relation to gastric ulcer, also in carcinoma of stomach associated with tenderness and pain in the liver, aggravated by lying on the right side and eased by taking hot drinks. Cutting pains may occur in the epigastrium; waterbrash may also occur, and nausea relieved by vomiting. May wake in the middle of the night with severe neuralgic pain in the lower part of the rectum and anus with spread to the perineum. The remedy has proved of value in rectal carcinoma associated with throbbing pain in the lumbosacral region, which is greatly aggravated on becoming warm in bed. There is also generalized abdominal discomfort with much rumbling and a constant urge to stool, resulting in the passage of a little blood-stained mucus or shreds of tissue.

Lymphatic and Glandular Systems
Enlargement of lymph nodes or glandular structures is characterized by induration. Lesions of the mammary glands are a special sphere of usefulness. Pains in the breasts during the process of suckling (pains radiating to the dorsum point to Croton Tiglium, and pains radiating to the uterus suggest Arsenicum Alb., Pulsatilla or Silicea). Milk is apt to coagulate and hang in strings from the nipple. Other breast symptoms may be cracked, sore nipples, and pain in the breast which is relieved by pressure of the hand. Breasts become sore and lumpy, especially at the menstrual periods or after exposure to damp cold. This condition may be associated with enlarged lymph nodes in the axilla and shooting pains all over the body. In acute mastitis the breast is swollen, stony hard, painful and tender. Emotional stress may be a causal factor in breast lesions.

Cardiovascular System
The remedy may be indicated in relation to anginal pain which is aggravated when walking and associated with pain in the right upper extremity. The heart seems to be throbbing in the throat.

Genital System
Sharp pain may shoot up the spermatic cords, followed by a more prolonged soreness of the parts. The remedy can be called for in relation to both gonorrhoeal and syphilitic infections and resulting lesions. Various uterine disorders have been recorded, including too frequent and too profuse menstruation and membranous dysmenorrhoea.

Urinary System
Pain and a sensation of weakness is felt in the kidney region, associated with symptoms of nephritis, especially post-exanthematous in type. Pain may be felt in the bladder both before and during urination. Urine stains linen yellow.

Locomotor System
Rheumatic pains and stiffness in muscles, cervical or elsewhere, are aggravated by movement and are worse at night. There is an urge to move but the sufferer is scared to do so. Joints become swollen, hard, tender and intensely hot. Severe pains in bones are worse in bed at night.

Sciatic pain occurs on the right side; the pain is specially located to the lateral aspect of the thigh and associated with a feeling of being bruised all over. Soreness of heels is very persistent, but relief is obtained if the feet are elevated above the level of the head. The remedy may also be of value in sudden short-lived attacks of cramp.

Skin

The remedy is to be considered in syphilitic eruptions and ulcers, as also in other skin lesions of pleomorphic character. Itching is made worse by scratching and is aggravated by the heat of the bed.

MODALITIES

There is aggravation from cold, especially damp cold; from thundery weather; from rain; from weather changes. Although basically chilly, symptoms are aggravated by the heat of the bed. Worse also from touch, when lying on the right side, at night and at the menstrual period.

The patient feels better in dry weather, when warm, when lying on the left side or on the stomach.

CLINICAL NOTES

It is noteworthy that in rheumatic conditions, when Bryonia and Rhus Tox. fail to give relief, Phytolacca may cure. Complementary remedies are Lueticum, Micrococcinum and Silicea.

Picricum Acidum

SOURCE

Picric acid is trinitrocarbolic acid. It occurs in the form of bright yellow crystals; solutions stain tissues yellow. At the beginning of the century it was employed in surgery and as a dressing for burns, but it was found to carry risk of damage to the kidneys and fell into disuse.

PHARMACOLOGY

Affinity with the central nervous system leads to grave asthenia, both mental and muscular; with the renal tissues it results in nephritis; with pancreas and liver it induces degenerative changes.

PROVING

Allen published a pathogenesis of Picric Acid obtained from three groups of provers.

APPEARANCE

Appearance of excessive langour; no desire to make any effort, or even to talk. May look jaundiced and cachectic.

PSYCHOLOGY

Is listless, torpid, indifferent to everything. The least attempt to study or concentrate produces exhaustion. May complain of a sensation as if the ground or the stairs were rising up to meet him.

PHYSIOLOGY

There may be aversion to all food. Thirst is for tepid water. Sleep is unrefreshing; often disturbed by constant dreams. Sweats are cold and clammy.

SYMPTOMATOLOGY

General
The chief characteristic is extreme muscular weakness, accompanied by a compelling desire to lie down and a complete absence of anxiety. Is utterly exhausted; can neither think nor study. Darting pains may be felt in various sites, possibly involving bones.

Head
Vertigo is worse on stooping, when walking, or ascending stairs. A throbbing headache is induced by the least mental effort; it is located in the forehead, at the base of the skull or in the occipito-cervical region. It is aggravated by movement and somewhat relieved by cool applications, in the open air, by rest, by recumbency, by tight bandaging. The head alternatively feels either heavy or empty. The occipital headache may spread to spine and lower limbs. Formication may be felt in the scalp.

Eyes
The pupils may be dilated. Lachrymation may be troublesome. Conjunctivitis, especially of right eye, is aggravated in a warm room and relieved by bathing in cold water or cold tea. Pain in the eyeballs is worse from movement, and better by closing the lids and by pressure.

Ears
There is a liability to boils in the external auditory canal. Sensations of puffy swelling, burning and formication may be present.

Respiratory System
Nose tends to be blocked with mucus; better in open air. Epistaxis may occur, especially from right nostril, with associated heat and congestion in head. Throat feels 'rough' or 'scraped'; is worse on empty swallow, when throat feels it would split. The throat feels better after sleep and after eating. Dry cough is associated with sensation of dust in the throat. Pain or throbbing may be felt in the chest, especially on the left side. Chest feels tight, as if encircled by a tight band.

Alimentary System
Lips tingle. There is much stringy, frothy saliva and a bitter taste in the mouth. Sour eructations and waterbrash occur. Nausea may be severe; worse at 5 a.m. and aggravated by rising and moving about. Fullness and weight in epigastrium are accompanied by ineffectual urge to belch.

Flatulence is associated with a variety of pains and discomfort. Diarrhoea occurs with thin, yellow, possibly oily, stools and burning and smarting at the anus.

Urinary System

Urine is concentrated, dark, ammoniacal and albuminous. Conditions such as frequency, glycosuria, anuria, nephritis, uraemia have been noted.

Genital System

Main features in this sphere are priapism; satyriasis; copious emissions followed by excessive exhaustion. Impotence may supervene. In the female there may be left ovarian pain. Leucorrhoea precedes menses, which are delayed. Nocturnal pruritus vulvae.

Locomotor System

Low back pain is worse by movement and after sleep. There is great weakness of lower limbs, associated with trembling, heaviness, numbness or formication. Legs feels like lead. A curious feature is a burning sensation felt along the spine, which is brought on by the least mental concentration. Legs may feel as if enclosed in elastic stockings, or as if being pricked by needles.

Skin

May show a yellow tint. Liability to papules on face and small boils in various sites. Pruritus may be troublesome, especially at night.

MODALITIES

The chief cause of aggravation is the least mental exertion. Is worse also in wet weather; from movement; when stooping; in a hot stuffy atmosphere; after sleep.

Is better when resting; from contact with cold air and cold water; in bright sunny weather; by firm pressure.

CLINICAL NOTES

Lesions of the spinal cord suggest the use of this remedy. It is also of value in prostatic hypertrophy.

Platinum Metallicum

SOURCE

The source of this remedy is the heavy metal platinum; the name derives from the Spanish word *platina*, 'like silver'. As in the case of gold and silver, the metal is malleable. It is classified as a 'noble' metal.

PHARMACOLOGY

There is affinity with the nervous system leading to emotional disorders on the one hand and also to neuromuscular disturbance evidenced by cramps and convulsions. Affinity with the reproductive system resulting in hypersensitivity of the sexual organs and increased libido; with the blood, causing anaemia; with bones, especially the nasal bones and the tarsus, inducing caries.

PROVING

Platina was proved by Gross, and listed in the second edition of Hahnemann's *Chronic Diseases*.

APPEARANCE

An arrogant, disdainful bearing is combined with a lean, tense appearance. Frequent changes of colour are noted in the face.

The subject is emotionally unstable; tears and laughter alternate; sings, whistles, dances, as the mood demands. Speech is characterised by exaggeration and mendacity.

PSYCHOLOGY

As suggested by the appearance, there is an outlook of excessive haughtiness; looks down on everyone and everything as the result of an overweening sense of self-importance.

Feels tall and stately, while everything around, people included, appear small, mean, contemptible. Familiar objects appear strange and different.

Suffers from lacerated feelings, a wounded spirit.

Is tired of life but has a dread of death, which may seem imminent; is full of fears and horrors.

Is markedly amorous; possibly hysterical or paranoic.

Cannot stand being contradicted; is very impatient; liable to destructive urges; laughs immoderately when should be serious and sympathetic, as when someone is relating a sad story.

Shows inordinate anxiety over loved ones in their absence.

Complains of odd sensations of constriction or formication. Hyperaesthesia alternates with feelings of numbness and deadness.

PHYSIOLOGY

Sensations of coldness are felt in patchy sites.

Sudden intense hunger is associated with gluttonous eating; conversely appetite may vanish after the first mouthful.

Sleep is restless; may lie awake for long periods, feeling sad and apprehensive. Lies on back with legs drawn up and one or both arms above the head. Liable to frequent spasmodic yawning. Sweating occurs only during sleep.

SYMPTOMATOLOGY

General

Somatic symptoms alternate with emotional distress; when the mind is at rest the body suffers, and vice versa. An outstanding feature is an exaggerated degree in either condition. Pains are constrictive, as if pinched or squeezed in a vice; both onset and decline are gradual; they are often accompanied by sensations of numbness and tingling.

Head

Periodic headaches are often accompanied by nausea and vomiting. A neuralgic headache, present on waking, is made worse by stooping but relieved by walking in the open air. Scalp feels numb. Intermittent cramping pain may be felt around the margin of the orbital cavity. Pain as if crushed in a vice may occur at the root of the nose; it is worse about noon and tends to ease off in the evening.

Eyes

Pain is felt in the eyes after gazing intently at some object. There is complaint of sparks seen before the eyes. Spasmodic quivering of eyelids, mostly affecting the right side. Objects looked at appear unduly small.

Ears

Cramp-like pains extend from ears to cheeks and lips, associated with numbness and coldness. Various types of tinnitus are described.

Respiratory System

An ineffectual urge to sneeze is associated with tingling inside the nose. Epistaxis occurs, with discharge of dark clotted blood. There may be sudden inability to breathe when walking against the wind. Dyspnoea occurs with a feeling of contraction in the chest and a desire to take a deep breath. Oppression is felt behind the sternum, accompanied by a short, dry cough. Spasmodic pain in chest comes on and eases off slowly.

Alimentary System

There is a cold sensation in the mouth, but the tongue may feel burnt. Much belching is likely after meals. Nausea may be associated with weakness and anxiety. Periumbilical pain extends to the back. Sensations of pressure and constriction occur in the abdomen. Constipation results from intestinal inertia. There is a frequent but ineffective urge to stool; the stools are small, hard as if burnt; if softer they seem to adhere to the anus like soft clay. The condition is common on voyages, and in the sedentary.

Genital System

Menstrual periods are early and the flow is profuse, thick, tarry and contains clots; duration is usually eight days and there are sharp shooting pains on the first day. Metrorrhagia occurs with a similar discharge and accompanied by violent pressure in the hypogastrium. Chronic ovaritis affects chiefly the right side, the associated pain being made worse by the least pressure. External genitalia are exceedingly sensitive; pruritus is severe; libido is increased, perhaps to the degree of nymphomania. Subject masturbates during sleep; vaginismus may be marked.

Nervous System

There is alternation of clonic with tonic spasms.

Locomotor System

Pain in the dorsal region is aggravated by bending over backwards. Pain in the coccyx while sitting is associated with a numb feeling as if the part had received a blow. Sensation as if a bandage was tied tightly round the thigh is accompanied by a feeling of great weakness. The lower extremities feel numb and stiff. Cramp-like pains and the described above sensations come on and ease off, both gradually. Fits of trembling may occur, affecting the whole body.

MODALITIES

There is aggravation in a warm room; when at rest, either sitting or standing; from bending over backwards; from touch and pressure; when fasting; at the menstrual period; at night.

Is better in sunshine; when walking out of doors; by stretching the limbs.

CLINICAL NOTES

The psychological picture will often provide the chief indication for the use of this remedy. The frequency of numb feelings and the gradual nature of the onset and decline of many symptoms are a recurrent characteristic, as is also a tendency to alternations.

Tuberculinum or Lueticum may be indicated by the history. Complementary remedies are Natrum Mur. and Sepia

Plumbum Metallicum

SOURCE

Plumbum, lead, is in many ways a remarkable metal. It is proverbially heavy, of a dull, grey, lifeless appearance. To touch it is softer and warmer than would be expected of a metal. It is singularly non-reactive to water, hence its value for roofing; an acid water supply is, however, plumbo-solvent. It is resistant to penetration by X-rays and other forms of radiation, hence its value for screens and containers in the use and storage of radioactive substances.

This seemingly inert metal is not as dead as it looks. It has 'fire in its belly', as is evidenced by the flaming colours, yellow, orange and red, seen in its ores. Moreover, the metal can be prepared in powder form by a process carried out in a vacuum. The powder is stable only so long as it is kept in a perfectly sealed vacuum tube; immediately air is admitted it bursts into flame and burns till consumed.

It is therefore not so suprising that the metal and its salts can be responsible for serious poisoning, both acute and chronic. A wide variety of symptoms can be caused and are included under the diagnosis of plumbism.

There is concern that petrol fumes high in lead content can cause decreased intelligence in young children.

PHARMACOLOGY

There are extensive tissue affinities. Prominent is the effect on muscle, both plain and striped, inducing spasm. Involvement of peripheral nerves leads to localized neuritis and flaccid paralysis of related muscles.

Sclerotic lesions may be produced in the central nervous system. If these involve the cerebrum they may produce a very severe degree of encephalopathy.

Lesions of the haemopoietic system result in anaemia of the secondary type with associated punctate basophilia. The kidneys may be affected, with production of a typical red granular nephritis.

PROVING

Plumbum was proved by Hartlaub and Trinks, and published in the *Arzneimittellehre*.

APPEARANCE

There is an anaemic, cachectic, ashen or icteroid appearance. The skin seems drawn tight over the bones, with a shrivelled look. Emaciation may be marked.

The expression is one of suffering or anxiety.

Gums are pale and swollen; a blue line may be seen at the junction of tooth and gum; foetor oris is evident.

The infant shows cold hands and feet, cold tongue, a very offensive odour and a greasy, shiny skin.

The belly is retracted and scaphoid, but in children may be distended.

Feet are cold, smelly, showing macerated skin between the toes.

Fibrillary twitching may be apparent in certain muscles.

Wrist-drop or other paralytic lesion may be seen.

PSYCHOLOGY

The subject is mentally sluggish and at the same time hyper-emotional – taciturn, indifferent, depressed, melancholic.

There is slowness of perception and impairment of memory, with inability to recall the 'wanted word'.

There may be a tendency to feign illness, especially of paralytic type. Fear of being assassinated has been noted.

PHYSIOLOGY

The subject is very chilly, feels the cold, needs a lot of clothing even in warm weather, but wants the head uncovered. When walking out of doors complains of cold feet and legs.

Appetite varies; may be lost with refusal of all food and drink. Or violent hunger may occur soon after a meal. There is a strong desire for bread, fried food, cakes, and tobacco.

Thirst for cold water may be excessive.

Drowsiness is prominent by day, but at night the subject is apt to be sleepless; may assume odd postures in bed and evince a great desire to stretch in all directions.

Perspiration is conspicuous by its absence.

SYMPTOMATOLOGY

General

Pains occur in various parts of the body; are cramping, constricting or radiating. The pains may be accompanied by trembling or shuddering; they can be relieved by hard pressure. Characteristic are slow insidious conditions which show no tendency to recover. Symptoms may be present in groups, e.g. a combination of anaemia, asthenia, pallor, persistent vomiting, gastralgia and constipation or, again, epilepsy associated with colic, dysmenorrhoea, constipation and a paralytic heaviness of lower limbs as aura.

Head

Vertigo is noticed on stooping or looking upward. The head feels heavy or confused. Violent pains occur in the scalp. A headache, either frontal or occipital, is associated with bilious vomiting and abdominal colic.

Eyes

The pupils may be contracted. Sclerotics show yellow discoloration. Eyeballs are painful and feel too large. Vision is obscured as if by a mist. Upper lids may be paretic, and lids may agglutinate at night. Possible lesions are optic neuritis and glaucoma.

Ears

Sudden deafness has been noted. Also tearing or shooting pain in the ear.

Respiratory System

Sense of smell may be disturbed. Nasal obstruction is associated with much tenacious mucus. Throat feels sore, as if plugged, constricted, or as if a ball was rising up in the throat. Voice may be hoarse or aphonic. Cough is accompanied by copious expectoration of viscid, transparent or yellowish green mucus, often in lumps. Dyspnoea may be troublesome. Fits of suffocation or spasmodic asthma occur.

Alimentary System

Mouth may be dry or salivation excessive. Tongue appears glazed and red or brown with fissures. Tongue may be paralysed, rendering speech difficult. Ulcers or purple blotches are seen in the mouth and at the tip of the tongue. There is a sweetish or horribly offensive taste in the mouth.

Swallowing may be difficult as the result of paralysis of the muscles of deglutition. Hiccough may be troublesome. Eructations are foul-smelling. Abdominal symptoms are predominant with nausea, vomiting and severe colic. The pains radiate from the region of the umbilicus and are accompanied by retraction of the belly wall, which may feel tethered to the spine by a string. Some relief is obtained by bending double, by firm pressure and by belching. Constipation may be very obstinate, accompanied by much ineffectual urging to stool, anal spasm and severe pain. Stools, when passed, are like sheep's dung. Rectum may feel retracted. A peristaltic tumour may be present in the ileo-caecal region, and severe pain may be felt in this site. The liver may be involved, with acute jaundice, constant severe nausea and vomiting, very acute pain in the organ, extending to the back, and extreme tenderness.

Cardiovascular System
The left ventricle may be hypertrophied and dilated. Anxious palpitation occurs. Pulse may be rapid and hard from hypertension, or slow and soft in association with myocarditis.

Urinary System
Strangury with drop-by-drop urination occurs in combination with the abdominal symptoms described above. Paresis of the bladder wall will result in retention of urine with distension and overflow. Pain may be felt in the ureter. Urine is apt to be very dark, with the presence of nephritis.

Genital System
Menses are delayed or absent. Abortion is likely. Vaginismus is caused by spasm and dysmennorrhoea is common. The testes become swollen and hard. Impotence is a concomitant symptom.

Nervous System
Neuritic pains often involve periarticular regions; the pains are tearing, bruising, stabbing and may be accompanied by sensations as if 'burning liquid coursed through the part' or 'the part was in contact with an ice-cold object'. The pains occur in bouts of a few minutes' duration; they are aggravated by the warmth of the bed, as well as from contact with extreme cold. Cerebral involvement is evidenced by delirium, both clonic and tonic convulsions, coma, and in some cases by epileptic attacks.

Locomotor System

Flaccid paralysis involves a single muscle or a muscle group, notably extensors, as in wrist-drop. This is preceded by weakness, coldness, and heaviness and impaired function in the part. Rapid atrophy of the affected muscles follows, and wasting in the neighbouring tissues. Sciatica is associated with great exhaustion on walking. Cramps in calf muscles are worse at night. Violent pains may occur in the limbs, possibly associated with numbness, for example, of feet.

Skin

The skin is discoloured, bluish or yellowish. Dark brown spots are distributed widely over the body. Foetid foot sweats, said to smell like old cheese. Painful ulcers which burn.

MODALITIES

There is aggravation from damp; in a crowded room; from mental exertion; from touch and movement; at night.

Relief is afforded by massage, by firm pressure; by lying down and by resting.

CLINICAL NOTES

Symptoms due on the one hand to muscle spasm, or on the other hand to muscle weakness, even atrophy, provide the main indications for this remedy.

Psorinum

SOURCE

This preparation was one of the early nosodes, attenuations of disease matter, and so-called from *nosos* (Greek for disease). It was the first of such products to be extensively 'proved' by Hahnemann and was found to have a very definite materia medica picture and to be a valuable therapeutic agent. Its origin was 'matter' contained in a 'scabies vesicle', obviously a mixed bag bacteriologically speaking, and in its way a precursor of the polyvalent vaccine. As the scabies vesicle also contained the acarus, the product might be classified as an insect remedy.

PHARMACOLOGY

The main affinity would appear to be with the circulation, inducing such interference with basal metabolism as to result in a state of non-reactivity and debility. There is also a marked affinity with the skin, producing a wide variety of eruptions and intractable pruritus.

PROVING

Psorinum was proved by Hahnemann. Its pathogenesis was published by Stapf in the *Archiv für die Homöopatische Heilkunst*, in 1833.

APPEARANCE

The Psorinum subject is said to present an inverted pyramidal-shaped head, a sharp long nose, a long upper lip and large ears.

Be that as it may, the characteristic physical feature is a dingy, dirty, dusky look associated with dry, lustreless, unkempt hair. The hands always look dirty, despite frequent washing.

The skin is rough and scaly or it may be coarse and greasy. Cracks and fissures may be present, with a tendency to bleed. All discharges have an offensive odour, as also do the body and breath.

A scarf is worn on the head for warmth; or a skull cap by men.

PSYCHOLOGY

Is depressed, sad and joyless; at the same time is irritable and easily angered; cannot stand noise; seeks solitude and may feel suicidal. There is despair of recovery, constant dwelling on dying; makes himself miserable and everyone else too.

Is full of fear; fear of failure in business; fear of poverty; fear of fire, of insanity and so on. Marked inferiority complex and tendency to give up.

Odd sensations are experienced, such as that the brain was pushing out through the forehead or that the head was detached from the body.

PHYSIOLOGY

The Psorinum person is phenomenally chilly; hates draughts and cold air; piles on clothes; wears a head-wrap, perhaps a fur hat, even in the summer; is unduly sensitive to air-conditioning.

Has a voracious hunger, especially at night, but may feel full after a few mouthfuls. Dislikes sweets and potatoes; has a loathing for pork; may show intolerance of fat, sugar, meat and coffee.

Is extremely thirsty, especially for beer and acid drinks.

Sleeps on the back with the arms held well away from the body; cannot bear the limbs to be in contact or the weight of the arms across the chest. If pushes off the bedcovers gets 'chilled'; if covers up again the skin may itch to distraction and prevent sleep. Sick babies worry, fret and cry day and night, or sleep during the day but toss and scream all night.

May wake from sleep grinding the teeth. Terrifying dreams.

Sweats easily and profusely; may stream with sweat at night; offensive sticky sweats occur on hands and feet.

SYMPTOMATOLOGY

General

There is an inherent lack of reactivity. Influenza or other feverish illness is followed by slow convalescence and prolonged debility. Response to well-chosen remedies may be wanting. There is a marked lack of energy and very easy fatigue, but an unusual sense of well-being may precede an acute exacerbation of illness. The left foot may be cooler than the right, just the reverse of a sign sometimes met with under Lycopodium.

Head

Headache is accompanied by hunger and relieved by taking food or following a nose-bleed. Migraine-type headaches recur every eight, fifteen or twenty-two days; these are preceded by black spots before the eyes and are aggravated by the least draught. Scalp affections are common; early patches of white appear in the hair; hair is tangled or matted and unmanageable.

Eyes

Photophobia is troublesome; face is turned into the pillow to avoid the light, and eyes are kept constantly half-closed. Recurrent attacks of conjunctivitis or pterygium are common.

Ears

Otitis media becomes chronic with extremely foul-smelling yellow discharge, which irritates and excoriates. A crusting type of eczema occurs behind the ears, with offensive exudation.

Respiratory System

Very chronic type of rhinitis is accompanied by crust formation causing nasal obstruction; accumulation of postnasal discharge may wake from sleep. Sense of smell is lost. Recurrent attacks of quinsy are accompanied by enlargement of cervical lymph nodes; on swallowing, pain extends to the ears. A plug sensation may be felt in the throat. Annually recurring hay-fever is often preceded by asthma or eczema. Asthmatic attacks are worse sitting up and in the open air, but relieved by lying on back with arms wide-flung. A winter cough alternates with skin eruption; the cough is worse on waking or on lying down in the evening; it is accompanied by great weakness in the chest and pain on the right side at the level of the tenth rib; there is much sticky green mucus, which is difficult to raise. Dyspnoea is noticed when walking in cold air, on sitting down to write, on rising, when using the arms; it is relieved by lying down with the arms wide apart. Excruciating pain may be felt in the chest, or a sensation of weight and oppression.

Alimentary System

The upper lip is often swollen; herpes labialis is common. Lips and mouth tend to be dry; the tip of the tongue feels dry, sore as if burnt; pyorrhoea alveolaris loosens the teeth. Eructations taste like rotten eggs; nausea occurs with vomiting of sour mucus at 10 a.m. and in the evening. Stools may be loose, spluttery and very offensive; diarrhoea may occur of fluid, dark brown highly offensive stools, often early in the morning between 1 a.m. and 4 a.m. Constipation may recur every third or fourth day, even the passage of a soft stool being rendered difficult by rectal atony.

Lymphatic and Glandular Systems

Chronic enlargements of lymph nodes is common, especially in the cervical region. Breasts become swollen, painful, and nipples flushed, burning and itching.

Urinary System
Bladder control is poor; incontinence is apt to recur at full moon. Papillomata on the prepuce itch and burn.

Genital System
Pain in the groin extends downwards along the spermatic cord, associated with soreness and heavy sensation in the testicles; libido is diminished; impotence common. The remedy may be called for in menopausal disorders associated with hot flushes. Leucorrhoea occurs with the passage of large lumps; the discharge has an unbearable odour; violent pains are felt in the sacrum.

Locomotor System
Joints and back are weak; falls and sprains occur easily; articulations feel as if they were dislocated.

Skin
Scaly eruptions disappear in summer and recur in winter. Itching, burning eruptions are especially common behind the ears, with a smelly, oozing discharge. Itching and burning may occur without any eruptions; must scratch till draws blood and without obtaining much relief. Skin conditions are aggravated when warm, especially by the warmth of the bed, also from contact with wool or with water. Eruptions vary, eczema, acne, boils, indolent ulcers, easy suppuration may need the remedy. There may be complaint of a sensation of rawness, tingling or formication.

MODALITIES

There is aggravation from cold, in cold air, out of doors, from weather changes, before and during a thunderstorm, in winter. Aggravation also from touch or pressure, at the menstrual period, when walking, from washing.

Is better from warmth, by wrapping up warmly, when lying down, in summer, while eating, after a free perspiration, after a nose-bleed.

CLINICAL NOTES

The remedy is indicated in states of low vitality, especially with involvement of skin or lymph nodes. Chronicity and periodicity of symptoms also call for consideration of Psorinum.

Pulsatilla Nigricans

SOURCE

The remedy is prepared from *Pulsatilla nigricans*, the wind-flower, meadow anemone, or pasque flower, a member of the Ranunculaceae family, which also includes *Aconitum*, *Cimicifuga* and *Staphisagria*.

This is one of the flowers of chalk-lands. It has strikingly beautiful bell-shaped flowers of a deep purple hue with a rich golden centre. The leaves are of two types – foliage leaves growing on their own stalks from ground level, deeply cleft and fern-like, and long finger-like leaves in three segments ringing the flower stems; these are modified bracts.

John Gilmour writes, 'In April the turf is sprinkled with the purple and gold pasque flower, the most famous chalk rarity. The first sight of it on a Chiltern slope, or decorating a certain bunker on an East Anglian golf course, is a baptismal moment in botanical experience – at any rate in that of an Englishman, for in Europe the plant has a wider range.'

Quelch describes the plant thus, 'It is a little plant, covered with long silky hairs, growing about six or eight inches high. Its large purple flowers open in April and May. Even the smell from the bruised leaves or broken flowers has been known to cause headache or fainting fits and to produce inflammation of the eyes. Handling many blooms causes a form of eczema on the hands, and if the juice enters any cut or scratch a very serious sore may develop.'

The flowers often bloom again in September and are found not singly but in little groups or clumps. The entire fresh plant is used in the preparation of the mother tincture. This has a yellow colour and possesses a somewhat sharp taste.

The name of this plant, wind-flower, suggests variability, which is incidentally a prominent characteristic of Pulsatilla symptoms. Its deep purple colour points to plethora reminiscent of the venous congestion associated with this remedy.

Hamilton writes, 'This plant has an extremely acrid taste when chewed, and corrodes the tongue and fauces; and the dried plant retains a considerable share of acrimony.' This is interesting, for one characteristic of the normally mild and amiable Pulsatilla subject is a capacity for becoming decidedly acrimonious if 'chewed' or 'fed-up'.

413

In its habit of growth the plant is not obtrusive as, for instance, *Belladonna* but quiet and retiring, and its tendency to grow in clusters manifests a correspondence with the gregarious nature of the Pulsatilla person, so fond of company and averse to solitude.

PHARMACOLOGY

This plant was formerly regarded as having considerable affinity with various parts and organs. Pliny recommends all kinds of the 'wind floure tree, in headache and inflammations thereof; cures the infirmities of the teeth; and laid to the eyes as a cataplasme, represseth the vehement flux of watery humours thither. The magicians and wise men attribute much to these hearbs, and tell many wonders of them . . .'

There is a very definite affinity with mucous membranes producing catarrhal responses evidenced by thick mucoid discharges.

The action on eyes, ears and skin causes irritation and inflammation. Joints are affected, giving rise to synovitis, swelling and pain. There is an affinity with the heart and circulation, notably the right side of the heart and veins, resulting in venous congestion and varicosity.

The action on the generative organs is to cause varying degrees of irregularity of function and inflammatory changes of chronic type, manifesting creamy discharges.

PROVING

Pulsatilla Nigricans was proved by Hahnemann, who published the results in the second volume of the *Materia Medica Pura*.

APPEARANCE

Light hair, blue eyes and a freckled countenance of rubicund hue are associated with the remedy.

The face may appear rather bloated with a tendency to puffiness, which may also affect the belly, feet and ankles. Obesity is common.

A certain clumsiness of movement may be observed in a tendency to stumble when walking or to drop plates and dishes.

The skin may appear red and hot to the touch without any abnormal rise in temperature. Inflamed mucous surfaces have a purplish hue; discharges are bland, thick and yellow or green in colour.

Speech is somewhat hesitant and answers may suggest peevishness. The sound of the child's cry is pitiful rather than petulant (as, for instance, with Chamomilla).

PSYCHOLOGY

The Pulsatilla subject is described as affectionate, gregarious, fond of company and very averse to solitude. It is noted, however, that the Pulsatilla child desires and absorbs affection, but does not return it in the responsive way that is characteristic of the Phosphorus child.

A French paediatrician has supplied a valuable picture: 'Pulsatilla is more timid than anxious. Melancholy and sad, the Pulsatilla child can stand in front of you dumb and blushing, obstinately refusing the sweet you offer him, petrified by a taboo the grown-ups cannot understand. And, while by every possible means you try to coax him out of his mutism, you feel that he is being tortured, that he wishes the end of the world would come, rather than that the conversation should continue.

'Suddenly, his resistance ended, his eyes fill with tears, and he throws himself into his mother's skirts, clinging with both hands and hiding his face. Then if she can find the soothing words he is waiting for the little wretch will dry his tears and you will see him smile.'

Variability seems to describe the Pulsatilla subject, variously described as tender-hearted, easily 'hurt', responsive to kindness; easily discouraged, but never sullen and never moping; good-tempered, placid, mild, yielding, craves sympathy; slow, phlegmatic, may become irritable and touchy, but not violent; changeable, moods vary like the wind; anxious, morose, hesitant, discontented, everything disgusts him.

Certainly this type is capable of inward grief, self-pity, and apt to suffer in silence. Tears come easily, with some relief to feelings. May weep when recounting symptoms, a feature shared with Kali Carb., Medorrhinum and Sepia.

There is desire for affection, attention, approbation, consolation. Fear of the dark is prominent, also possibly fear of insanity, and the urge to suicide by drowning. Fear is 'felt' in the epigastrium and described as 'the stomach turning over'. The sensation may be accompanied by hot flushes and palpitation, even by actual vomiting.

Unfounded imaginings about food, sex, religion, germs and so on may reach the stage of psychotic obsession.

PHYSIOLOGY

The Pulsatilla circulation is extremely labile. Heat and chilly feelings alternate, or occur synchronously in different sites, coming and going in a patchy manner.

Although perhaps feeling chilly, even in a warm room, yet cannot tolerate a stuffy airless atmosphere and craves open windows and plenty of fresh air. Draws away from the fire, gets too hot in bed, and flags in really hot weather.

Appetite is capricious, but there is often a fondness for pastries, fat, ice-cream, rich foods, all of which disagree. Food may lack flavour, and there may be a definite dislike of various things such as meat, milk, butter and especially pork.

Thirst is usually minimal, even in fevers, but a craving for lemon drinks has been observed.

The Pulsatilla person is usually sleepy on retiring, but is apt to lie awake from ebullition of blood, get too hot, throw off the bed-covers, become chilly and haul them up again. There is a tendency also to wake in the early hours and stay awake for a prolonged spell. May change posture while asleep and is likely to put the hands up above the head.

Sweating is common and may be localized to certain areas or involve only one side of the body. Sweats break out on the face in association with waves of heat. Night sweats may be profuse; the sweat may have a musty odour.

SYMPTOMATOLOGY

General

The Pulsatilla pains are shifting and variable, often of bursting or expanding type, the soreness of congestive states. Pains are apt to appear abruptly and decline gradually, or the reverse; they are often diffuse, poorly localized or felt in ill-defined locations. They are worse when at rest and on first movement after rest. Symptoms in general are variable, no two attacks alike; they come and go in an unexpected and unpredictable manner. Only one side of the body may be affected.

Head

Vertigo may be severe, even so far as to staggering or falling. It is worse when rising from lying down, when stooping, also when sitting and when walking in the open air. It may also be increased after a meal and by looking upwards, and is more marked in the evening. Headache is often frontal and associated with digestive or menstrual disorders. It is aggravated by using the eyes for close work, by stooping, when sitting quietly or when lying down. Relief is obtained by tight bandaging of the forehead and by walking slowly out of doors. There is often great heaviness in the head and sensitivity in the scalp, which may itch and be sore to the touch.

Eyes

Severe eye symptoms are associated with this remedy, notably those involving the cornea, possibly with ulceration. Conjunctivitis is accompanied by thick yellow discharge, with agglutination of the lids in the morning, although redness of the lids is not noticed. Various sensations may be complained about – burning, itching, 'a gauze veil before the eyes', and there is a constant urge to rub the eyes in search of relief. Styes occur, especially on the lower lid. Cataract may ensure. Photophobia may be accompanied by lancinating pain in eyeball.

Ears

The remedy is of great value in relation to earache, especially if brought on by exposure to cold or in association with an exanthem. Established otitis media is accompanied by thick creamy pus, possibly offensive in odour. Tinnitus may occur, of the pulsating type. Inflammation of the pinna is accompanied by much heat, redness, swelling and pain, suggestive of erysipelas. Catarrhal deafness may occur, the ear or ears feeling 'stuffed up'.

Respiratory System

Catarrhal rhinitis tends to persist, accompanied by thick, yellowish or green, profuse, bland discharge. The discharge may contain large blood-stained crusts. The nose may become sore and swollen. Discharge may alternate from side to side; tends to be freer out of doors; in a warm room and in the evening the nose becomes blocked. Loss of smell and taste are common and there may be complaint of a 'bad smell in the nose'. Epistaxis occurs, often vicarious in nature, and the blood lost is thick, easily clotting and dark in colour, almost black. Involvement of the maxillary antrum is not infrequent, especially on the right side, accompanied by an orange-yellow discharge.

Hayfever in the Pulsatilla person is usually accompanied by amelioration of all the other symptoms which had been present. Sore throat is accompanied by a swollen sensation or by intolerable dryness, but in spite of the latter the patient is not thirsty. Involvement of the larynx is associated with scraping, dryness, pain as from excoriation and aphonia. Soreness may be felt below the clavicles, possibly extending to shoulder or arm. A dry teasing cough becomes more loose in the daytime or vice versa. The cough is worse when lying down, and a suffocating sensation forces the sufferer to sit up and 'get more air'. Or, on the contrary, the cough may trouble all day and cease at night. Sputum varies in amount and in character.

Alimentary System

There is often a bitter, slimy or even putrid taste in the mouth. The mouth may be unpleasantly dry, yet without any appreciable thirst. The tongue feels numb or as if burnt, and may be thickly coated with rough white fur. Painful gums are associated with toothache of a gnawing, shooting type, accompanied by chilly feelings and pallor, and most noticeable in the evening. The condition is aggravated in a warm room or when getting warm in bed; some relief is obtained from the impact of cool air. The pain is not increased by chewing food, but is activated by the use of a toothpick. When eating, the food may seem to stick in the throat or it feels as if the food regurgitates half way up the oesophagus, sticks there and then goes down again. Hiccough may be induced by smoking.

Easy vomiting may result from emotional upset or excitement. Attacks of nausea and vomiting are accompanied by a horribly chilly feeling, but in a warm stuffy room the suffering is increased with sweating and flushing of the face. Walking quietly in the open will afford relief. Gastric symptoms may be accompanied by the sensation of a lump behind the sternum, and much fullness and heaviness in the epigastrium, coming on some one to two hours after a meal. Eructations taste of food. The burning sensation in the stomach is increased by taking warm food, but relieved temporarily by cold food or fluids. Bloating of the belly and cutting pains are noticed more especially in the evening after supper, and are worse after rich food. Belching gives some temporary relief. Heartburn is characteristic of Pulsatilla, and waterbrash of Nux Vomica.

Constipation may occur, of the Nux Vomica type, with much ineffectual urging and the sensation of inadequate emptying of the rectum after going to stool. Diarrhoea may be violent, often nocturnal, with much burning in the bowel and mucus in the stools. These are loose and watery, accompanied by much flatus, tend to be greenish in colour and vary from stool to stool. Diarrhoea of this type may result from exposure to cold, from taking iced food or drinks, or from eating too much fruit. Piles tend to be protruding, painful and pruritic, worse by warmth of bed, when sitting still or lying down, and eased by gentle motion out of doors. The liver may be involved, as evidenced by heavy dragging pain in the hepatic region. The pain tends to spread through to the back between the shoulder-blades. There may be a slight degree of jaundice, associated with a heavily white-furred tongue, and a tendency to acute giddiness on attempting to get up in the morning.

Cardiovascular System

The chief features in this sphere are a tendency to dilatation of the right side of the heart, to venous congestion, varicose veins and chilblains. Palpitation and hot flushes accompany anxiety states, or emotional upset, and may occur after a heavy meal.

Lymphatic and Glandular Systems

Swellings of transient nature may occur in the breast or other sites. The remedy is often called for in an attack of mumps, especially if associated with swelling in breasts or testicles.

Urinary System

Diminished sphincter control resulting in a leaky bladder is especially liable to give trouble when sitting, walking or coughing. Irritability of bladder may occur with much frequency of urge and incontinence if there is delay in emptying the organ. Dysuria gives distress, and soreness persists even after passage of urine. The remedy may be of value in relation to nocturnal enuresis, especially when it is impossible to lie on the back without urge to urinate. It may also be called for when bladder symptoms occur during pregnancy.

Genital System

Pain in testicle extending to spermatic cord and groin. Varicocele, hydrocele, orchitis may be indications for the remedy, as well as gonorrhoea in either sex. Various uterine disorders are described, associated with thick, green, creamy non-irritating discharges. Dysmenorrhoea may be associated with inframammary pain. Menstrual periods are apt to be delayed and the flow scanty. Milk may be present in the breasts apart from pregnancy. There may be a constant sensation as if a menstrual period was imminent. Amenorrhoea may occur from fear of pregnancy. There may be a tendency to early abortion at the fifth week. The remedy has proved of value in disorders of pregnancy, with abnormal presentations, in uterine inertia and feeble labour pains.

Locomotor System

In this sphere have been noted varying complaints of heaviness, weariness, weakness, bruised feelings, pains and swellings in various sites. Shooting pains in shoulders or arms occur in the morning and are aggravated by use of the limb. Legs feel queer with tottery gait. Legs feel very heavy by day and ache at night. Gouty pains wander from joint to joint and alternate with digestive upsets; the pains are worse from heat and somewhat relieved by gentle motion. Shooting pains occur in the nape, accompanied by soreness to touch. There may be cracking in neck and shoulders on movement. The remedy may give relief when scoliosis is associated with lumbosacral pain. With synovitis or articular rheumatism the pains are worse on first movement but are eased somewhat by gentle motion and by pressure.

Skin
Various eruptions may occur with burning or itching, made decidedly worse by heat in any form and relieved by cold applications. Ulcers tend to bleed or exude yellow or green discharges.

MODALITIES

These are such as would increase or alleviate the disturbances in the circulation. There is aggravation from heat, close atmosphere, humidity, even cold; also from too many clothes or too heavy bed-covers. The sufferer feels worse when at rest, when lying on the left side; also in the evening and during the first part of the night.

Relief is felt in fresh air, especially cold dry air, by gentle motion out of doors (too active movement generates heat and causes discomfort); also from cold food, cool applications, pressure, or lying on the painful part, and uncovering. Ailments brought on by becoming suddenly chilled when hot, or from getting wet through, may call for Pulsatilla or possibly Dulcamara.

CLINICAL NOTES

As will have been obvious above, this remedy has a wide sphere of usefulness in affections of chest, digestive tract, pelvic organs, joints and skin in the Pulsatilla type of individual.

The remedy is often called for when the troubles from which the patient is suffering date from adolescence.

Pulsatilla patients may need Graphites or Sepia in middle age; they often require Nux Vomica as an intercurrent remedy.

Silica is said to be the chronic of Pulsatilla. Other complementary remedies are Lycopodium and Sulphuric Acid.

Unpleasant effects of Pulsatilla can be antidoted by Chamomilla, Ignatia or Nux Vomica. Pulsatilla antidotes overreaction to Sulphur.

Pyrogenium

SOURCE

This rather odd remedy might be described as a polyvalent nosode. It was first prepared by Drysdale in the 1870s from putrid matter obtained by exposing chopped lean beef in water 'in a sunny place' for three weeks. The resulting material was put through various processes, including two boilings, and the final watery extract was named Sepsin. This product mixed with an equal part of glycerine was termed Pyrexin Ø or Pyrogen. At a later date potencies were prepared from this product or from the pure extract without the addition of glycerine. It is an extremely active and most valuable remedy.

PHARMACOLOGY

The tissue affinities appear to be mainly with the blood, causing a degeneration such as is met with in septicaemic states with resulting fever, rigors, interstitial and intestinal haemorrhages.

PROVING

Pyrogen was proved by Drysdale, Wyborn and others, and described by Burnett, as well as in Allen's *Materia Medica of the Nosodes*.

APPEARANCE

The face and ears are red and hot or may change to the Hippocratic facies, with an ashy hue of the skin.

Hands are cold and clammy. The subject is icy cold with evident air hunger. Fan-like movements of the alae nasi are seen, a sign that is also seen with Lycopodium patients.

Restlessness is very noticeable, the sufferer being in constant movement despite the condition of prostration and weakness.

There is a tendency for over-talkativeness with rapid speech, but dryness of the tongue may make articulation difficult. This may pass on to a muttering type of delirium, especially on closing the eyes. The head is rolled from side to side on the pillow.

The temperature/pulse ratio is totally out of rhythm. With quite a low temperature the pulse may be very rapid, small and thready. With high fever the pulse rate may not be as rapid as would normally be expected.

All discharges are horribly offensive. Foetor oris is very evident.

The tongue is large, flabby, clean and smoothly glazed as if with a coat of varnish; it is fiery red in colour and in sharp contrast to the heavily coated tongue of Baptisia. It becomes dry and fissured.

PSYCHOLOGY

Mental confusion is extreme, a variety of odd sensations being described in relation to body-image. Feels as if 'she covered the whole bed'; as if 'he were two people'; as if 'crowded with legs and arms'; as if the bed lain on were too hard and full of lumps – a symptom shared with Arnica and Baptisia. There may also be delusions of wealth.

A sensation of numbness starts in hands and feet and spreads all over the body.

PHYSIOLOGY

There is complaint of extreme chilliness that no fire can warm, and at the same time a craving for fresh, cool air.

Anorexia is usual. Thirst for cold drinks is marked. These are usually not retained but vomited as soon as warmed up in the stomach – a symptom also found in Phosphorus.

Sleep is shallow; seems to dream all night.

Sweats are profuse, very offensive, cold and clammy.

SYMPTOMATOLOGY

General

The picture is one of septicaemia with dry tongue, chills which start between the shoulder-blades, rigors, irregular fever, cold sweats and disturbance of temperature/pulse ratio. Fever may be high, up to 41°C, with dry burning skin in alternation with sweats. Violent burning may occur, for instance in an abscess. Severe aching pains may be felt in the bones. The whole body feels bruised and over-sensitive. Hence the constant restlessness and moving about in search of ease. There is a tendency for symptoms to relapse, or for recovery to be incomplete.

Head
Vertigo is noticed when attempting to rise up in bed. A bursting, throbbing headache may be present, associated with a feeling as if 'the skull was being tightly constricted by a cap'. Firm pressure gives some relief. The head sweats profusely.

Eyes
The eyeballs are sore to touch, and looking upwards or outwards causes pain.

Respiratory System. The larynx is involved, causing the voice to be weak and husky. A cough is accompanied by the production of large quantities of mucus from the larynx, and sputum which may be purulent or 'rusty'. It is worse by movement and in a warm room.

Alimentary System
There is a horrible sweetish taste in the mouth, like pus. Nausea is relieved by taking very hot water, but cold water, though desired, is usually vomited up again as soon as warm. Vomiting is often persistent, the vomitus being brownish, offensive, even faeculent. The abdomen is distended and acutely tender; taking a deep breath causes pain; cutting colicky pains are felt especially on the right side with a spread through to the back, but there is some relief when lying on the right side. Horribly offensive diarrhoea occurs, the stools being brown or black, painless and even involuntary. Constipation may also be present as the result of rectal inertia; the impacted faeces when passed are like small black balls and of carrion-like odour. Severe rectal tenesmus may cause distress.

Cardiovascular System
There is also undue awareness of the heart, which feels tired; palpitations are of a violent thudding character; the heart beats can be heard a foot away from the chest. There is much throbbing of the carotids, and pulsation felt in the ears tends to prevent sleep.

Urinary System
There is urgency to micturate when fever is imminent; the urine may be scanty with an adhesive red deposit of urates, and is likely to contain albumen and casts. Tenesmus is felt in the bladder.

Pyrogenium

Genital System

Prolapsus uteri occurs with much bearing-down sensation, somewhat relieved by holding the breath and actively bearing down. Septic fever following abortion or labour is characterized by thin brownish lochia, which may be scanty or suppressed and is very foetid.

Skin

Ulcers tend to become chronic, foul, freely discharging and are extremely painful. They may be of varicose origin.

MODALITIES

There is aggravation from cold, especially damp cold; the sufferer is worse when attempting to sit up.

Temporary relief is obtained by constant alteration of posture.

CLINICAL NOTES

This remedy is often called for in septic, toxaemic or pyaemic conditions, perhaps when some other apparently indicated remedy has failed to cure. It may also be of value when there is a history of previous sepsis, say puerperal fever, from which there has never been a full and satisfactory recovery of health. Arsenicum Alb. is a complementary remedy.

Ranunculus Bulbosus

SOURCE

Ranunculus bulbosus, the bulbous buttercup, crowfoot, St Anthony's turnip, goldcup, is perhaps the commonest of the Ranunculaceae, covering the meadows in May with dazzling yellow. It is the small buttercup of lawns and fields, swollen at the base to form a round, solid bulb about one inch in diameter.

The flowers and fruits resemble those of the common buttercup, *Ranunculus acris*, while the leaves, which are divided into three stalked segments, are more like those of the creeping crowfoot. Notably the three vivid green sepals of the flower are folded back along the grooved hairy stem, which reaches a height of one foot. The rich yellow of the petals is remarkable for a mirror-like sheen, claimed by some botanists to be a unique feature.

Like other members of the family it was used by the ancients; for medicinal purposes the entire plant is employed, gathered at the time of flowering in May and June.

PHARMACOLOGY

That the plant is by no means devoid of toxic properties was recognized by Gerrard, who wrote, 'There be divers sorts or kinds of these pernitious herbes comprehended under the name of Ranunculus or Crowfoote, whereof most are very dangerous to be taken into the body. Not any of them are to be taken alone by themselves, because they are of the most violent force, and therefore have the great nede of correction.' However, he does admit that, 'These dangerous simples are likewise many times of themselves beneficiall and sometimes profitable.'

Writing in special reference to the bulbous variety he quotes from Pliny that 'when drunke with wine and myrrh, it causeth a man to see divers strange sights, and not to cease laughing till he hath drunk pine-apple kernels with pepper', and adds, 'I think he would have said until he be dead; because the nature of laughing Crowefoot is thought to kill laughing; but without doubt the thing is clean contrary, for it causeth such convulsions, cramps and wringings of the mouth and jawes, that it hath seemed to some that the parties have died laughing, whereas, in truth, they have died with great torment.'

Furthermore Gerrard notes, 'Cunning beggers do use to stampe the leaves, and lay it until their legs and armes, which causeth such filthy ulcers as we daily see (among such wicked vagabondes), to moove the people the more to pittie.'

Such somewhat crude provings reveal an affinity of toxic nature with skin and other tissues, notably the nervous system. The effect on the skin is one of violent irritation, causing redness, burning, smarting, itching and a vesicular type of eruption.

Central nervous effects are seen in mental disturbances and a tendency to convulsions with grimacing. Peripheral effects, or rather involvement of nerve roots, give rise to severe neuralgic pains and the peculiar type of herpetic eruption which follows the distribution of the affected nerve (herpes zoster).

There is also affinity with serous membranes, producing inflammatory reactions which result in either adhesions of opposed surfaces or effusion. Muscles, especially those of the trunk, are involved, giving rise to pains of 'rheumatic' type.

An affinity with gastric mucosa was evidenced by 'four persons who had eaten the root of the *Ranunculus bulbosus* boiled in chicken-broth, and manifested the following symptoms; violent burning in the region of the cardiac orifice of the stomach, with great anxiety about the heart; pressure at the pit of the stomach, with painful soreness at the stomach when touched.'

PROVING

The provings of Ranunculus Bulbosus first appear in Stapf's *Additions*.

APPEARANCE

Redness of the cheeks is noticeable, and a tendency to rigidity and immobility, owing to the fact that any movement is liable to increase suffering (as is also the case with Bryonia).

PSYCHOLOGY

There is much disturbance in this sphere. Fear of ghosts may be present. Over-excitability, hasty temper, tendency to be .irritable and quarrelsome in the morning, may contrast with depression and a desire to die.

The mental condition may be due to alcoholism, and actual delirium tremens may ensue, calling for treatment with the remedy in potency.

PHYSIOLOGY

There is great sensitivity to cold, and cold air, whether out of doors or in a draught. Sometimes there may be complaint of a sensation as if part of the body is swathed in a cold, wet cloth.

Hunger may be increased in the morning and thirst be very evident in the afternoon. Drowsiness by day is followed by sleeplessness at night, or a tendency to wake and lie awake for prolonged periods. There may be inability to remain lying on the left side.

SYMPTOMATOLOGY

General
Pains are of 'rheumatic' or neuralgic type, stitching, burning or pressing, and are often brought on by exposure to cold or damp.

Head
Severe headache may occur, especially felt over the right eye; it is worse when lying down but relieved when standing erect or walking about. It may be associated with a whirling giddiness, a feeling of dejection and a desire to weep. A pressive headache in the forehead or on the vertex is notably aggravated by a change in temperature, either from cold to warm or the reverse. It is also worse in the morning.

Eyes
Eye symptoms are severe and distressing, with pressive and smarting, stabbing pains, sometimes in one eye, sometimes in the other. These pains are made worse by moving the eyeballs. The pupils are dilated and vision is dimmed, with a sensation of mist before the eyes, associated with photophobia and lachrymation. Herpes zoster may involve the lids and also the conjunctiva and cornea.

Respiratory System
The remedy may be indicated in hay fever, accompanied by smarting and burning in the eyes, with soreness of the lids. The nose is stuffed up, especially in the evening, and there is a relentless tingling and crawling sensation inside the nose or in the naso-pharynx, which causes constant but ineffectual hawking in the endeavour to obtain relief. Severe pain in the chest is a prominent symptom. This is of the nature of a myalgia of the pectoral or intercostal muscles, or an intercostal neuralgia with sharp stitching pains in the thorax and between the shoulder-blades. Charac-

teristically there is also a marked soreness to touch as if the tissues had been pounded or bruised. Movement aggravates the pain, as do also pressure of clothes or hands. A stabbing pain may be located in the lowest intercostal space on the right side, associated with a sensation as if a weight were pressing on the top of the right shoulder. Breathing is interfered with, especially inspiration, and it is impossible to lie on the right side. Pleurisy, possibly diaphragmatic, may be dry or accompanied by effusion, and is associated with great anxiety, dyspnoea and distress, and with pains which shoot from front to back.

Alimentary System
Spasmodic hiccough may be induced by alcoholic drinks. Belching is prominent. Nausea is especially noticed in the afternoon. Pain is felt in both hypochondria as if bruised, or as if one had been lying in a wrong position. Painful soreness is felt under the short ribs on the left side; pressure is felt deep in the region of the liver after a meal; a pinching pain is felt below the umbilicus; violent stitches spread from the left lumbar region through the belly and towards the left groin. There is marked flatulence and soreness to touch, especially in the epigastrium. Watery diarrhoea or dysentery may occur. Often a morning stool is passed with considerable difficulty, and a natural easy stool in the afternoon.

Lymphatic and Glandular Systems
A stabbing pain below the left nipple, aggravated by contact or movement, deserves mention.

Cardiovascular System
Sudden circulatory weakness may lead to actual syncope.

Nervous System
The remedy is often called for in herpes zoster, shingles, where the involvement of nerve roots is evidence in the first instance by severe pain along the area of distribution of a nerve path, to be followed by the typical burning, itching eruption of small vesicles. These may coalesce and form horny scabs or scurf.

Locomotor System
Severe pains are felt along the spine, especially between the shoulder-blades or along the medial border of the left scapula. The latter pain may spread to the whole left side of the chest. Tearing, shooting pains occur in the limbs. These may be paroxysmal in character and are increased by

cold and movement. Joints may be involved, and extreme weakness may be felt in the lower limbs when walking, especially during the morning hours.

Skin

Symptoms are prominent in this sphere. Eruptions tend to be vesicular and the small blisters often have a dark blue colour. They may appear on the palms and fingers or in other sites. After bursting, scabs of a tough horny consistency form. Other forms of skin affection may be pemphigoid or xerodermatous. Crawling and creeping sensations may be felt in scalp, nose or fingers. Cracks occur at the tips of the fingers. Corns smart, burn and are very sensitive to touch and pressure.

MODALITIES

There is aggravation from any exposure to cold air and from change in the weather, especially from warm or cold. Humid and thundery weather also tend to aggravate the symptoms. Pain is increased by touch or pressure, also by stretching the limbs or by any movement. A definite aggravation in the evening is a marked feature.

Relief may be felt when sitting down with the body inclined forward, as is the case with Kali Carb.

CLINICAL NOTES

The above-mentioned conditions, alcoholism included, may call for the use of the remedy, which is perhaps prescribed too infrequently. The lower potencies, up to 30c, have given good results.

Rhododendron Chrysanthum

SOURCE

Rhododendron chrysanthum, rosebay, yellow snowrose, is a small bush found in Siberia as well as in the Alps and the Pyrenees. It grows only to a height of 1 to 1½ feet and is often so concealed by moss that only the tips of the shoots are visible. Its leaves are alternate, like those of the laurel, ovate, rough above, paler and smoother on the under aspect. The flowers are large, showy, golden-yellow, in clusters, emerging from large downy scales. The mother tincture is prepared from the fresh leaves.

PHARMACOLOGY

There is affinity with fibrous tissues, notably ligaments, periosteum, tunica vaginalis testis, resulting in inflammation and rheumatic type pain. The plant also contains a narcotic principle.

PROVING

Rhododendron was proved by Dr Seidl and published in Stapf's *Additions*.

APPEARANCE

Possible observations may be inequality of pupils or the presence of 'rheumatic nodules'.

PSYCHOLOGY

The subject is apt to be anxious, depressed, nervy, with a peculiar sensitivity to electric storms and fear of thunder.

Memory is impaired; whole words are omitted when writing; loses the thread when talking.

May be apathetic, with aversion to making any kind of effort.

PHYSIOLOGY

There is coldness of the extremities, especially the feet, even in a warm room. Hands may feel hot but are cold to touch.

Is apt to complain of feeling full after taking only a small amount of food. Food has no flavour. May be quite thirsty.

Liability to be sleepless after midnight; cannot sleep unless legs are crossed. Appears terrified while asleep but wakes quite cheerful. Pains may drive from bed.

Sweats are profuse and debilitating; sweat may have an odour of spice; sweats while walking in open air. Perspiration is accompanied by itching and tingling.

SYMPTOMATOLOGY

General

Pains are described as tearing, aching, jerking and are apt to shift from one site to another. They are usually accompanied by much stiffness. Pains seem deep, and sites most commonly affected are forearms, hands, fingers, legs and toes. The pains may intermit for indefinite periods. The right side is often mainly involved.

Head

Vertigo assails when lying in bed; is better when moving about. Violent headache in bed in the morning is relieved to some extent by rising and moving about, also by warm wraps; it is worse in wet and cold weather, also from taking wine. The pain may be felt in the bones of the skull. Pain may be felt in forehead and temporal regions. Head feels sore, as if bruised. Trigeminal and dental neuralgia is worse in wet windy weather and before a storm; is better from warmth and by taking food.

Eyes

Ciliary neuralgia involves eyeball orbit and head, and the pains are described as darting like arrows; it is worse before a storm and better from heat and movement. Eyes tire easily. There may be spasm or twitching of eyelids. One pupil may be contracted and the other dilated.

Ears

Violent earache is worse before a storm and relieved by heat. Intense roaring, whizzing, ringing tinnitus may be associated with a degree of deafness.

Respiratory System
Fluent coryza is associated with obstruction in one or other nostril. Epistaxis may occur. Violent pleuritic pains are accompanied by severe dyspnoea and possibly by aphonia. The throat feels burning and constricted. A dry paroxysmal cough is caused by a persistent tickle in the trachea. A stitch may be felt in the left hypochondrium when walking fast.

Alimentary System
Toothache affecting the molars is liable to occur in wet cold weather or before and during a storm. Change of weather or sharp east winds may also be causal factors. Tongue may be coated and of greenish hue. A bitter putrid taste may be noticed in the mouth. Salivation is apt to be profuse. Gastric complaints include nausea with inclination to vomit; waterbrash; pyrosis; fullness after meals embarrassing respiration; relief from belching. Shooting pains occur in the upper abdomen associated with flatulent distension. Urgent call to stool is accompanied by difficult evacuation, even of quite soft stool, and with much straining. Diarrhoea or dysentery may be induced by cold wet weather, approach of a storm or eating fruit. Liable to occur on rising in the morning. Crawling or throbbing sensations may be felt in the anal canal.

Urinary System
Frequency of urination is accompanied by discomfort in bladder and groins.

Genital System
Pain in testicles extends to spermatic cord, upwards into the abdomen and downwards into perineum or thigh. Testicle feels 'squeezed' and is very sensitive to touch. Testicles may become enlarged and indurated. Hydrocele occurs in children. Menses liable to be irregular. Fever and headache accompany menstrual period.

Locomotor System
In acute rheumatic attack, pains and swelling wander from joint to joint; are worse at rest and at night and are often accompanied by copious urination; liable to recur with change of weather. Chronic rheumatism affects mainly the smaller joints and their ligaments. Fibrous nodular deposits occur, especially in the great toe, often described as 'gouty'. Pain and stiffness affect muscles of nape and neck. Wrenching pains are felt in hip and knee. Wrists feel as if sprained.

Skin

Itching and burning occur with or without eruption.

MODALITIES

Aggravating factors are cold, wet cold, before rain, windy weather and, most important of all, approaching and actual thunderstorms. Aggravation also from touch and pressure; wine; when at rest; at night.

Is better from warmth; by moving about; by belching; after the storm has passed.

CLINICAL NOTES

The main indications for the remedy are the meteorological modalities, especially the undue sensitivity to stormy or windy weather. A complementary remedy is Natrum Sulph.

Rhus Toxicodendron

SOURCE

The name *Rhus toxicodendron* covers both poison ivy and poison oak. The latter is also known as *Rhus diversiloba* or *Toxicodendron quercifolium*, the leaves being oak-like, and is found on the Pacific coast of North America. Poison ivy, on the other hand, occurs on the east coast and is very common in Canada. It grows either as a shrub or as a woody vine, climbing by aerial rootlets. The climbing variety is also known as *Rhus radicans*.

It is an essentially restless plant, unwilling to stay put, spreading all over the countryside. Hence the liability of workers clearing the bush, or berry pickers inadvertently coming in contact with the leaves to their subsequent sorrow. It is of note that a chief characteristic of the Rhus Tox. drug picture is unease when at rest, with the urge to get moving for relief.

Both poison ivy and poison oak are members of the Anacardiaceae or Sumac family, and it has been found in provings that they induce almost identical responses. The mother tincture is prepared from the leaves, freshly gathered just before the time of flowering, and preferably at or just after sunset on a cloudy, sultry day, from plants growing in shady places. The tincture possesses a red colour, a somewhat astringent taste and a peculiar odour.

The distinguishing mark of poison ivy is the arrangement of its three leaflets. These form a triangle, the two leaflets at the base being almost sessile with very short stalks, whereas the third at the apex has quite a long stalk. Curiously enough, this leaf formation is also shared by *Ptelea trifoliata*, a small Rutaceous tree, commonly known as wafer ash or hop tree. The fruit, however, is quite different, being a cluster of papery seeds very reminiscent of the seeds of the wych-elm. Whereas the fruit of poison ivy is a cluster of small, round, smooth, white or ivory-coloured berries.

The flowers are small, five-petalled, greenish yellow, with a central golden cone of upright stamens, and bloom in June and July. They occur in a spike.

The leaves are placed alternately, supported on long petioles, their three dark green shining leaflets being about three inches long, ovate in shape, strongly veined, more or less downy on the under-suface. In the fall the foliage is dangerously attractive, when the leaves take on vivid flaming red and crimson tints. The root sends up a great many stems, which seldom grow erect but trail along the ground. They divide into slender woody branches, covered with a brown bark. The roots contain even more of the poisonous substance than any other part of the plant, and are just as dangerous in the depth of winter if contacted in the course of bush clearance or other activity.

Human sensitivity varies a great deal, as with other forms of allergic sensitivity to contact poisons. The horse, mule and goat can apparently eat the plant with impunity. The berries are eaten by birds.

PHARMACOLOGY

There has been much controversy as to which ingredient of the plant is responsible for its extreme toxicity. Investigation points to a polyhedric phenol, named by one worker lobinol and by another urushiol, as the chief offender. One author states that 'there are probably no other plants in existence which cause so much human distress and suffering as the four Toxicodendrons, all of which are responsible for so-called poison ivy dermatitis.'

This seems a somewhat sweeping statement, but the symptoms of poisoning are certainly no joke. They are described in a Canadian medical journal thus:

'After a period of twelve to forty-eight hours following contact, the skin becomes red and itchy. A few hours later small papules are formed, close together, and cover the area touched by the plant. Later these become vesicles with colourless serum which does not contain the poisonous substance, for it is quite harmless when transferred to other parts of the body. The itching is intense.

'Vesicles appear on the third day and last a week, then gradually dry up. In severe cases the skin is discoloured for a month, but itching is usually gone in ten days from its first appearance.'

Wheeler and Kenyon point out further that, 'The vesicular eruption may spread to mucous membranes. Mouth and throat swell; nausea and vomiting and irritating cough apeear. Pains develop about the joints with great lumbar stiffness. Arms and legs become numb. Fever may be accompanied by delirium and mental confusion, and often ends with copious sweating. Urinary secretion is increased and diarrhoea is usual. Great general soreness and prostration are prominent symptoms.'

Certainly a gamut of distress and suffering. Evidently the tissue affinities of this plant are extensive. To sum up: with the skin inducing an intense irritant dermatitis, characterized by itching, burning, swelling, erythema and vesication; with lymphoid tissue and various glands, e.g. the parotid, giving rise to inflammation and hypertrophy; with the brain, tending to depression and mental confusion; with muscles and ligaments, causing both pain and temporary paralysis; with fascial and connective tissues, giving rise to oedematous swelling and stiffness.

PROVING

Rhus Tox. was proved by Hahnemann, and the second volume of *Materia Medica Pura* contains its pathogenesis.

APPEARANCE

The sufferer needing this remedy may present a pale, sickly appearance with sunken eyes surrounded by blue rings, or the face may be suffused with a red flush and a flaming red nose. Sometimes the countenance is distorted, being drawn to one side or the other, and exhibits a furtive suspicious expression.

The patient is in obvious pain and distress yet cannot stay still; keeps tossing and turning if in bed, or will move restlessly about in search of relief if up.

The lips tend to become cracked and dry. The tongue also is dry and may be cracked or fissured, the cracks tending to gape and bleed. The tongue looks dark brown in colour, often with a triangular red area at the tip.

Herpetic eruptions are common, especially around the mouth and on the chin.

Movements tend to be awkward and clumsy. In fact stiffness and consequent lameness may produce a condition bordering on paralysis. This results in a reeling, staggering type of gait, suggestive of intoxication, with a tendency to swerve to the right. Actual tremors are apt to ensue in the limbs after active exertion.

PSYCHOLOGY

Extreme restlessness of spirit accompanies the physical unease, and this is accentuated at night. The sufferer cannot get unpleasant thoughts out of his head; gets very worried about the future, about his family, about his business; becomes depressed and despondent.

There may be actual confusion of thought, disinclination for any mental effort, forgetfulness of what he set out to do, even while doing it.

The mental anxiety may take the form of actual suspicion and fear of being poisoned, resulting in a refusal to take any medicine offered and a tendency to get out of bed at night in an attempt to escape.

There is frequently a desire for solitude, much weariness of life, sadness, with a tendency to 'weep without knowing why'. Fever is apt to be accompanied by actual stupor or muttering delirium.

PHYSIOLOGY

Great sensitivity to open air or to uncovering. Even putting a hand outside the bed-covers may bring on a fit of coughing.

Empty hunger may occur without any real appetite. Desire for cold milk and sweets may be noted, also a dislike of meat and bread.

Notable is an unquenchable thirst for cold drinks, especially at night, but at the same time the drinking of cold fluids may increase the sensation of chilliness and may aggravate cough. The thirst is associated with dryness of mouth, tongue and throat.

Sleep is restless, patchy, disturbed, especially in the second half of the night. There is a tendency to dream of activities involving great exertion. Violent spasmodic yawning may occur.

Sweating may be a prominent feature. Sweats from pain; sweats even while sitting still; very persistent sweats, the perspiration acquiring an unpleasant odour; sweating accompanied by trembling; sweating at night in association with a pruritic miliary eruption; sweating as the result of taking a warm drink.

SYMPTOMATOLOGY

General

Symptoms requiring this remedy are likely to be induced by getting wet, especially after being overheated; also by undue exertion, especially if muscle groups are involved in some form of unaccustomed activity. Another aetiological factor may be stress due to undergoing a surgical operation. Pains are described as shooting or tearing, or perhaps as a dull gnawing or burning ache; when at rest – the 'rheumatic' type of pain. Pains tend to be worse when resting, resulting in an irresistible urge to shift position or get up and move about in search of relief. Pains are commonly accompanied by a sensation of stiffness, which is also relieved temporarily by movement, but worse after a period of inactivity. The first movement after rest is usually quite painful. Muscular weakness is also a prominent feature and may be associated with a feeling of numbness. Fever is accompanied by a sensation of chilliness; the chill often starts in one lower limb, perhaps in the thigh, or is first noticed in the dorsum between the shoulder-blades; it causes fits of shivering with a feeling as if 'plunged into a bath of cold water'.

Head
The peculiar feeling of giddiness associated with this remedy is noticed on rising from the lying posture, and is a sensation as if one would fall over, either forwards or backwards. Headaches of great variety are described under Rhus Tox. in the literature, as well as a dull stupid feeling in this region. A frontal headache is mentioned, worse from cold and aggravated by every step when walking, as also by shaking the head. The headache may be accompanied by a curious sensation as if the brain was loose and swashing about inside the skull. A severe occipital headache may occur, relieved by warmth and also by bending the head backwards – a headache modality shared by Belladonna, Cactus, Chamomilla and Hepar Sulph. The Rhus Tox. headache is apt to recur at the least feeling of chagrin or frustration. It is often accompanied by extreme sensitivity of the scalp. Furthermore the sufferer on stooping down feels unable to straighten up again. Mention is also made under this remedy of a migraine-type headache which is relieved by taking a long walk out of doors. Moist itching eruptions may occur on the scalp with the formation of thick crusts and the presence of an offensive odour.

Eyes
Eye conditions calling for this remedy are acute and severe, such as acute swelling of lids; chemosis; orbital cellulitis; ptosis; suppurative iritis. Soreness of the eyeballs is marked, with stiffness of the lids which stick together at night. Corneal ulcer may occur with marked photophobia. Styes and profuse lachrymation are also mentioned.

Ears
A peculiar sensation may be complained of as if 'wind was blowing into the ear'. In the case of otitis media the pus is likely to be blood-stained.

Respiratory System
A severe type of nasal coryza is worse on first rising in the morning, is accompanied by much sneezing, violent in character, and associated with a tendency to epistaxis of dark coloured blood. Hoarseness is noticed on attempting to sing, but perseverance in the attempt results in improve-

ment. This is in distinction from the hoarseness associated with Arum Triphyllum. In the latter case persistence in the attempt to use the voice results in complete aphonia. A dry teasing cough resulting from a tickle behind the upper part of the sternum is apt to occur with shivering or as the result of putting a hand outside the bed-covers. It is associated with a raw, scraped sensation in the air passages, and often with the taste of blood in the mouth. Much hawking of mucus with a salty taste is common. Coughing hurts the chest and may also cause a 'shattering' type of headache. It is aggravated by contact with cold air. The sputum may be rust-coloured. Asthma, when the attacks alternate with herpes labialis, may require this remedy.

Alimentary System
The remedy may be indicated in affections of the temporomaxillary joint, easy dislocation of the lower jaw, arthritis accompanied by the constant desire to yawn (in order to move the tissues around the joint in search of relief). Cracking in the joint when chewing. Ulcers occur at the corners of the mouth. Lips and mouth are very dry and the lips often cracked. The tongue is dry and sore, coated white or brown, with a red triangular area at the tip. A bitter or putrid taste may be present and in place of dryness the secretion of much viscid saliva. Aberrations of appetite may be experienced – anorexia with repugnance to food; empty hunger without any relish for food; bouts of ravenous hunger passing off after sitting for a while; nausea and vomiting associated with loss of appetite. 'Fullness' and 'weight' may be noticed in the epigastrium after meals. Severe colicky pains in the belly are relieved by bending double or by moving about. The remedy may be called for in inflammatory conditions in the abdomen, also in Typhoid fever marked by great restlessness and mild delirium, the symptoms being much worse at night. Involuntary stools are accompanied by extreme exhaustion. With dysentery, tenesmus is marked, with tearing pains in the thighs during passage of stools; there is often also a craving for cold milk. Chronic painless morning diarrhoea may require this remedy, the stools being brick-red or brown in colour and very foul-smelling.

Cardiovascular System
Dilatation of the heart accompanied by palpitation, distress and trembling when sitting still may call for the remedy, especially when the symptoms are aggravated by over-exertion, and perhaps associated with a feeling of numbness in the left shoulder and arm. It may be indicated when cardiac hypertrophy has resulted from over-strain.

Lymphatic and Glandular Systems
Inflammation and enlargement of lymph nodes, of the parotid or the submaxillary salivary glands, possibly with suppuration, is a frequent indication for this remedy.

Genital System
An inflammatory dermatitis of erysipeloid type is especially likely to involve the scrotum and external genitalia, accompanied by much oedema and severe itching.

Urinary System
A sphere of usefulness here is in relation to post-operative retention of urine from paresis of the bladder. Bladder symptoms resulting from getting soaked in the wet may need the remedy. It has on occasion proved of value in connection with nocturnal enuresis in children.

Locomotor System
Here the remedy is of paramount worth, and has proved its value in conditions such as the following:
Strains and sprains from muscular stress, especially in the performance of some unusual activity, or from sudden violent movement. Low back pain, pain between the shoulder-blades on dry swallowing, stiff neck – the pain being of jerking or tearing character, worse in the morning and on first movement. As mentioned before, the pains tend to be relieved by movement but only for a time, recurring with fatigue. Stiffness of severe degree is a marked concomitant of the pains and shares in the same modalities, relief from warmth and from movement for a time. A further feature is weakness accompanied by trembling in the limbs following excessive exertion; this may almost reach the pitch of paralysis, and the limbs feel inordinately heavy. Almost complete temporary paralysis may ensue after severe exposure to cold and wet. A sticking drawing pain in the left arm has been described, extending to the finger tips. Also paraesthesia – pins and needles – felt in the tips of the fingers, especially on grasping an object. This is presumably a form of compression neuritis. Also mentioned are: tingling pain in the shin bones, curiously made worse by warmth; hot, painful swollen joints; 'rheumatic gout' in the big toe joints; shooting pains in tendons and ligaments; left-sided sciatic pain.

Skin
The drug picture of this remedy naturally enough shows a variety of skin affections. Acute severe conditions of erysipeloid, vesicular, even bulbous, types associated with much oedema. When there is involvement

of the face the sufferer may be unrecognizable. Eruptions tend to itch and burn, especially at night and if exposed to heat or warmth in any form; scratching is compulsive but affords little relief. Eruptions may be pustular, or raw and weeping, or possibly covered with thick crusts and oozing offensive discharge. Again they may show periodic exacerbation, perhaps recurring every spring. The remedy is of value in some cases of herpes zoster.

MODALITIES

Symptoms are aggravated by cold, especially the combination of cold and wet; also by cold winds, in thunderstorms, and when rain is on the way. Again, the symptoms are worse when at rest, sitting, lying or standing still. Pain is aggravated by the first movement after sitting still for a while, and again when activity which has given temporary relief has reached the point of fatigue. This results in a vicious circle, thus: unease at rest compelling movement→relief: continued movement→fatigue→ fresh pain, compelling rest; rest→fresh unease and pain. Symptoms are also aggravated when lying on the right side, in the evening, especially about 7 p.m. and at night, particularly the second half of the night.

Relief is usually afforded by warmth and local hot applications, by warm dry weather, by wrapping up warmly. Movement also gives relief, if not persisted in to the point of fatigue.

CLINICAL NOTES

A survey of the above symptoms will show that Rhus Tox. has a very wide range of usefulness. A complementary remedy is Bryonia, but it should be noted that Apis Mellifica, which has some somewhat similar symptoms, should not be given in immediate sequence, either before or after Rhus Tox. Where the remedy, although apparently indicated, does not give the desired result, Radium Brom. has been found of value.

The remedy is called for in low fevers when stupor and delirium are mild but very persistent, and when restlessness is a prominent feature.

Tuberculinum is often called for as an intercurrent remedy.

With regard to actual ivy poisoning, if contact is known to have taken place the first measure is to wash the parts involved promptly, or within the hour, by thorough scrubbing with laundry soap lather. The scrubbing can be followed by rubbing with 65% alcohol.

If the condition has developed, various remedies have been found useful, notably Rhus Tox. (30c or higher – one authority gives the 10M), Croton Tiglium, Grindelia Robusta, Sepia. Crude preparations of Rhus Tox. only make things worse and should never be used.

Ruta Graveolens

SOURCE

This remedy is prepared from rue, a plant well known as a medicinal herb from ancient times. It is a striking-looking plant with its grey-green, somewhat glaucous foliage and its four-petalled bright yellow flowers in their cup-shared calices, which persist after the blooms have withered.

The four flower petals are wide apart, giving the bloom a rather untidy appearance, and the flower heads are arranged in a raceme of umbellate type. The stamens are interesting, numbering ten in the first flower of the group and eight in the others, inasmuch as their anthers move in turn to the pistil, shed their pollen and then retire.

The stem is woody at the base; the leaves, appearing alternately on the stem, are so deeply subdivided as to give an almost reticulate look. The plant prefers a dry, shady location and definitely dislikes cold and wet.

It possesses a strong, not very pleasant scent, and bitter taste-'Sour herb of grace' as Shakespeare calls it in *Richard III*. This name, Herb of Grace, may derive from the fact that a bunch of rue was commonly used by priests in ritual sprinklings.

In Pliny's day rue was popularly supposed to be a cure for no fewer than eighty-four maladies. It was thought to make a warrior invulnerable if he heated his sword-point in the fire and then smeared it with the juice of the plant. It was also held to nullify poisons, and the Speculum Mundi has this to say of its properties, 'Excellent is that medicine approved of Mithridates, King of Pontus, in Asia, viz. that if any do eat fasting two drie walnuts, as many figs, and twenty leaves of rue, with one grain of salt, nothing which is venomous may that day hurt him.'

It was formerly used as a remedy against the plague, and Gerrard avers that 'the leaves of rue eaten with the kernels of walnuts or figs, stamped together and made into a masse or paste, is good against all evil aires, the pestilence or plague.'

This may link up with the property of the plant to inhibit the activities of fleas, lice and other insects, which gave rise to the practice of placing a bunch of rue on the judge's bench and strewing the plant on the floor of the courtroom at the Assizes as a prophylactic against gaol fever – typhus – a louse-borne disease.

The association of the herb with visual acuity was formerly recognized, and it was frequently consumed in salads by painters to strengthen and improve their sight. One writer, Swan, has this to say, 'For those who are feeble in their sight, let them distill rue and white roses together, and putting the water thereof into their eies, it will open their windows and let in more light.'

Culpeper recommended the herb for sciatica and pains in joints. In more recent times the essential principle of the plant, rutin, a yellow crystalline substance, has been isolated and has had a certain vogue in the treatment of hypertension. Homoeopathic preparations are made from the whole plant gathered before the flowers have developed.

PHARMACOLOGY

The name Herb of Grace is in contradistinction to that of poison ivy, yet this latter plant, *Rhus toxicodendron*, has many symptoms in common with *Ruta*. Although the reputation of rue was benign and medical rather than toxic, the plant if much handled has been known to cause 'redness, swelling and vesication of the skin'. Further, in a number of instances where rue was administered with a view to procuring abortion, definite toxic effects were induced, namely, 'epigastric pain, violent and persistent vomiting, swelling of tongue, salivation, colic, fever, thirst, staggering gait, muscular twitching and spasms, vertigo, disturbances of vision, drowsiness, and after an interval of some days miscarriage'. Quite a list!

From such evidence and from planned provings it appears that the tissue affinities of the plant are mainly with the eyes, especially the ocular muscles, with muscles and tendons, especially those of flexor muscles, with the rectum and with skin.

It is the synovial sheaths of tendons which are chiefly affected, as well as the sites of insertion into the periosteum. The joints mainly involved are wrists, knees and ankles, wherein lies a difference from Rhus Tox. which has special affinity with the lumbosacral region, the larger joints and fibrous tissue all over the body. Inflammatory changes are produced, leading to pain and stiffness.

PROVING

The proving of Ruta is in the fourth volume of Hahnemann's *Materia Medica Pura*.

APPEARANCE

There are no special facial appearances associated with this remedy, but the eyes may look tired, red and watery. Sometimes a red rash is present on the forehead or pimples are seen on the lips.

There is evidence of restlessness and inability to sit still for any length of time, but on getting up from a chair there is a tendency to flop back again at the first attempt. This is due to a feeling as if the knees would give way. Even after rising at a further attempt the limbs feel stiff and the gait is unsteady and staggering.

PSYCHOLOGY

Restlessness of mind is accompanied by feelings of anxiety, as from a troubled conscience. There is a marked tendency to peevishness, with the inclination to contradict and pick a quarrel. Despondency may afflict, especially at dusk, and possibly with a disposition to weep over recent actions or occurrences, tears of aggravation rather than repentance.

PHYSIOLOGY

Feels the cold and wants warmth; indoors preferred to outside. Chilliness may affect hands and feet or be felt all over.

Poor appetite; easy satiety or anorexia. Thirst is insatiable, with desire for ice-cold water.

Is drowsy after meals but liable to frequent waking at night, disturbed by vivid confused dreams, or a feeling as if it was time to get up.

Yawning is frequent, with desire to stretch the limbs.

SYMPTOMATOLOGY

General

The Ruta pains are associated with weariness rather than weakness, and lack the paralysed feeling which often accompanies the Rhus Tox. type of pain. With Ruta a bruised or beaten-up or strained sensation is experienced. Sometimes pain is described as located to one small spot, as if a nail were driven in. Often there is great unease of the limbs, especially the lower limbs – 'does not know where to put them for relief'.

Head

Various head symptoms are recorded, mainly of persistent dullness or heaviness, with confusion of thought. Giddiness on first rising in the morning, with need to clutch something for support, or perhaps while walking in the open air.

Eyes

This is an important sphere for the therapeutic action of Ruta. It relieves eye-strain resulting in pain in the eye when reading or doing fine work of any kind. Blurring of vision also ensues with a sensation of heat and burning, rendered worse by using the eyes and also worse in the evening. Other eye symptoms are lachrymation, twitching of lower lids, itching at the inner canthus and of the lower lid, and a green halo seen round an artificial light. Rubbing the eye leads to smarting and watering.

Ears

A prover noticed a feeling as if a blunt piece of wood were being pushed into the ear; another felt a pain below the mastoid process as from a blow or contusion.

Respiratory System

Gnawing or stitching pains may be felt in the chest, often increased by walking upstairs. These may be due to soreness at the insertions of the muscles of the thorax. A cough is described, worse by lying down at night and associated with copious, thick yellow sputum. Pain may be felt in the sternum.

Alimentary System

A variety of abdominal symptoms are recorded, mainly pinchings and gnawing sensations, especially affecting the hypogastrium. Pains in the stomach are relieved by taking milk. The rectal symptoms would appear to be more important, namely stitching and tearing pains in the rectum, especially noticed when sitting still. Anal prolapse, piles and rectal stricture are also mentioned, often associated with a constant urge to stool and the passage of quite soft faeces.

Urinary System

A tearing sensation may be felt in the urethra, quite apart from urinating. Constant urge to empty the bladder may be accompanied by difficulty in relaxing the sphincter if opportunity is delayed. Poor sphincter control may result in nocturnal enuresis or involuntary urination in the daytime, especially when walking.

Locomotor System

This is the main sphere of usefulness of the remedy. Pains up and down the spine or in the paraspinal muscles, usually of a bruised-feeling type and worse when sitting. Low back pain, however, may be relieved by lying on the back. Tenderness in the muscles or at the point of tendon insertion into the periosteum. This is often the result of repeated occupational strain rather than of a single injury, e.g. tennis elbow. Joints feel weak and knees tend to 'give' on rising from sitting or when going up or down steps. Painful wrists, knuckles, knees and ankles with or without associated swelling. Contractures of tendons, especially flexors, occur with limitation of movement in fingers and toes, accompanied by stiffness. Fibrous bands or nodules may develop in hands and feet. Sciatic pain is associated with a desire to walk up and down for relief, the pain being worse when sitting or lying. The thighs, on one aspect or another, may feel bruised and be painful to the touch; this may make walking difficult and the gait unsteady.

Skin

The chief symptom here is a tendency to generalized itching with relief from scratching. Despite relief at the site actually scratched, the itching tends to start up in another site.

MODALITIES

There is aggravation from cold and wet, when at rest, when lying down or lying on the painful part. The symptoms are also worse when walking out of doors. This is different from Rhus Tox. which shows relief when walking out of doors, until fatigue sets in. Ruta symptoms are also aggravated by looking fixedly at an object, by touch, by stooping, and as the result of eating raw food.

Some relief is obtained by warmth and by moving about indoors.

CLINICAL NOTES

This remedy is not so generally useful as Rhus Tox. but it is of special value in relation to the ill-effects of overstrain of muscles and trauma, often unsuspected, at tendon insertions. This may be the result of repeated postural or occupational stress, and tending to inflammation or fibrosis. Areas affected may be the shoulder region, elbows, wrists, and the anterior aspect of the upper part of the tibia, also the palms of the hands. Ruta has proved of value in relation to ganglion.

Complementary remedies are Calcarea Phos. and Silica.

Sabina

SOURCE

The source of this remedy is *Juniperus sabina*, or savin. The plant is an evergreen found in central and southern Europe. It may spread horizontally or rise erect to a height of eight to ten feet. The trunk is covered with reddish brown bark and may be a foot in diameter. It gives rise to numerous branches spreading in all directions and covered completely for the most part by very small, very numerous, erect, pointed bright green leaves. The leaves are in opposite pairs and are strongly aromatic when bruised.

The pollen-bearing flowers are conical with three florets; the ovary flowers have three rigid petals and three stigmas. The fruit is a rounded fleshy berry, ¼ inch in diameter, dark brown in colour and covered with a blue bloom. It contains three irregular shaped hard seeds.

The mother tincture is prepared from fresh leaves pounded in an iron mortar to express the juice.

PHARMACOLOGY

Oil of Sabin is a powerful poison. It acts on the skin as a rubefacient and vesicant. Its effects on the body are widespread; in the alimentary canal it causes vomiting and purging with severe colic; in the liver it increases the flow of bile, possibly through venous engorgement; there is an irritant action on kidneys and uterus – the drug was formerly much used as an emmenagogue, and its mistaken and unwise use as an abortifacient resulted in many cases in death. The irritant action extends also to serous membranes and fibrous tissues, hence its use in relation to arthritic lesions, notably gout.

PROVING

Sabina was proved by Stapf and published in *Additions*.

PSYCHOLOGY

The subject is extremely irritable, ill-humoured and hypochondriacal. Cannot stand music, which sets the nerves on edge.

PHYSIOLOGY

Appetite is poor. There is a desire for juicy things, especially lemonade, also for sour things. Sleep is apt to be restless; there is a tendency to sweats at night.

SYMPTOMATOLOGY

General
Pains are violent and piercing. Haemorrhages are of bright blood admixed with clots. Violent pulsations may be experienced. Hot flushes are common, accompanied by a desire for open windows.

Head
Vertigo is associated with suppressed menses. A bursting headache in the forehead is of sudden onset but fades out slowly.

Respiratory System
There is great dryness of the throat, accompanied by a sensation as if a foreign body were lodged there.

Alimentary System
Drawing pains may be felt in the masseter muscles. Teeth are apt to ache when masticating. Pain in the epigastrium stabs through to the back. Intermittent colicky pains occur in the region of the umbilicus with a feeling as if about to vomit, but without the sensation of nausea. Tympanites may be present with colicky pain in the hypogastrium. There is a sensation of fullness in the rectum. Constipation is associated with hard stools, the passage of which causes pain. Haemorrhoids bleed copiously, with bright red blood.

Urinary System
Burning and throbbing sensations are felt in the region of the kidneys. There is frequency of urination with much urging and haematuria. Throbbing also in the region of the bladder.

Genital System
In the male, urethritis, gonorrhoeal or other, with purulent discharge, may call for the remedy. There is burning and soreness in the glans; the prepuce is sore and retraction painful. Condylomatous warts may be present on the prepuce. Libido is increased.

In the female, menses are early, abundant and prolonged. The period may last eight to ten days; the blood is bright red and admixed with clots. The period is accompanied by violent pains, spreading from sacrum to pubis, and cutting pain from below upwards in the vagina. This pain extorts cries from the sufferer who is unable to bend forward, especially when seated. Uterine haemorrhage is aggravated by the least movement, by getting heated, in a warm room, accompanied by the characteristic pains. Metrorrhagia of this type is associated with increased libido. The period may be followed by profuse, irritant and very offensive leucorrhoea. The remedy may be considered in threatened abortion, also in ovarian and uterine symptoms following abortion. Is mentioned also in relation to retained placenta and intense after-pains. A further indication is the presence of warts or condylomata in the genitals, accompanied by intense pruritus and burning sensations.

Locomotor System
Shooting, transfixing pains extend from the sacro-lumbar region to the pubis and radiate to the anterior thigh regions. Acute pain is felt in the wrists, extending to the elbows, aggravated by movement or by contact. Shooting pains occur in the heels and in the metatarsal bones, made worse by heat and relieved by cold applications. Arthritic pains, gout, with red shining swelling or gouty nodosities, all are worse in an over-heated room.

MODALITIES

Heat aggravates, especially a hot room; also the least movement and physical contact. Is worse at night.

Feels better in cool air and out of doors.

CLINICAL NOTES

The tincture may be used locally for warts. The complementary remedy is Thuja.

Sanguinaria Canadensis

SOURCE

Sanguinaria canadensis is a plant with many local names, bloodroot, red puccoon, Indian red paint, tetterwort, red root, snakebite. It is found growing in deciduous woods in North America. Early in spring, when the sunlight can still reach the soil through the bare leafless branches, a solitary leaf arises from the underground root stock. This leaf, at first kidney-shaped and later palmate in form, is wrapped around the flower bud; it is yellow green on the upper aspect and whitish with violet veins and an overall bluish tint underneath. It attains a length of six to ten inches, and at its apex appears a large white wax-like flower with golden stamens.

The root stock, with which medicine is more concerned, is thick, round, soft and fleshy, one to four inches in length and bearing orange-red rootlets. Both root and rootlets are replete with a yellow-red milky juice, sharp, bitter and aromatic in taste and capable of use both as a dye and as a medicine. The mother tincture is prepared from the fresh root.

The plant belongs to the poppy family, as do also *Chelidonium* and *Opium*. Its constituents are listed as: alkaloids – sanguinarine, chelery-thrine, protopine, beta- and gamma-homochelidonine; resin, citric and malic acids, and starch. Sanguinarine, the chief active ingredient, crystallizes in colourless needles and forms reddish salts with sulphuric and nitric acids. The plant has been employed as an expectorant, an emetic and an emmenagogue; the powdered root causes sneezing and nasal irritation; the seeds are slightly narcotic.

PHARMACOLOGY

There is an affinity with the circulation, tending to localized congestion and circumscribed areas of erythema; also vertigo, faintness, depressed cardiac action and muscular prostration.

Mucous membranes are affected, giving rise at first to dryness, rawness and burning, and later to catarrh.

Acts on uterus and ovaries; with formation of uterine polyps and tendency to profuse haemorrhage.

Effects on the nervous system are shown by tonic spasms and wild excitement, or on the other hand by torpor with dilated pupils.

PROVINGS

Some homoeopathic experiments with Sanguinaria are given in the *Materia Medica of American Provings*.

APPEARANCE

Circumscribed redness of cheeks, malar flush may be observed, also red, burning ears. Dilated veins are seen in the temples, which are tender to touch. Palms and soles are hot to touch and appear dry and wrinkled. Discharges are offensive; foetor oris may be noticeable.

PSYCHOLOGY

Quite marked anxiety accompanies symptoms. The mood varies; is morose, irritable, peevish or excitable.

In general the condition is one of langour, torpor, with indisposition to make any effort, either physical or mental.

Sensations are described as of 'streams of heat flowing from one part of the body to another'.

PHYSIOLOGY

Palms and soles feel so hot that they must be pushed outside the bedcovers in search of coolness. With headache, however, the sufferer may feel chilly.

Unquenchable thirst is associated with a desire for acid and spicy things. A sinking, all-gone feeling occurs without any real desire for food. There is aversion to butter and sweets; in fact there may be disgust for all food, especially in the morning.

Lies awake at night, or wakes from sleep in fright with a sensation of falling; sleep is disturbed by the least sound.

Cold sweats accompany nausea and vomiting.

SYMPTOMATOLOGY

General

Gastrointestinal disturbance often accompanies other symptoms. Pains are described as cutting, tearing, lacerating, and leave tender spots behind. Weakness and debility are concomitants. There is a great proneness to take fresh colds. Discharges are acrid. Polypi are haemorrhagic. Symptoms tend to be right-sided or spread from right to left. Periodicity is a feature, e.g. headache every seventh day.

Head

Vertigo occurs, especially in the morning, on rising from sitting posture, on turning head quickly, on looking upward; it is accompanied by a rush of blood to the head. A number of types of headache are related to this remedy. A bilious headache may result from overeating, from taking rich food or drinking wine; it may also be related to fasting. The head feels as if it would burst, or there is a sensation as if the eyes were being pressed out. Some relief is obtained when walking in the open air. Important is the migraine-type headache, usually right-sided, and often recurring at seven day intervals. The attack starts early in the morning, increases in intensity till noon, begins to ease up about 3 p.m. and has spent itself by sundown. The pain is throbbing and lancinating, spreads from occiput to above the right eye, and is accompanied by chills, nausea and vomiting of food taken the previous day. The sufferer has to lie down and stay perfectly still in a darkened room. At the peak of the attack there is aggravation from any jar or jolt, even the footfalls of someone walking across the floor of the room, and hypersensitivity to noise, light and odours. Vomiting and the passage of flatus both up and down is followed by sleep, and after sleep the headache is relieved. There is also a neuralgic type of headache involving the face; it is severe but can be relieved to some extent by kneeling down and pressing the head firmly against the pillow, the floor or other firm object. Menopausal headaches are associated with a surge of blood to the head, hot flushes, tinnitus, nausea and vomiting; open air and sleep afford relief.

Eyes

A number of symptoms are mentioned here, e.g. acute conjunctivitis with ecchymoses; pain in the eyeballs on movement; dimness of vision as if looking through a cloud.

Ears

Earache may accompany headache. There is acute sensitivity to noise, especially sudden sounds, associated with a feeling as if surrounded by rapid, confused chatter. Aural polypi may form. Heat and redness of the external ear may be accompanied by humming and roaring tinnitus and a sensation of vibration all over the body; this may be so severe that the sufferer asks to be held firmly to control the tremors.

Respiratory System

Fluent coryza is accompanied by much sneezing, pain in the forehead, eyeballs and root of nose, and stinging sensation in the nostrils. Sense of smell may be hyperacute – feels sick and faint from odour of flowers; or on occasion there may be loss of both taste and smell. This may be associated with hayfever in June, accompanied by much burning and dryness in nose and throat. Laryngitis is accompanied by a sensation of rawness and intense choking feeling; throat feels swollen as if it would suffocate; worse talking, on swallowing and worse on right side. Presence of nasal or laryngeal polypi. Cough accompanies gastric or menstrual disorders. A tickling cough is associated with irritation in pharynx and a 'crawling' sensation behind the sternum. Sputum is thick, mucoid, tenacious and may be almost impossible to raise; may be rusty or blood-streaked. A loose cough is associated with badly-smelling sputum and foetor oris, evident to the patient; wakes at night into a fit of coughing and has to sit up, belch and pass flatus for relief. The remedy may be needed when a spasmodic cough persists after an attack of whooping cough. Chest feels contricted with stitching pains and a desire to take a deep breath. Burning pain may be felt in chest, behind the sternum, deep to right breast and extending to the right shoulder region.

Alimentary System
Pain is described in carious teeth when in contact with food or cold fluids. Gums are likely to be spongy and haemorrhagic. Tongue may be white-coated, with a slimy fatty taste in the mouth. Tongue, mouth, pharynx feel scalded, especially the tip of the tongue. Or a prickling sensation may be noticed in the tongue and palate. Waterbrash, pyrosis occur with much belching; nausea is common with vomiting of altered bile, bitter, green or yellow fluid. The gastric symptoms are not relieved by vomiting but are better on taking food. Burning sensation is a concomitant. A dull burning pain may be felt in the right hypochondrium. Various cutting pains and discomforts affect the abdomen, including flatulent distension and escape of flatus per vaginam. There may be urge to stool, followed by passage of only flatus. Improvement in gastric condition or cessation of nasal catarrh may be followed by sudden onset of acute gushing diarrhoea with bilious, very offensive stool and much flatus. A sensation of 'something alive moving about in the belly' has been described.

Cardiovascular System
Stitching or pressive pains may be felt in the cardiac region; also palpitation with slow, weak, irregular pulse. Circulatory imbalance may give rise to localized congestion or subjective sensations of heat.

Urinary System

Nocturia may occur with frequent passage of copious amounts of pale urine. Dull heavy pain in loins has been described.

Genital System

Menorrhagia is associated with headache and gastric upset. Pain and stitches in the breasts accompany menstruation. Menopausal disorders may be accompanied by metrorrhagia with loss of bright red blood, easily clotting and offensive in odour. Heat flushes occur at the menopause associated with burning in palms and soles; bed covers must be thrown off at night for relief. Uterine polpypi bleed very easily. Ulceration of cervix uteri is associated with foetid, corrosive leucorrhoea.

Locomotor System

Rheumatic type pains affect the nape of the neck, the right shoulder and right arm; the right arm may be fixed to the side or cannot be raised above shoulder level; the pain is worse at night, in damp weather and on turning over in bed. Similar pains are felt in areas where bone is only thinly covered, e.g. backs of hands and shins. Pain is felt in the sacral region on lifting and is relieved by bending forward.

Skin

Acne occurs in young women, often in association with scanty menses. Red blotchy eruptions may appear in the spring.

MODALITIES

Aggravating factors are cold, damp weather, any change in weather; the least draught, touch, jar, movement, exertion, lying on right side, eating sweets, swallowing; the climacteric; night.

Relieved by lying on the left side, being in the dark, and sleep.

CLINICAL NOTES

The remedy has proved of value in cough and respiratory trouble in influenza. It is said to antidote Rhus Tox. poisoning.

Secale Cornutum

SOURCE

The remedy is prepared from ergot, *Secale cornutum*, the dark purplish cylindroid sclerotium formed in the ear of rye by the fungus *Claviceps purpurea*. When fully developed this is a flattened, crescent-shaped body about 5mm in diameter and 4.5cm in length. A number of these may be found in the ripened ear of rye, or of wheat or barley as the case may be.

This plant parasite has a most interesting history medicinally, as its inadvertent ingestion in contaminated flour has caused outbreaks of serious disease to which the name ergotism has been applied. The history is a long one. An Assyrian tablet of 600 B.C. refers to a noxious pustule found on ears of grain, and a sacred book of the Parsees (400-300 B.C) speaks of noxious grasses that caused pregnant women to 'drop the womb and die in childbed'. In France, epidemics of ergotism can be traced back as far as A.D. 857, and in the tenth to the thirteenth century there were numerous outbreaks in that country. It was in the eleventh century that the affliction began to be known as St Anthony's fire, from the custom which had grown up of sufferers from the disease making pilgrimages to the shrine of St Anthony located 'near Vienne, in Dauphiné', in the hope of cure. One of the symptoms is a sensation as if ants were running about under the skin, associated with a generalised erythema and much burning.

In addition to prominent symptoms such as convulsions and gangrene of the limbs, the condition was often accompanied by hallucinations, delirium, mania or mental feebleness. A number of alkaloids are present in the sclerotium – ergonovine, the oxytoxic principle, ergotoxine, ergotamine, ergotinine. A further constituent is lysergic acid, which is probably responsible for the psychotic effects. Amongst other ingredients are histamine and acetylcholine. The mother tincture is prepared from fresh spurs gathered just before harvest.

PHARMACOLOGY

There is an affinity with the neuromuscular system, inducing violent spasm of muscle, especially plain muscle in the walls of the arterioles, and the muscle of the gravid uterus. The prolonged use of ergot preparations, for instance in the treatment of migraine, carries a serious risk of circulatory disturbance in the extremities or even in the mesentery, where gangrene of the intestine may supervene as the result of vasospasm.

Affinity with the nervous system leads to varying degrees of paraesthesia or anaesthesia of the skin. Symptoms of mental deterioration, ataxia, rombergism, lightning pains and convulsions may also occur.

Vasospasm is, of course, followed by a rebound vasodilatation; this may account for the tendency to haemorrhage of passive type. Moreoever the blood is lacking in coagulability, which results in persistent oozing and may involve serious loss of blood.

PROVING

No formal proving has been made of Secale, but a collection of symptoms by Hartlaub and Trinks was published in the *British Homoeopathic Journal*, Vol.IV.

APPEARANCE

The face appears pale and drawn. Pupils are large. Facial muscles may show twitching. Skin looks dry, shrivelled, sallow. The picture may be one of collapse with sunken eyes, blue rings around the orbits, lips pale or blue, and cold extremities. The gait, if up and about, is trembling and staggering.

Foetor oris is present; discharges have a putrid odour.

PSYCHOLOGY

There is an air of timidity, sadness and discouragement, even anguish. Anxiety may progress to actual fear of death. Semi-stupor may occur, or a maniacal state with an urge to bite. The sufferer may complain of sensations of numbness or formication, relieved by rubbing.

PHYSIOLOGY

A feature is marked coldness to touch over the whole surface of the body. In contrast to this objective coldness, the patient complains of burning heat internally and a sensation as if burning sparks were falling on the skin. This produces a great aversion to being covered and a desire for coolness.

Appetite is often ravenous with aversion to fat and meat. Thirst is unquenchable with a craving for lemon or acid drinks.

Sleep can be deep and prolonged, but in drug addicts and alcoholics insomnia is more common. Profuse cold clammy sweats involve the whole body, especially above the waist-line.

SYMPTOMATOLOGY

General

Pains are described as burning in character and are made much worse by heat. Haemorrhage is a prominent symptom, from mucous surfaces, ulcers, even from small wounds. The bleeding is of the oozing type with dark non-coagulating blood, accompanied by burning pains and chilliness. It may be persistent to the point of causing collapse.

Head

A confused feeling in the head is associated with vertigo and a tendency for the head to sway from side to side like a pendulum. This is worse when moving about. A burning violent pain in the forehead spreads over the vertex to the occipital region.

Eyes

Eye symptoms are various and often accompanied by headache and vertigo. Mentioned are squint, double vision, sparks before the eyes, incipient cataract.

Ears

Quite slight noises may re-echo in the head and cause alarm. Roaring and humming tinnitus may be present.

Respiratory System

The nose feels stuffed up, but a watery discharge flows from the nostrils. Severe epistaxis occurs, with dark blood which does not coagulate; the bleeding may be difficult to stay, with resulting prostration and thready pulse. The voice may become weak and aphonic. Breathing may be shallow with a feeling of oppression in the chest and diaphragmatic cramp. Spitting of blood may occur with or without cough. A boring pain may be felt in the chest.

Alimentary System
Trismus may occur. Gums may bleed easily. The tongue becomes dry, fissured and coated brown or black, and may exude inky blood. It feels stiff and tingles at the tip. Nausea is very persistent and made worse by taking food. It may be accompanied by much retching and vomiting. Bleeding may occur with coffee-ground vomit. The abdomen becomes distended like a drum, with cutting and tearing pains. Profuse watery diarrhoea occurs, with olive green foul-smelling stools expelled like a jet; this is accompanied by great prostration and icy coldness, but the sufferer wants coolness and throws off the covers. Stools may be involuntary with patulous anus. Melaena may be present.

Cardiovascular System
Anxiety, even pain, may be felt in the precordial region, associated with tenderness on pressure. The pulse may be small, rapid and intermittent. Involvement of the circulation may give rise to such conditions as Raynaud's disease, intermittent claudication, erythromelalgia, dry gangrene.

Urinary System
There may be much ineffectual urging to urinate. Incontinence may also be present, or retention with distension and overflow. Haematuria may be a symptom.

Genital System
Menses are profuse, irregular and accompanied by severe bearing-down pains which are relieved when the flow starts. A persistent loss of thin dark blood may continue till the next period; this is aggravated by the least movement. The remedy may be indicated in abortion at the third month. Other uterine symptoms are irregular, weak labour pains; prolonged after-pains; offensive, greenish purulent lochia; puerperal fever, suppression or non-appearance of lactation.

Nervous System
Twitchings and jerkings begin in the facial muscles and may spread to involve the whole body. Intermittent tonic spasms chiefly affect extensor muscles; if the hands are involved, the fingers are spread wide apart. There are complaints of formication, numbness and tinglings, especially in fingers and feet.

Locomotor System

Limbs feel heavy, tremulous, even paralytic. There may be associated pallor and icy coldness, but with burning pains and desire for coolness. Violent cramp may occur, especially in the lower extremities.

Skin

Small boils occur which are extremely painful and contain a green core. Gangrenous carbuncle may require the remedy. Large ecchymoses or blood blisters may be present. Ulcers become black and exude dark blood. Suppuration occurs in nail-beds with shedding of nails.

MODALITIES

There is aggravation from being warmly covered, in fact from heat in any form; also from touch, exertion, round about 3 a.m., and both before and during menstruation.

Relief is obtained in cool air, by uncovering, when lying doubled up in bed, by being rubbed.

CLINICAL NOTES

Haemorrhagic and uterine complaints provide the main indications for the remedy; also conditions resulting from vasospasm. Psorinum is a complementary remedy.

Sepia

SOURCE

The source of this remedy provides a most intriguing example of the relation between the nature and behaviour of the plant or animal from which the remedy is obtained, and the nature and characteristics of the individual patient for whom it is therapeutically indicated.

The remedy Sepia is a potentization of the liquid found in the ink sac of the cuttlefish, *Sepia officinalis*. The common cuttlefish or squid is found in the N.E. Atlantic, Mediterranean, North Sea and English Channel. It was observed and described by Aristotle twenty-two centuries ago.

Next to the common octopus it is the best known cephalopod in the world. It is a mollusc, lying midway between the nautilus with a shell and ninety tentacles and the octopus with its enormous eyes and extremely lengthy tentacles to the number of eight. The cuttlefish has eight short tentacles and a pair of longer ones. When the tentacles are extended the overall length is about three feet.

The secretion in the ink sac of the cuttlefish is of its very essence and nature. Its main constituent is melanin, a brown pigment containing up to 3.24 per cent of sulphur compounds. Calcium and magnesium are also present. It has been suggested that the ink sac of the cephalopod is analogous to the gallbladder in the vertebrates. Bile, gall and biliousness are synonymous with black depression in the human. Depression is a prominent feature of the Sepia state. Of all the cephalopods, cuttlefish have the largest supply of ink for their size and are the most ready to use it.

Like all of its class the *Sepia* is very intelligent. It may at times be the picture of immobile inertia, but it can flash into instant activity should occasion arise, either to grab its prey or to escape from danger. The Sepia subject, for all her appearance of apathy, is not dull or stupid – just utterly weary and worn and sad. Moreover the readiness to flash back into activity and sociability is there lying latent. A smile can often be elicited from the most apathetic Parkinsonian Sepia countenance.

Again, we are told that in addition to their more abundant ink supply,

460

cuttlefish also have a greater power of changing colour than other cephalopods, surpassing even the famed chameleon in the speed and variety of their colour changes. Morover the cuttlefish, are more apt to bite than octopuses and will readily take a bite at a finger. 'Moods' are typical of the Sepia subject, tears may alternate with fits of petulant anger. Like the colour changes in the cuttlefish, emotional responses may be provoked very readily by annoyance, contradiction, noise, bright light, odours, in fact any strong stimulus or irritation.

Perhaps the most characteristic feature of the Sepia depression is a desire to escape – 'if only one could get away from it all'. This urge to escape is remarkably exemplified in the cuttlefish in two ways. Ages before man discovered jet propulsion, cephalopods were jetting through primaeval seas. This power of jetting rapidly through the water and actually out of the water is vividly described by Thor Heyerdal in *The Voyage of the Kon-Tiki*, when he and his companions had a front-seat view of the phenomenon. To quote: 'Young squids continued to come aboard. One sunny morning we all saw a glittering shoal of something which shot up out of the water and flew through the air like large raindrops, while the sea boiled with pursuing dolphins (the brilliantly coloured tropical fish, dorado). At first we took it for a shoal of flying fish. But when they came near and some of them sailed over the raft at a height of four or five feet, one ran straight into Bengt's chest and fell slap on the deck. It was a small squid. It was thus shown that young squids can escape their pursuers by taking to the air. They pump water through themselves till they get up terrific speed, and then steer up at an angle from the surface by unfolding their side pieces of skin like wings. They make a glider flight over the waves as far as their speed can carry them. We often saw them sailing along (airborne) for fifty to sixty yards.'

But this desire for protection and escape is also manifested by the cuttlefish in another way. It has developed a highly effective method of camouflage, not only by rapidly changing colour but also by emptying its ink bag into the surrounding water, thus laying a species of smoke screen under cover of which it can become virtually invisible and proceed to make good its escape. The Sepia subject finds some relief by active movement, may even indulge in solo dancing in the privacy of her own apartment, but more often lapses into depression, becoming enveloped in a stygian gloom of her own manufacture, seeking therein escape from the overwhelming boredom and oppression of her circumstances.

Another interesting fact about the cuttlefish is that although it is an extroverted oyster and has dispensed with an external shell, it has beneath its skin the remains of its remote ancestor's shell, namely a hard

461

core of bone. This is the white boat-shaped cuttle-bone often found lying in quantities on the sea shore in certain latitudes. It is to be noted that the Sepia patient beneath the guise of apparent apathy and inertia has nevertheless a hard core of will and determination and desire to get well.

We are told that 'cuttlefish are animals which shamefully neglect their young'. This item of information lines up with the strange indifference to dear ones, children, wife, husband, which is often a noticeable feature of the Sepia state.

A final observation – in its shape and form the cuttlefish bears an extremely suggestive resemblance to the human uterus and its appendages. And it is an established clinical fact that as a remedy Sepia has a special relation to the female pelvic organs.

PHARMACOLOGY

The main tissue affinity of Sepia is with the endocrine glands, resulting in hormonal imbalance of the adrenocortico-gonadal-pituitary system. Relative adrenal insufficiency is associated with preponderance of androgens over oestrogens.

This results in widespread loss of tone and general weakness, with induced inertia of both mind and muscle. The pelvic tissues and organs are specially affected, as is also the circulation. In the latter case the hypotonia leads to stasis, congestions and hypoxia of tissues.

Preponderance of androgens conduces to excessive pigmentation, hirsutes and seborrhoeic skin eruptions, alopecia and acne.

PROVING

Hahnemann published a pathogenesis of Sepia in the first edition of *Chronic Diseases*. It is said that he first became aware of the potential of this remedy through treating an artist who developed certain symptoms after using Sepia, the ink of the cuttlefish, in his work. No doubt he sucked his brushes.

APPEARANCE

The appearance of the Sepia patient may be described as sallow, sessile, sweating and sagging. Weak, trembly, she is obviously worn out and on the verge of tears or a hysterical outburst. The eyelids appear heavy and drooping.

The face looks doughy and devoid of sharp lines and angles, wearing an expression of apathy and a 'browned-off' look. Pallor like that of the 'wax of old church candles' may be set off by dark crescents below the eyes.

In stature the type is apt to be either tall and angular or puffy and pale, with a tendency to portliness.

Pigmentation is common, a saddle of brown discoloration across the bridge of the nose, or freckles. Patchy pigmentation may be present on the cheeks or scattered all over the body.

A crack may be seen in the middle of the lip, as is often present in connection with Drosera or Natrum Mur.

The posture is not merely sagging but one leg is apt to be crossed over the other, as the result of a feeling of pelvic weakness and insecurity.

Discharges are thick, bland and copious.

PSYCHOLOGY

The emotional attributes already mentioned result in a sad, silent, solitary individual entirely lacking in zest.

There is a desire to get away from people, but at the same time a dread of complete solitude. Although utterly apathetic and indifferent towards everything and everyone, nears and dears included, there is still a latent capacity for reaction to contradiction and frustrations, an ability to take offence and become argumentative, a tendency to restlessness and irritability.

Tears are not far below the surface, tears from sadness, tears when telling symptoms, tears from consolation or attempts at consolation, even tears without any obvious cause.

Feels desperate, losing control, 'must hold on to herself or will scream', just can't cope; wants to get away from it all and have a little peace.

There is a desire to be occupied but is too tired to make any effort, to meet strangers, to get on with the chores. There may possibly be an urge to repeatedly perform some futile act. Fear is often a prominent feature – fear of 'some intangible evil' – fear of incurable disease – fear of going crazy.

Odd sensations abound, as if 'ribs were broken and sticking into the flesh', as if 'a strap the width of a hand were drawn tightly round the waist', as if 'a knife were being thrust into the top of the left lung', as if 'a mouse was running round the lower limbs', to give a few examples.

PHYSIOLOGY

Sepia is a decidedly chilly remedy as would be expected with a circulation in such a hypotonic state. Feet and hands feel cold, especially feet, with a sensation as if 'standing in cold water up to the ankles'. Sometimes the hands feel hot with cold feet, or vice versa.

There may be patchy coldness, e.g. a sensation like 'an icy cold hand pressing between the shoulder-blades'. Although so chilly, becomes faint in a hot, stuffy room, which intensifies the already existing hypoxic condition of the tissues.

Appetite varies from one extreme to the other, canine hunger or, perhaps, complete anorexia. There may be a craving for vinegar, pickles, spicy things, sweets, wine. This may be associated with a dislike of meat, fat and milk. There may be actual intolerance to fats, milk, bread and acids. Even the smell of food may be repugnant.

Sleep is most unsatisfactory. Although sleepy during the day and in the evening, there is difficulty in getting off to sleep at night. There is a tendency to frequent waking, to waking early and staying awake for a long time; wakes finally unrefreshed and feeling as if had not had sufficient sleep. Bodily distress of various types or anxious frightening dreams may seriously interfere with sleep, and result in restless tossing around in bed.

Sweats are brought on by only slight exertion, are profuse and often preceded by flushes of heat – as if 'hot water were poured over her'. Cold sweats are common in armpits and on the feet, and may be malodorous. Profuse sweating may occur at night on head, chest, back and thighs. The sweats are not accompanied by thirst.

SYMPTOMATOLOGY

General

The marked debility and lassitude of Sepia is not due to inherent laziness or indolence, far from it. It is the result of prolonged strain and of having had, finally, to admit defeat, perhaps subconsciously, and give up the unequal struggle.

Is easily tired to the point of prostration by quite trifling causes. The condition is often accompanied by considerable distress of body, throbbings, pulsations, bursting feelings, sensations of emptiness or hollowness, easy 'pins and needles', cramps or jerkings in muscles. Pains and flushes tend to spread from below upwards. Pains vary in type and site and are usually relieved by warmth. Owing to the inefficiency of the circulation, sensations of giddiness are liable to occur in the morning, when walking, or on movement of the arms. This may be accompanied by a feeling as if 'something was rolling around inside the skull'. Headache is of severe type, often unilateral, with darting, tearing, throbbing or shooting pains, shooting upwards or outwards. The head tends to jerk backwards and forwards with the pain. Light, noise, movement, thunder all aggravate the pain, but it is relieved after a prolonged sleep. Vigorous exercise out of doors also gives relief. Another type of Sepia headache is associated with extreme anorexia, and even the smell of cooking causes a deathly nausea. The remedy is also effective at times in facial neuralgia associated with pregnancy, which is relieved by contact of cold air or when out of doors. Sensitivity of the scalp to touch, patchy alopecia, itchy eruptions, usually dry, on vertex or occiput, are also mentioned.

Eyes
The eye symptoms of Sepia are worse in the morning and in the evening. Some relief is obtained by rubbing the eyes, by pressing the lids together, by bathing with cold water. Mentioned are a sensation of grit in the eye, burning as if 'eyes were balls of fire', lachrymation, sudden vanishing of sight, and fiery sparks, zigzags, flickerings seen before the eyes, this latter symptom shared with Natrum Mur.

Respiratory System
There is a tendency to take cold easily. Dry coryza may supervene; the nostrils become sore with internal ulceration and crust formation. Large green plugs may be discharged from the nose. The organ may be swollen and inflamed, especially at the tip. Olfactory sense may be acute or lost. Violent epistaxis may occur, especially during the menstrual period. Sepia has a hacking cough, worse on waking and also from bedtime to midnight. The cough is accompanied by retching and vomiting, and often by a desire for food. Sputum is variable, may be profuse, is mucoid and may be blood-streaked. Various discomforts or pains in the chest are relieved by pressure of the hands on the thorax.

Alimentary System
Sepia has some rather peculiar symptoms. One is a complaint of a horrible sinking, all-gone, empty feeling in the epigastrium, associated with faintness, often brought on by trifling cause. It may be induced by the kneeling posture in church, or by such effort as 'doing the wash'. It is not relieved by taking food. On the other hand a sensation of nausea

present on waking is often better after eating something or taking a hot drink. The Sepia patient may complain of 'acidity', of 'something alive moving about in the belly', of stitches in the left hypochondrium, of aching or shooting pains in the hepatic region (associated with congestion of the liver). Stools tend to be dry, hard and inadequate, and defaecation is slow and difficult, even with a soft stool. There is often a complaint of a sensation of fullness or of a ball in the rectum, not relieved by the passage of a stool. Stitching pains in the rectum shoot upwards. Rectal prolapse may be present from loss of tone in the anal sphincter muscles. Bleeding piles, anal warts, diarrhoea from taking milk are also mentioned.

Cardiovascular System

This is affected by the Sepia hypotonus, manifesting irregularities of the circulation, throbbings, pulsations, one part hot, another part icy cold, hot flushes with sudden faintness and prostration, and various 'queer feelings'. The hot flushes start on the trunk, surge upwards towards the head, are accompanied by a feeling of apprehension and end in profuse perspiration.

Urinary System

Sepia is associated with tension in the bladder and a sensation of 'outward pressure', causing great discomfort. There is frequency of urination as the result of this, often just ineffectual urging, and frequency also at night. The urine is liable to be highly coloured, offensive, depositing a yellowish pasty sediment, or is turbid with a sediment of red sand. The sediment consists mainly of uric acid or urates. It tends to adhere to the surface of the toilet, in contrast to Lycopodium with its red sandy deposit, which is non-adherent. Lack of tone may result in enuresis, especially in the first part of the night. Urethral warts also may be present.

Genital System

This provides an important sphere for the usefulness of this remedy, as would be expected from the tendency to oestrogen insufficiency, hypotonus, venous congestion and ptosis. Disorders of menstruation are common, usually with delayed periods and scanty flow, and great exhaustion is experienced during the period, especially in the morning. Uterine displacements are accompanied by a typical intense bearing-down sensation, as if 'everything in the pelvis would be expelled'. This is aggravated by standing or walking, causing the sufferer to sit down and cross one thigh over the other for support. There may be actual prolapse of uterus and vagina. Leucorrhoea is commonly present with a yellow or yellow-greenish, irritating, acrid and sometimes offensive discharge. There may be an associated erosion of the cervix uteri and great tenderness on examination. This will intensify the tendency to aversion to intercouse, diminished libido and frigidity being further factors. Dryness of vagina and vulva may cause distress when walking and may be associated with severe pruritus. Disorders of pregnancy may call for this remedy when associated with much nausea and vomiting. In some cases persistent sterility may yield to treatment with Sepia.

Locomotor System
Here also is a sphere in which the remedy can prove most useful. Limbs feel heavy and weak, especially the lower limbs; joints seem weak and unreliable, knees 'give out' when walking. A condition affecting the knees may occur at the menopause, namely a doughy swelling of the joint with pain which is especially aggravated when going down stairs or steps. The limbs may feel actually sore, bruised and unwieldy, almost paralysed, and are worse after sleep. Sepia is often indicated in low back pain, especially with the complaint of a pain as if the small of the back was breaking, or as if struck with a hammer. A special feature is that the pain is relieved by firm pressure in the small of the back by a hard cushion or some other means. This postural modality is shared also by Bryonia, Kali Carb. and Natrum Mur.

Skin
Circinate eruptions, notably those on the scalp, herpes tonsurans, ringworm, which tend to be worse in the spring. This type of eruption on the trunk will more likely yield to Tuberculinum. Eruptions which are vesicular, such as herpes in the region of the mouth and chin, also common in the Natrum Mur. picture. Also mentioned are acne in puberty, acne rosacea and urticaria in association with menstrual disorders, and eczemas occurring at the menopause. The urticaria is aggravated out of doors and, oddly enough, better in a warm room. It is worse, however, when warm in bed. Itching is common, changing to burning on scratching. The skin tends to be delicate, with easy ulceration from slight injury. Cracks, horny growths, papillomata, psoriasis may call for the remedy if other indications are present.

MODALITIES

There is aggravation in dull cloudy weather, also before thunder. Worse also when sitting still, before the menstrual period, and when vexed or emotionally upset. The worst times are in the forenoon and at dusk.

The Sepia subject, if not too exhausted to make the effort, gets relief from violent movement, especially in the open air; enjoys facing the wind; feels better when warm in bed and from taking food. Better also after sleep, even a short nap, from hard, firm pressure, and during the afternoon.

CLINICAL NOTES

Sepia is of special service from puberty to the age of twenty-five, and again at the menopause. While in the main a female remedy, it can also be of value in male patients. It is prescribed largely in relation to the characteristic psychosomatic picture. Has proved useful with children who are easily tired and 'tiring' to handle.

Sepia and Lachesis are said to be incompatible, but Natrum Mur. is often called for in the Sepia type of individual.

Silica

SOURCE

This remedy is an example of a substance apparently inert in the crude state becoming therapeutically active when dematerialized by the processses of trituration, dilution and succussion. Silica is silicon dioxide, occurring in nature in quartz, flint, sandstone and many other minerals. Silicon is, next to oxygen, the most abundant of all the elements in the earth's crust. It is also a constituent of emeralds, aquamarines and the semi-precious stones amethyst, opal and zircon.

The correspondence between the nature and character of the source of the remedy, and the characteristics of the type of patient for whom it may be the 'similar', is of course less obvious with a mineral of this sort than with a plant or animal source. Nevertheless it is of note that compounds of silicon are of wide use in modern industry because of their non-reactivity. They are resistent to oxidation and extremely water-repellent. One of the chief characteristics of the Silica patient is extreme inertia, lack of response, lack of fire and very poor resistance.

The grain of sand is content to drift, subside and settle motionless on the surface of the desert or on the seabed, away beneath the waves of bother and strife. The Silica patient just wants to sit around or lie down in apparent unconcern. But if provoked he may blow up over trifles and become quite violent, even as the sand of the desert, if stirred up, may become a whirl of violence and destructiveness.

PHARMACOLOGY

The tissue affinities of the remedy become apparent when it is potentized. The digestive system is affected, resulting in malabsorption and consequent malnutrition and debility. Connective tissue becomes liable to inflammatory and fibrotic changes, and skin to trophic changes and chronic sepsis.

PROVING

The original pathogenesis of Silica appeared in the first edition of Hahnemann's *Chronic Diseases*.

Silica

APPEARANCE

The Silica child appears sallow, sickly, shivery, sweaty, suffering and small for its age. Fontanelles remain unclosed too long. The head seems too large for the body and the belly too prominent. On exertion goes deathly white.

Complexion is fair or dark. Teeth look in good shape. Hands are cold and clammy. Gait is stooping with toes turned in.

In general a thin, sessile, tired-looking individual liable to boils and sores. Agrees to everything that is said; if cross-questioned gets confused and begins to sweat about the head and face – would make a bad witness in a court of law.

Nails are often rough, yellowish and brittle. Articulations appear knob-like.

PSYCHOLOGY

The Silica child is self-willed, touchy, cannot bear to be touched or even looked at. Is usually quite intelligent, but shy at parties. An apt description of the type is given by a French paediatrician: 'The little Silica patient is full of apprehension. He lacks confidence in himself and always thinks that he will be incapable of writing a composition or learning a lesson. The Silica subject's lack of self-confidence plays its part in the difficulty he has in fixing his attention. He is too tired to stick to a task which he is anyhow too timid to undertake. With his back to the wall he can be annoyed, can grumble and can get angry.'

There is a lack of 'go', of 'drive', of 'grit', of initiative. He is so tired that he just wants to sit around or lie down all the time. Scrupulously conscientious, however, but lacking in application as thoughts tend to wander. May possibly develop an 'idée fixe'.

Is timid, full of fears, especially a dread of failure from a feeling of incapacity. There is a peculiar fear of pointed objects; this is shared by Spigelia. So sensitive and nervous that he starts at every sound, jumps if touched and 'comes all over hot'. Is easily irritated by trifles, and if provoked 'goes beserk'. This unexpected reaction on the part of such a spineless specimen of humanity is well exemplified by Leon Vannier's description in *Typologie*:

'Silica is the remedy of depth for the over-worked individual whose nervous resistance is used up. 'Depressed, the subject becomes faint-hearted, fearful and lacking in self-confidence. The least thing seems a mountain. He has no confidence in himself and is discouraged by the least failure. 'Little by little the subject becomes incapable of consecutive thought'. The least mental effort fatigues him. He makes mistakes in speaking. Talking is a burden, he gropes for the right word, and when writing he has the greatest difficulty in expressing his thought.

'He lacks even the drive to come to the decision to stop over-working in order to take the complete rest which he needs'. One recognizes these patients who, profoundly depressed, are resigned to their physical and mental deterioration and are unwilling to listen to their family's exhortation to lay off and rest.

'Often agitated with an agitation both useless and disorderly, constantly shifting about, he cannot stay put and jumps at the least noise. Thus, while at table, if a knife is dropped or a glass suddenly knocked over, he starts to shake and flies into a rage. His nervous system, which he has overstrained and over-taxed for weeks and months, cannot stand anything more and the least thing provokes a veritable crisis which does violent hurt to his poor tired brain. He may be so exhausted that his one desire is to lie down.' Another French author notes that the Silica patient lacks serenity, is apt to get unduly worried over having committed some small offence, is in two minds about everything, finds intellectual effort a 'pain in the neck'.

In many ways the emotional state of the Silica patient resembles that of Sepia, but the hard core of will to recover, which characterizes the latter remedy, is lacking. The Sepia subject just cannot cope, owing to sheer exhaustion; the Silica patient has no desire to cope, owing to his feeling of utter inability.

The Silica picture may be precipitated by experiences which involve serious fright or grave emotional shock.

A curious feature is a tendency on the part of the Silica subject to preoccupation with pins, is afraid of pins, hunts for them, counts them over and over.

PHYSIOLOGY

The thermal reactions of Silica are somewhat contradictory. Owing to lability of the circulation, extreme chilliness may contrast with apparent warm-bloodedness at times. Though desiring to be loaded with bed-covers at night may go out on an icy day with relatively light clothing.

Chilliness, however, predominates – even moving about in bed may increase the chilly feeling; may complain of being 'cold to the marrow'; feet and legs especially liable to feel as cold as ice.

Appetite is poor or nil. The child may eat hair or sand or chew nails. There is a desire for cold food and cold milk, especially mother's milk. Paradoxically the appetite may in some cases be increased and ravenous. Excessive thirst is the rule.

Sleep is disturbed by frightful dreams and there is a liability to sleep-walking, especially at new and full moon.

As would be expected in a subject suffering from serious debility, drenching sweats are common, especially on the head and the feet. The foot sweats especially are extremely offensive in odour. The head sweats are mainly on forehead, vertex and neck, in contrast with Calcarea Carb. sweats, which are mainly occipital, soaking the pillow.

SYMPTOMATOLOGY

General

The Silica symptoms appear to be the result not of atonia and hypoxia, as is the case with Sepia, but of defective food assimilation with consequent undernourishment, debility and asthenia. Both physical and mental debility are marked; the child is slow in starting to walk; the adult is 'tired all the time', takes 'cold' very readily, complains of great muscular weariness and is fatigued by the least exertion. This again is in contrast to the Sepia patient who feels better and is bucked up by vigorous exercise. There is a marked tendency to sepsis, with thinnish pus of the strep-tococcal type, sluggish both in onset and in healing, leading to chronicity and fistula formation. This remedy is particularly rich in peculiar sensations, some sixty of which are mentioned in one textbook alone, distributed widely all over the body, and due presumably to the generalized hypersensitivity of nerve endings.

Head

The Silica vertigo is worse on looking up, on closing the eyes and when lying on the left side. There is a liability to suffer from a sudden rush of blood to the head, especially affecting the right temporal region and the vertex. The Silica headaches are violent, often of chronic type. They are apt to start in the occiput and spread forwards over the whole head to the supra-orbital region, often accompanied by a sensation as if 'the head would burst'. They are aggravated by moving the head, by mental exertion, by light, noise and contact of cold air; relief is obtained by wrapping the head warmly, by local heat and also by tight bandaging round the forehead.

Eyes

Symptoms include a sensation of dryness, of 'sand' or 'splinter' in the eye, profuse lachrymation out of doors, seeing sparks or specks before the eyes, dimness of vision accompanying headache. The remedy may be called for in relation to corneal ulcer, hypopyon, also for recurring styes.

Ears

Here the indication for Silica will be suppuration of chronic type with thin, offensive, purulent discharge and possibly associated caries of bone in the middle ear or in the mastoid process.

Respiratory System

Nasal symptoms are associated with a chronic type of dry rhinitis, frequent severe bouts of sneezing, intra-nasal itching, alternate fluent and dry coryza, soreness and tenderness of nasal bones, obstinate obstruction. Silica may be indicated when there are recurrent attacks of tonsillitis with a tendency to quinsy formation. In the more acute forms, Hepar Sulph. and Mercurius will call for consideration. The Silica subject is prone to colds involving the air passages. One type of cough is dry, associated with a tiresome tickle at the level of the supra-sternal notch and often accompanied by hoarseness, possibly aggravated by taking a cold drink or by talking. In more chronic cases the cough is productive, with thick, yellow, purulent sputum with an offensive odour. The cough is often persistent and fatiguing with suffocative spasms. Taking a warm drink gives some relief.

Alimentary System

Sores at the corners of the mouth may accompany the other symptoms of debility. Sometimes there is the complaint of a sensation as if a hair was lying on the forepart of the tongue. Apical abscess of a tooth causes pain which is aggravated by contact with cold air, but relieved by holding warm water in the mouth. The gums also are very sensitive to cold air or cold water. Stomach symptoms include much nausea and vomiting, which tend to be worse in the forenoon. Water has a nasty taste and drinking brings on fresh vomiting. There is a disgust for warm dishes and a desire for cold things. Abdominal pains are accompanied by much tenderness and board-like induration, especially in children. Local applications of heat give relief. Flatus is extremely offensive in odour. A diarrhoea with frequent foul stools and tendency to become chronic is brought on by dentition in children or by exposure to cold, as when sleeping out on the ground. Constipation results from rectal atony associated with anal spasms. The stools are apt to be hard and lumpy and only passed with much difficulty. Much straining is required even with a soft stool and it may slip back into the rectum when only partially extruded – the 'bashful stool'. This latter symptom is shared by Sanicula and Thuja. Rectal symptoms include very sensitive piles, fissure or anal fistula, sticking pains in rectum, perianal moisture.

Lymphatic and Glandular Systems
This is an important Silica sphere. With inflammation in the throat or elsewhere involvement of the lymph nodes may call for the remedy, especially if there is much induration in the enlarged nodes and a tendency to sluggish suppuration. Tuberculous lymphadenitis with broken caseating nodes and sinus and ulcer formation, a condition formerly described as scrofula and still quite common in the Far East, specially affecting the cervical region, is a case in point. Salivary glands may be similarly involved, especially the parotid. Mastitis too, especially on the right side, with hard indurated lumps in breast, sharp stinging pains and tending to formation of abscess and fistulous ulcers.

Urinary System
Chronic suppurative conditions of the urinary tract may call for this remedy, especially if the Silica picture of debility is present. Enuresis is likely to be a concomitant of the other symptoms in a Silica child.

Genital System
Irregularities of menstrual function are common, perhaps complete amenorrhoea. There is a tendency to easy uterine bleeding, for instance before periods from excitement, or between the periods, or in nursing mothers when the child is put to the breast. Other conditions mentioned under this remedy are hydrosalpinx, pyosalpinx, serous cysts in the vagina, a profuse, acrid, milky leucorrhoea, associated with cutting pains in the region of the umbilicus and tending to flow in gushes. In keeping with the general weakness and debility there is a tendency to easy abortion or actual sterility.

Locomotor System
Various pains and aches are met with in both upper and lower limbs and in the back from nape to coccyx, associated with almost paralytic weakness, much stiffness and aggravation on first movement and by uncovering, but with much relief from warmth. The fingers especially become stiff and the finger-tips feel 'like paper', a symptom shared by Antimonium Tart. Parts lain on also easily go numb, with sensation of pins and needles. Cramps occur in arms and legs, from deficient circulation, and joints may give way when walking or running.

Skin
Silica is a most valuable remedy in affections of the skin, especially those of a chronic suppurative nature. Every little scratch tends to become

septic. Boils or carbuncles tend to recur. Abscesses form and discharge thin, sanious pus, leading to fistula or sinus formation and showing no tendency to heal. The remedy may be called for in caries of bone, especially long bones and spine; also with malformation and splitting of the nails.

MODALITIES

Aggravation is caused by contact with cold air, in cold weather and by change to damp weather from dry, also before and during thunderstorms. (In contrast, the Sepia patient feels worse before a thunderstorm but better when the storm breaks and quite enjoys it.) Silica symptoms are aggravated by pressure, as when lying on the painful part. They are worse during the menstrual period, and tend to be aggravated in the forenoon and also at new and full moon.

In the main, relief is obtained by being warmly wrapped up, by hot applications, when lying down, and in the summer.

CLINICAL NOTES

The special sphere of Silica is in chronic disease, fibrotic or septic. It has proved of value in tuberculosis of lung, skin, bone, abdomen, lymph nodes, but in advanced disease should not be given in too high a potency. The remedy possesses an ability to stimulate an absorption of fibrosed and scar tissues. It should, therefore, be avoided in old cases of pulmonary tuberculosis where there may be encapsulated pockets of tubercle bacilli which might be released to cause fresh active disease.

A remarkable feature of Silica is its ability to promote the expulsion, exteriorization, of foreign bodies from the tissues. Many are the records of splinters, thorns, pieces of glass, gravel or metal which have been extruded from various parts of the body after the administration of the remedy. There are sites where surgical removal, or attempts thereat, are fraught with considerable risk of adding trauma to trauma, and the extrusion of a foreign body by natural means, aided and abetted by Silica in potency, is a preferable procedure, albeit involving some delay.

Silica is the complement and 'chronic' of Pulsatilla. It may often be preceded or followed by Natrum Mur. It is quite incompatible with Mercurius, and the two remedies should never be given near one another in point of time.

Spigelia Anthelmia

SOURCE

This plant is also known as pink root or annual wormgrass, the latter obviously from its anthelmintic properties. It belongs to the Loganiaceae; it is a perennial herb, the underground portion of which is a slender knotty rhizome with long fine roots. The root is blackish on its outer aspect. The stem reaches 1½ feet in height and is branched. The leaves are placed at the tips of branches in two opposite pairs in cruciate formation; they are darkish green, ovate and pointed. The small flowers of pale pink appear in July in short clustered spikes.

When fresh the plant has a poisonous, foetid odour which in an enclosed space may have a narcotic effect. The taste is nauseous and may remain a long time on the tongue. It was known to have poisonous qualities similar to those of Strychnos, and was employed in the seventeenth century as an ingredient of mixtures known by the suggestive title as 'Poudres de Succession', a poison employed by Exili, St. Croix and Madame de Brinvilliers.

The name accorded by Linnaeus was in commemoration of an old botanist of note, one Adrian Spigelius, born in Brussels in 1578. The plant was first introduced as a medicine by a Dr Browne in 1751; he claimed that it could induce sleep almost as certainly as opium. The plant is indigenous in the West Indies and South America. The mother tincture is prepared from the freshly dried plant.

PHARMACOLOGY

The main affinities are with the brain and spinal cord, causing at first irritation and later depression; these effects are chiefly manifested in spasmodic movements of the face and eye muscles, and in neuralgic pains in the areas supplied by the trigeminal nerve, in the chest and cardiac region; there is also depression of respiration and cardiac action.

PROVING

Spigelia was proved by Hahnemann and reported in *Materia Medica Pura*, Vol. V.

APPEARANCE

The subject is often a pale, sickly-looking, debilitated individual, or perhaps a child of scrofulous type infested with round or thread worms.

Pupils may be large; face may be flushed and swollen. The subject may sit gazing into space as if lost in thought.

Skin is apt to be yellowish, wrinkled, and earthy in hue.

PSYCHOLOGY

There is marked intolerance of pain and extreme sensitivity to touch; contact may actually send a shudder through the whole body.

Probably associated with this hypersensitivity is a peculiar fear of pointed objects, pins, needles and the like.

The subject is restless, anxious, disinclined for effort; worried about the future; gloomy, even suicidal; easily irritated or offended.

PHYSIOLOGY

Anorexia is common, associated with violent thirst. There is aversion to coffee, tobacco smoke and snuff.

Drowsiness in the daytime is followed by difficulty in getting to sleep at night. Sleep is disturbed by confused dreams; wakes tired in the morning.

Clammy, cold sweats may occur.

SYMPTOMATOLOGY

General
Pains are very widespread, neuralgic in type; hardly a nerve in the body escapes. The pains are described as sharp, shooting, cutting, burning; they are worse from light touch but relieved by firm pressure. The pains often start at some definite spot and radiate fanwise; the longer the pain lasts the more unbearable it becomes. Painful areas are hypersensitive to the least contact. The pains tend to be left-sided, and to shoot from within outwards and from below upwards. They affect especially the head, face and chest.

Head
Vertigo may occur on rising in the morning, or as a result of looking down the nose, so that the subject sits looking straight ahead; another cause can be movement of the eyes. Neuralgia, usually left-sided, involves head, face and eyes; the pains increase with sunrise and diminish at sunset; the eye on the affected side pours clear water. The pain is

477

worse in stormy weather and aggravated by the least jar, noise or facial movement. It may end in an attack of vomiting or get steadily worse till noon, and then decline gradually towards evening. Headache may occur on the right side or in the occiput and is better in open air; one type starts in the occiput and extends over the vertex to the left eye or down the neck to the shoulder. Painful tenderness is felt in the occiput and the nape feels numb and stiff.

Eyes

Intolerable stabbing pains in the eyes seem to be running through to the back of the head. The pain is made worse by the least movement of the eyes, so that the sufferer must turn the whole body in order to look round. Pain is felt deep in orbit. The eyes feel too large. Vision is constantly changing, making the prescription of glasses most difficult. Medial strabismus may be present. Pupils may be enlarged. Twitching of lids may occur, or blepharitis. The eyes may appear red, inflamed, congested.

Ears

Earache is accompanied by an ichorous, scalding discharge. Several varieties of tinnitus are recorded. The ears may feel plugged.

Respiratory System

Intranasal itching may be present, or a tickling sensation as if 'lightly touched by hairs or by the contact of a gentle breeze'. Frequent sneezing; fluent coryza is apt to recur, especially after the least chill. Copious postnasal discharge causes choking at night. Sore throat is associated with swelling of the soft palate, sticking pains and involvement of cervical lymph nodes. Cutting, tearing pains are felt below the left nipple, extending to shoulder and arm, worse on taking a deep breath, worse also in cold, wet weather. Dyspnoea occurs when talking, accompanied by anxiety and redness of cheeks and lips. If present at night, the subject has to lie on the right side for relief. With intercostal neuritis the pain spreads to the arms. Cough, if present, is relieved out of doors.

Alimentary System

There is an offensive taste in the mouth. Toothache is aggravated by inhaling cold air, by drinking cold water and after a meal; it is better while actually eating and when lying down, but not if lying on the right side. The tongue shows fissures. Foetor oris occurs, but is only apparent to other persons. Various cuttings, stitches, colicky pains are felt in the abdomen. Tight clothing is resented, especially around the waist.

Borborygmus occurs and painful distension in the hypogastrium, as if something would burst. Stools are irregular; there may be frequent ineffectual urge to pass a stool. Flatus is foetid. Scirrhus carcinoma in sigmoid or rectum is accompanied by atrocious, unbearable pain.

Cardiovascular System
Both acute and chronic cardiac affections may call for this remedy. Particularly violent palpitations shakes the whole chest, is both visible and audible, and worse when lying down or if bending forward and associated with dyspnoea. In acute attacks can only lie on right side or with the head very high. Pain may be felt deep to the sternum, associated with numbness of the left arm; the pain may spread to both arms, especially the left. It is aggravated by activity, by cold, by eating and by emotional upset. Pericarditis may be present with sticking pains.

Urinary System
Frequency occurs, even at night, with the passage of copious quantities of urine. Involuntary dribbling may be present, with a burning sensation in the urethra.

Locomotor System
Pains in the neck and shoulders are relieved by heat. Shooting pains in the extremities, like hot wires piercing the flesh, are worse when eating; any movement, even gentle exercise such as going up or down stairs, renders the pain unbearable; rest affords relief.

Skin
Contact with the oversensitive surface of the body may not only produce a feeling of coldness but may even result in the appearance of a red papular rash.

MODALITIES
Aggravation results from change in weather, especially to stormy weather; when lying on back; from movement, especially of the arms; from turning the eyes, shaking the head; from touch and the least jar or jolt; from noise; from contact with tobacco smoke; at sunrise.

Relief is afforded by rest, by lying on the right side with the head high, and at sundown.

CLINICAL NOTES
The main indications for the use of this remedy are cardiac lesions and neuralgias, trigeminal and other types.

Spongia Tosta

SOURCE

The remedy is prepared from the roasted and powdered skeleton of *Euspongia officinalis*, the marine sponge, which is found in the Mediterranean and other seas. It is important that it should be roasted to a brown colour and not burnt black.

Two prominent ingredients are iodine and bromine, the former of which was demonstrated as being present in the drug by Fyfe, in Edinburgh, in 1819. But five hundred years before this, the remedy was in use as a specific for disease of the thyroid gland, as recorded in the writings of one Arnaldus da Villanova.

PHARMACOLOGY

There is an affinity with the respiratory tract, especially the larynx and trachea, causing severe irritation; also with lymph nodes, thyroid gland and testes, giving rise to inflammation or hyperplasia with resulting enlargement and induration; with the heart, tending to degeneration of heart muscle. The effect in the thyroid gland appears to be a stimulation of the function of the gland to form and store the organic iodine compounds.

PROVING

Spongia was proved by Hahnemann, and the result published in *Materia Medica Pura*, Vol. VI.

APPEARANCE

As with Bromium, the Spongia type is usually of fair complexion with light-coloured hair and blue eyes.

PSYCHOLOGY

Anxiety, even terror, may accompany cardiac or respiratory distress. A state of excitement tends to aggravate cough. Anxiety may alternate with exhilaration, accompanied by a desire to burst into song.

Spongia Tosta

PHYSIOLOGY

Chills are felt, especially in the back; tends to shiver even when close to the fire. The chilly feeling is apt to give place to a glow of heat all over the body, except in the thighs, which remain numb and cold. May wake from sleep in terror with a feeling of impending suffocation, a flushed face and rapid embarrassed breathing.

SYMPTOMATOLOGY

General
Symptoms are accompanied by extreme exhaustion and heaviness of body, after even slight exertion. This may be associated with a feeling of dejection. In general, more relief is obtained when lying down than in any other position.

Head
A headache may come on after entering a warm room. Pain may be felt at the base of the brain when lying down, causing the sufferer to sit up and hold the head perfectly motionless for relief.

Respiratory System
With laryngitis the throat is peculiarly sensitive; even turning the head will bring on a suffocative seizure. The larynx feels plugged or constricted, with a scraped or burning sensation. Indicated in laryngeal croup with difficulty on inspiration. (Impeded expiration suggests Hepar Sulph.) Chronic hoarseness may be present; the voice gives out when talking or singing. The air passages feel excessively dry. A harsh, dry, barking or ringing croupy cough is associated with rasping, 'sawing' respiration. Sputum is absent or very scanty; if there is any it is usually swallowed. Bronchitis is associated with suffocative spells, worse on breathing cold air, if lying with the head low, by talking or attempting to sing, and by drinking cold fluids. Taking food and drinking warm fluids afford relief. The dry cough is said to be worse from a cold, dry wind; also in a warm room, from talking, eating sweets, breathing tobacco smoke and in the first part of the night. Acute dyspnoea is relieved by sitting up and leaning forward, a modality shared with Kali Carb.

Cardiovascular System
Violent palpitation is accompanied by pain in the precordium, a rush of blood to the chest and gasping respiration. Wakes suddenly soon after

midnight in a suffocative attack with acute anxiety and fear. The condition is worse when lying with the head low and when bending forward, though actual dyspnoea is relieved in this posture.

Lymphatic System
Lymph nodes and salivary glands become enlarged and indurated. The thyroid gland becomes enlarged and hard, possibly causing suffocative spells by pressure on the trachea, enlargement of veins and embarrassment of the pulmonary circulation and the right heart. The remedy may also be called for in the presence of a soft, parenchymatous goitre associated with palpitations, heat flushes and precordial pain.

Genital System
Painful swelling of the testes and spermatic cords is accompanied by induration and a sensation as if the affected parts were being pinched or squeezed. Movement aggravates.

MODALITIES

Symptoms are aggravated by touch, pressure, movement; also when thinking about them, at night and on waking from sleep (a characteristic modality also of Lachesis).
There is relief from taking warm food or drink.

CLINICAL NOTES

The remedy may be indicated if there is a family history of tuberculosis, if there is evidence of a tubercular diathesis, or in active tuberculosis of lung. In thyroid lesions low potencies are recommended, say 3c; in croup, either 3c or 30c.

Staphysagria

Delphinium staphysagria, stavesacre, palmated larkspur, is an erect herb belonging to the Ranunculaceae. It is a biennial plant and flowers from April till August. The stem is one to two feet in height, downy and of a purplish hue. The leaves are large, palmate and divided into seven lobes which are oblong, ovate, veined, downy and of a pale green colour; the upper leaves are five-lobed, and supported on hairy footstalks of the colour of the stem. The flowers are bluish purple on terminal racemes, with pedicels twice as long as the flowers and bractioles inserted at the base of the pedicel; the upper sepal is extended behind into a long tubular spur. The fruit consists of three downy follicles containing many rough, brown triangular seeds. The latter are used to prepare the mother tincture.

PHARMACOLOGY

Staphysagria is an ancient remedy, employed as early as the time of Hippocrates and used mainly as a cathartic or emetic. Pliny considered it a dangerous drug – 'The said kernels I would not advise to be used as a purgation, considering the doubtful event and danger that may ensue of choking and strangulation; . . . I would not counsel the use of the seed, so exceeding hot it is, and of so fierce a nature.' The drug has affinity with the nervous system, acting both peripherally on the nerve endings and centrally on the cord. An initial irritant effect is followed by depressant action; hyperaesthesia and excessive sensitivity give place to paralysis. In cases of poisoning, slowing of the pulse and respiration precedes paralysis and death from asphyxia.

PROVING

Staphysagria was proved by Hahnemann, and appears in *Materia Medica Pura*, Vol IV.

Staphysagria

APPEARANCE

There is a marked action on the genito-urinary system. Children show a scrawny pot-bellied appearance. The subject may have a sickly look, with blue-ringed, sunken eyes.

PSYCHOLOGY

The Staphysagria subject has been described as 'one of the cultivated gentlemen of the earth; controlling his feelings at any price, but silently brooding over his wrongs, real or imaginary'. Suffers in silence; rages and fumes within and, finally, as the result of pent-up emotion and repressed feelings, goes all to pieces – trembling from head to foot, aphonic, unable to work, unable to concentrate, apathetic by day, sleepless by night. There is indifference, depression, impairment of memory, desire for solitude.

Constantly takes offence without due justification; broods on 'wrongs' persistently. When walking quickly has a sensation of 'being followed'.

Inclined to dwell on matters sexual; disinclined for any effort.

The child is cross and 'ugly'; demands things and then, when brought, pushes them petulantly away.

PHYSIOLOGY

A chilly subject; shivers when eating, wakes in night feeling chilly.

Is excessively hungry, even just after a meal. Craves bread, milk, fluids, tobacco. Thirst is usually absent.

Violent yawning brings tears to the eyes. Tends to be drowsy in the afternoon with heaviness of eyelids. May be sleepless at night and, if does sleep, wakes cross and sulky.

Sweats profusely, and perspiration has the odour of 'rotten eggs'.

SYMPTOMATOLOGY

General

Complaints are often the outcome of wounded pride, suppressed wrath, or sexual excess. There is general hypersensitivity of mind and body, often evidenced by burning or pricking sensation in various sites, or a generalized itching and pricking all over the body, which drives the victim out of bed at night. There is a general weakness; knees feel uncertain when walking; there may be a tired aching in the bones, worse at night. The remedy may be indicated in shock and pain following injury, especially incised wounds and stretching of sphincters.

Head

A whirling vertigo occurs when sitting or lying down, relieved by getting up and turning round in a circle. A stupefying headache mainly affects the forehead; the head feels numb, hollow, wooden, compressed. Itching, pricking sensations occur in the head from within outwards.

Eyes

Blepharitis occurs with dryness of margins of the lids. Lids feel heavy and itch at the lid-borders. Upper lids may be painful. Styes apt to recur. Chalazion may be present. Pupils often dilated.

Respiratory System

Coryza occurs; discharge at first thick and mucoid, later fluent. Stitches occur in the throat, flying to the ear on swallowing.

Alimentary System

Burning and pricking sensations are felt on the tongue and lower lip. There is a constant accumulation of mucus in the mouth. Ulcerative stomatitis occurs; the gums bleed easily, retract and are tender to touch. Dental caries is accompanied by blackening of the teeth, which become brittle, apt to fragment and grow loose. Toothache pain shoots into the ear; is worse holding cold fluid in mouth, on inspiring cold air, after eating and from light touch; also worse at menstrual period. Clenching the jaws gives relief. There is a sensation as if the stomach was loose and sagging; this is much worse after food has been taken; it is also aggravated by tobacco, which nevertheless is strongly craved. Nausea may occur with a sensation of burning and pressure in the stomach, possibly accompanied by retching. Drinking cold water brings on colic; getting in a rage has the same effect; it is aggravated by heat and by both food and drink. Flatulence is marked, and also tympanites. Painful pressure occurs in the right iliac fossa with urge to stool, hot flatus and pruritus ani. The presence of piles which are 'exquisitely tender'.

Cardiovascular System

Stitching pains occur in the region of the heart and there is complaint of palpitation.

Urinary System

There is frequent urge to urinate, either ineffectual or accompanied by the passage of scanty dark-coloured urine. Frequency is common in the newly-wed. There is burning in the urethra during the passage of urine, which is apt to persist after the bladder has been emptied. Chronic prostatitis may be present. There may be a sensation of a drop of urine persisting in the urethra continually.

Genital System
Excessive masturbation; frequent seminal emissions; tendency to early onset of impotence. Stitches and aching affect the scrotum and testicles. In the female there is great sensitivity of genitals, pruritus vulvae and increased libido. Lumbago may occur or be aggravated by coitus; also bruised pains occur in the calves.

Locomotor System
Pains occur in the right shoulder, which feels 'dislocated', especially on movement. Aching pains are felt in the extremities, associated with a paralytic sensation, worse both touch and movement. Joints feel stiff and tired. Nodosities may be present. Pain in dorsum as if back was broken, worse when at rest and at night. Pain in bones; limbs feel bruised and semi-paralysed.

Skin
Moist, offensive eruptions occur, especially behind the ears, often accompanied by soreness of scalp. Itching eruptions which burn, scratching may afford local relief but itching starts up in some other site. Wounds do not heal but sprout unhealthy granulations; the condition is accompanied by stinging pains. Eczema is associated with thick crusts and an irritant discharge, especially affecting the hairy scalp and the margins of the eyelids. Pedunculated warts of cauliflower type may be either dry or moist.

MODALITIES
Condition is made worse by mental exertion, from anger or indignation; from least touch or pressure; from sexual excess; the use of tobacco; in the early morning.

Feels better after a meal, when warm, by a night's rest, unless suffering from lumbago.

CLINICAL NOTES
The remedy is indicated when rheumatic symptoms alternate with skin affections. Hahnemann lists 438 symptoms in his *Materia Medica Pura*; important are those relating to the temperament and the genito-urinary system. Complementary remedies are Causticum, Colocynth and Thuja.

Stramonium

SOURCE

Datura stramonium or thorn-apple is a rank-smelling weed, forming a large, coarse-looking bush some three feet high and about the same size in diameter. It is found in most parts of the world and, although it flourishes in warmer climates, has been found as far north as Sweden. It frequents barnyards, timber-yards, docks, dung-heaps, roadsides and commons – any places where a rank soil is created by deposits of refuse from human habitations.

It is quite a striking-looking plant. The stem is stout, erect, leafy in rather a ragged fashion, smooth, pale yellowish-green in colour and branching freely. In the fork of the branches arises a leaf and a single erect flower.

The leaves are large, of a dark lurid green on the upper aspect but paler underneath. They reach four to six inches in length and have wavy, sharply-toothed margins and show well-developed branching veins. Their taste is bitter and nauseous.

The flowers are dead white, tubular, about three inches long, with a half-opened corolla the folds of which end in sharp points, like a pale trumpet with out-flaring rim. Flowering continues throughout the summer. The flowers open in the evening when they attract night-flying moths and emit a powerful odour. At night the leaves, particularly the upper ones, rise up and enclose the flowers.

The fruit is an egg-shaped capsule about the size of a walnut. It splits open when ripe to reveal the dark black kidney-shaped seeds. It is covered externally with sharp spines, as menacing in appearance as a prickly curled-up hedgehog.

The whole plant exhales a very heavy, somewhat narcotic and nauseating odour which arises from the leaves. The flowers are sweet scented but produce stupor if sniffed for too long.

The whole plant, including the long, thin, whitish root covered with fibres, is poisonous, the seeds especially so. The seeds possess a sweetish taste but have a disagreeable odour repellent to animals.

That this is a menacing and repulsive plant is evident by its names – devil's apple, devil's trumpet, stinkweed. Its pallid blanched funnel-shaped flowers instil fear. Its ragged untidy leaves suggest wildness. Its spiky fruit could scarcely be more hostile, both in appearance and also when it explodes like a hand-grenade, scattering black seeds of death.

Its dark sombre leaves enwrapping the pale flowers at night are suggestive of the black cloud of nightmarish nonsense that envelops the befuddled mind of its victim. Its overpowering soporific smell suggests stupor and loss of rational control over mind and muscle.

All down history the various species of *Datura* have been used as medicaments and intoxicants. The medieval witches' salves consisted primarily of black henbane and thorn-apple; the hallucinations they produced were considered to have been real even after the intoxication and mental derangement had worn off. The mother tincture is prepared from the fresh plant when in flower, or from the powdered seeds.

PHARMACOLOGY

Like other members of the Solanum group, notably *Belladonna* and *Hyoscyamus*, *D. stramonium* contains the poisonous alkaloids atropine, hyoscyamine and hyoscine or scopolamine. Its toxic action therefore is very similar to that of these other plants, tending to stimulation of the sympathetic system and depression of the parasympathetic. There is marked disorder of cerebral coordination both in the realm of thought and motor control.

This is well exemplified in a 17th century account of the 'black madness' which resulted from eating thorn-apple:

'The servants ate a dish of lentils into which thorn-apple seeds had accidentally come. Afterwards they all became foolish. The lace-maker worked with unusual diligence, throwing the bobbin vigorously to and fro but getting everything into a frightful muddle. The chambermaid came into the room shouting at the top of her voice, 'Look, all the devils from hell are coming in.' One servant carried the wood piece by piece into the secret chamber, announcing that he must burn brandy there. Another struck two hatchets or wood axes together, saying he had to chop up wood. Another crawled about on all fours scratching up earth and grass with his mouth and grubbing about in it like a pig with its snout. Yet another imagined himself a cartwright and wanted to bore holes in every piece of wood he could lay hands on. Another went into the smithy and called for people to come and help him catch fish, for there were huge shoals of fish swimming in the smithy. To others this fools' plant gave yet other crazy ideas, so that they engaged in all kinds of labour without being paid for it and acted a proper comedy. The next day none of them knew what ludicrous antics they had got up to. Not one of them would believe or allow himself to be persuaded that he had had these fancies.'

There seems here to be an absence of the violence associated with Belladonna or the lewdness and disorganization of body-image associated with Hyoscyamus. Absurdity of behaviour is a prominent feature as well as the amnesia for what had been experienced. More severe cases of poisoning with the seeds, however, have manifested a picture very similar to that of grave Belladonna poisoning. Much probably depends on both the size of the dose and the individual susceptibility of the recipient. Indeed, satyriasis and delusions related to body-image may also occur with Stramonium.

PROVING

There is a pathogenesis of Stramonium in the third volume of Hahnemann's *Materia Medica Pura.*

PHYSIOLOGY

The Stramonium case presents a scared frightened appearance; draws back in alarm from the first object seen on opening the eyes. The brow is wrinkled, the face furrowed, red and hot. The pupils are widely dilated and the conjunctiva injected. Face and ears are both bright red. This is in contrast to the pallor of Hyoscyamus. Facial contortions are persistent.

There is a tendency to jerk the head from the pillow and to the right, or to bore the head into the pillow. Grinding the teeth may also be present.

Movements may be very disorderly or, perhaps, of a graceful gyratory rhythmic character, suggestive of chorea. One side of the body may show paralysis while the other side is convulsed.

Loquacity is often a marked feature and takes various forms, entreating and beseeching, cursing and joking, with immoderate laughter, singing and talking absurdities.

The actual form of speech is stammering and often unintelligible, or the sufferer may become inarticulate – dumb.

Gait too is ataxic with a tendency to stumble in the dark or if the eyes are closed, and to fall backwards or to the left.

PSYCHOLOGY

Sadness is a prominent feature associated with a desire for company and sunshine. It may afflict especially in the evening in bed, and be accompanied by thoughts of death and copious weeping. The subject is very adversely affected by darkness and solitude, but curiously enough manifests a fear of brightly glistening objects, such as light reflected from a mirror, or anything suggesting water.

Rages reach the point of loss of control. Delirium is particularly wild and often associated with terror. The subject wants to clutch hold of companions, uttering frantic cries; holds out the arms as if seeking solace; adopts a kneeling posture; makes constant chewing movements.

Delusions are present; hears voices during sleep; believes herself all alone, abandoned; child jumps up with a start, believes he is going to fall and clings desperately to his mother.

Terrifying hallucinations obtrude; sees snakes, cats, bugs, dogs and so on at his side, coming out of the ground, or seen 'double'. Seems to have two bodies or an extra limb.

In all this the picture is, in fact, very similar to that presented by Hyoscyamus and may even on occasion approximate to that of Belladonna. One authority states: 'Stramonium is like an earthquake in its violence.' This after all is not surprising, inasmuch as all three of these plants contain the same toxic alkaloids, and the psychosomatic effects will vary as one or other poison predominates in any particular case.

PHYSIOLOGY

Although head and face are hot, the limbs tend to be cold, owing to circulatory imbalance.

The sense of taste is lost or perverted, food tasting like sand or straw. There may be a desire for bitter things.

A burning thirst is common but is likely to be associated with a dread of water, inasmuch as the attempt to swallow provokes a spasm in the muscles of deglutition causing both alarm and distress.

The subject is scared to go to sleep in the dark, but soon falls asleep in a dimly lighted room; may, however, wake from sleep in acute terror.

Sweats are liable to be frequent, copious and cold.

SYMPTOMATOLOGY

General

Despite the intensity of the disturbance in both mental and physical spheres many of the symptoms are characteristically painless. Considerable fever is likely to accompany the symptoms, unlike Hyoscyamus which manifests very little fever. Septic inflammations tend to progress to abscess formation and be accompanied in this case by excruciating pain.

Head Region

Vertigo is worse in the dark and lying on the side; the head may feel 'drawn back'. A violent throbbing headache may be brought on by walking in strong sunlight, made worse by any movement or jar, and often located in the occiput. The head is hot and burning and may be deflected to the right. Relief is obtained by lying down and keeping still.

Eyes

Inflammatory conditions occur with photophobia, much lachrymation and agglutination of the lids at night. Disturbances of vision are many and varied.

Respiratory System

The throat is desperately dry and the dryness is not relieved by any sort of drink. The voice becomes hoarse and croaking or squeaking. Up-and-down twitching of the laryngeal cartilage may be very prominent. A dry, shrill, periodic screeching cough is worse in both morning and evening. It is painless and paroxysmal, and accompanied by a feeling of constriction and suffocation in the chest.

Alimentary System

Lips, mouth, tongue are all excessively dry and the lips may become glued together. As mentioned above, the tongue is extremely tremulous and may be swollen. A feeling of 'anxiety' may be located in the epigastrium. The belly tends to be tender but soft. Bloating and violent tearing pains may be present and much flatus may be passed. A typhoid state may supervene with loose, blackish, foul stools smelling like carrion, accompanied by fever with peak at noon, loss of sight, hearing and power of articulation, dilated immobile pupils, drenching sweats, suppression of urine and the appearance of imminent death. This termination may however be averted by the timely administration of Stramonium.

Cardiovascular System
The heart and circulation are caught up in the general turmoil. Heart action may be very irregular, and almost anginal sensations of constriction may be felt in the chest.

Urinary System
Suppression of urine may occur, or paralytic incontinence due to distension of the bladder with overflow.

Nervous System
The variegated disturbances and disorders in the sphere of nervous control have been referred to above. Twitchings may affect single muscles or groups of muscles, or generalized convulsions may occur.

Locomotor System
There is a liability to undue sensitivity of the spine, especially in the cervical region. Drawing pains occur in the spine and also in the thighs. Limbs 'go to sleep' and legs tend to 'give way'.

MODALITIES

Cold water aggravates, as does also wind; touch is resented and sudden confrontation with a glistening object has a most adverse effect. There is aggravation in the dark, after sleep, in the evening and during the night.
    Warmth, light and company all afford relief.

CLINICAL NOTES

The indications for the use of this remedy are much the same as for Hyoscyamus or Belladonna, with slight variations in symptoms as mentioned above. Acute maniacal states, puerperal mania, delirium tremens may call for the remedy. It is said to be of special value in chorea, especially if involvement of the face muscles is a prominent feature.

Sulphur

SOURCE

'Bring me fire, that I may purify the house with sulphur' wrote Homer in the Odyssey. This yellow rock, which burns to form choking fumes, has been known since the earliest days of civilization. Medicine has always made use of sulphur, which is an important constituent of Epsom salts, many mineral spa waters and the more recent group of sulpha drugs.

Sulphur, like Phosphorus, is a remedy associated with burning, both literally in a physical sense and clinically in symptoms of 'burnings' and heat in various parts and organs.

But Sulphur possesses opposite propensities to Phosphorus. Unlike the latter element which, when ignited by spontaneous combustion, disappears upwards in vapour form by force of levity, Sulphur, when ignited, burns with a blue flame and its vapour recondenses at normal surface temperature to form a yellow crystalline powder. This is a manifestation of gravitational force and the tendency on the part of the element to become re-materialized, even when oxidized by heat into vapour.

Sulphur, in contradistinction to Phosphorus, exhibits an earthward tendency, a preoccupation with material things rather than art, a penchant for down-to-earth schemes rather than for poetic fancy, a predisposition for physical awareness rather than imaginings and extra-sensory perceptiveness. Sulphur is essentially related to the processes of metabolism.

PHARMACOLOGY

Sulphur is one of the constituents of protoplasm. It thus possesses affinity with all the tissues of the body and can evoke symptoms in a wide variety of organs and tissues. This is demonstrated by the toxicity of sulphur dioxide and sulphuretted hydrogen and by the very long list of side effects reported in the literature of the sulpha drugs.

Skin and mucous membranes are especially involved in the circulatory disturbances, which are of congestive type and give rise to sensations of heat, inflammations and pruritic eruptions.

493

Sulphur has been described as the homoeopathic centrifuge, driving to the surface (exteriorizing) deep seated toxins – the remedy of chronic toxicosis.

PROVING

The pathogenesis of Sulphur appeared first in the fourth volume of Hahnemann's *Materia Medica Pura*.

APPEARANCE

While Sulphur as a remedy may be called for in a variety of individuals and over a wide range of bodily ills, the Sulphur subject does often present some fairly characteristic physical features.

There are, perhaps, three main types. One is the lean, lanky, hungry-looking, dyspeptic individual with stooped shoulders and slouching gait. Another tends to be fat, rotund, well-fed, with red face and red ears and a generally unkempt appearance. A third is a shrivelled, dishevelled type of person with an unwashed look and carrying an unpleasant body odour which persists even after washing.

Hair tends to be coarse, lustreless and not well groomed. The face is described as pale or yellowish with a rather sickly look, and deep sunken eyes surrounded by a blue circle; but the face may become suffused and deep red, especially when exposed to damp or cold air. Freckles are common.

The skin is dry, rough, scaly with a tendency to eruptions, sores and pustules. A notable feature is obvious redness at all the orifices of the body – eyelids, lips, nostrils, urethra, vulva, anus. All discharges tend to be offensive and cause excoriation of the surrounding skin.

The hands tend to be hot and sweaty, and to show tremors when employed for fine work. Posture is characteristic with a tendency to slump into a chair or sprawl on a sofa or 'support the doorpost'. Gait shows a forward stoop.

In manner the Sulphur subject is off-hand and indifferent to the small amenities – omits to doff his hat on coming indoors, flops into a chair without invitation, dresses untidily, especially about the neck.

Speech tends to be voluble and affable, replete with explanations more verbose than lucid, and philosophical ideas lacking substance or sound logic. He obviously enjoys the sound of his own voice and revels in argument or anecdote. One author describes the Sulphur individual as much given to spitting, fond of whistling, and liable to dribbling of saliva from the mouth during sleep.

PSYCHOLOGY

The Sulphur subject is selfish and self-centred to an extreme degree. Because of this he is quick-tempered and touchily ready to take offence – to ignite, in other words. He thinks his own performances and possessions of paramount worth and excellence, despite their self-evident worthlessness; he is in fact a paranoic type.

He is apt to appear quite bright, even brilliant, for a spell and then lapse into indolence or incoherence, revealing a sad lack of persistence.

The Sulphur subject manifests a peculiar aversion to water, to washing, also to work or any sustained effort, and to standing for any length of time.

All this probably derives from inefficiency of the circulation and consequent inadequate oxygen supply to the tissues of the body.

He is apt to be extremely sorry for himself – 'feels so wretched he would like to die'; worries about the future; becomes hypochondriacal; shows a great tendency to tears; gets so worried that he keeps forgetting what he was going to do.

The child becomes unbearable and difficult to quieten; cannot get what he wants quick enough; may become sulky and averse to talking.

A peculiar feature is an undue sensitivity to any nasty odour, though possibly quite unaware of his personal aroma. Aberrations of smell may occur, with awareness of imaginary odours.

Memory is apt to be poor; he forgets names and recent events. There may be complaints of odd sensations such as 'swinging in space', standing on wavering ground', 'the bed is surging up and down', all the result of fluctuations in blood-flow.

PHYSIOLOGY

The Sulphur subject is essentially a warm-blooded person extremely intolerant of heat in any form. There is, however, a dislike of extreme cold, which presumably affects the circulation adversely. Uneven distribution of blood-flow may cause the complaint that while the top of the head is uncomfortably hot the feet are unpleasantly cold. There is, moreover, a definite craving for the open air and an aversion to a hot stuffy atmosphere.

There is a tendency to be always hungry, except at breakfast time, but on sitting down to a meal the desire to eat may vanish. Nevertheless, if meals are delayed a feeling of weakness, even nausea, is common; also an empty sinking feeling comes on in the middle of the forenoon, demanding a snack for relief.

There may be a strong craving for fat and a fondness for salt, pickles, acids and also sweets, but aversion to these things may supervene. Children often have a definite dislike of fat. There may be intolerance for eggs as well as for milk, which may cause vomiting.

Thirst is marked, with inclination to drink a lot of water; there is also a partiality for alcohol.

Drowsiness is common in the afternoon, but at night is apt to be wide-awake and feel too hot in bed. The soles of the feet also may get so hot that they are pushed out from under the bed-covers to cool off – a symptom shared by Chamomilla, Medorrhinum and Pulsatilla.

Again, the bed may feel 'too small', and this remedy shares with Belladonna the liability to jerk violently just when dropping off to sleep. Sleep is apt to be disturbed by anxious or horrific dreams which wake the sleeper with a start. Sometimes sleep is actually prevented by a cataract of unpleasant thoughts. After waking about 3 a.m. no further sleep may be obtained till it is time to get up, and in consequence there is often a desire to 'sleep in'.

Perspiration is not a marked feature – the skin tends to be dry.

SYMPTOMATOLOGY

General
In general this remedy shows a tendency to either generalized or patchy burnings and smartings, both on the surface and internally, although patchy areas of coldness may be felt at the same time. Irregularities of blood flow and distribution often produce flashes of heat and may cause serious distress and embarrassment, especially in women at the time of the menopause. Similar hot flushes may occur during the course of any illness or during convalescence. They may be just dry heat or else be followed by a generalized sweat which is a moist clamminess rather than a dripping perspiration.

Another common tendency is to develop catarrhal conditions of mucous membranes, often resulting in foul-odoured discharges which are acrid and cause redness, burning, rawness and soreness of the neighbouring skin surfaces.

Another feature is periodicity, symptoms recurring every seven or fourteen days, or perhaps at the same time every day, for instance a weekend headache or urgent call to stool at 5 a.m. every morning.

Head Region
Sulphur subjects are very liable to attacks of dizziness, which may come on at any time, both indoors and in the open air, especially if compelled

to stand for any length of time. The attacks are often accompanied by a feeling of weakness and nausea and may result in syncope. Dryness of the scalp is common, as well as malnutrition of the hair, which comes out in handfuls when using the comb. The Sulphur headache is often situated above the right eye, but may be on the vertex or other site. It is associated with redness of visage and a sensation of heat on the top of the head. It is aggravated when out of doors and is made worse by stooping; resting quietly in a warmish temperature may afford relief. A periodic sick headache is noted, especially liable to come on at the weekend, when presumably a state of congestion occurs as a rebound effect after the activities of the preceding five or six days. A variety of unpleasant or confused sensations in the head are mentioned, e.g. 'tight band round forehead', 'brain beating against inside of skull', 'head going to burst', 'scalp seems loose', 'sounds penetrate through forehead rather than ears'.

Eyes
Pain is felt in the eyeballs and extends to the head, being made worse by movement of the eyes and exposure to sunlight. Profuse lachrymation may occur with burning sensations. Itching and burning is felt, especially affecting the canthi and the lids. Actual blepharitis is common with copious secretion, agglutination of the lids in the morning and marked redness of the lid margins. The condition may progress to corneal involvement. Disturbances of vision are frequent, sparks, spots and so on being seen in front of the eyes, or objects may acquire a yellow halo. Such aberrations of vision often precede a headache, as is also the case with Natrum Mur. and Psorinum.

Ears
Hearing is apt to be unduly acute, and sensitivity to sounds such that certain noises may be so unbearable as to cause nausea. The liability of the middle ear to catarrh may so affect the lining membrane and the ear drum as to cause both tinnitus and deafness. Otorrhoea if present is very offensive.

Respiratory System
The sense of smell may be very over-developed, or else lost through atrophy of the nasal mucosa. There is an undue liability to constantly 'take fresh cold'. This results in coryza, much burning and itching inside the nose, with offensive mucous discharge, possibly blood-streaked. The coryza is worse out of doors; in the house the nose tends to be stuffed up.

The tip of the nose may become red and shiny. Persistent soreness and dryness of the throat is a common complaint, associated with much hawking and a sensation as if there was a ball stuck in the throat, which cannot be shifted by swallowing. On inspection the pharynx is seen to have a purplish look. Dyspnoea occurs with a feeling of tightness or oppression in the chest. Actual suffocative attacks may occur at night, associated with violent palpitations of the heart and an insistent desire to have the door and windows opened. This is the result of overloading of the right side of the heart and may be accompanied by haemoptysis. Actual asthmatic attacks may occur and are likely to alternate with the appearance of eruptions on the skin. Again, there may be bronchitis associated with an urgent craving for air and much white, frothy, possibly blood-stained sputum. The remedy may be indicated in unresolved pneumonia or in the presence of pleural effusion.

Alimentary System

The mouth is often unhealthy, with a tendency to sepsis, bitter taste and unpleasant breath. The mouth and tongue are often sore with or without the presence of small nodules on the margin of the tongue or actual ulcers. Heartburn, pyrosis, loud eructations, regurgitation of food may all be present and cause distress. Various discomforts are noted in the abdomen, flatulence of severe degree, acute stitching pains, perhaps located especially on the left side. The belly may be greatly distended, in marked contrast to the emaciated-looking neck, chest and limbs, as for instance in marasmic infants. Involvement of the liver with congestion and inflammatory changes gives rise to enlargement of the organ and jaundice. The gallbladder may also be affected and gallstones be present. An important feature is early morning diarrhoea, which drives from bed at 5 a.m. The urgent stool is usually painless and very variable in consistence, but offensive in odour. Actual dysentery may occur with violent tenesmus. Constipation and diarrhoea may alternate, the former characterized by hard, knotty stools which are very painful. The anus becomes red and sore. Ineffectual urging to stool is often present as with Nux Vomica. Piles tend to prolapse, ooze moisture, itch and burn and often bleed. Sulphur may be called for in cholera infantum when the child is stuporous, with facial pallor and bathed in sweat.

Cardiovascular System

Embarrassment of the right side of the heart leads to suffocative dyspnoea and palpitation, possibly associated with sharp pain in the region of the heart extending through to the back between the shoulder-blades. The heart may feel 'too large'. Cardiac symptoms are worse at night and in bed; they are aggravated by walking uphill or ascending stairs. A sensation of unease in the cardiac area may be accompanied by faintness and trembling in the upper limbs. There is a tendency to develop varicose veins with various complications, and possibly ulceration with foul-smelling discharge. These symptoms are aggravated by going from a cold into a warm atmosphere.

Lymphatic and Glandular Systems
Sulphur tends to involvement of lymph nodes or glandular structures, leading to inflammatory changes and abscess formation. It is indicated in tuberculous lymphadenitis complicated by caseation, breakdown and multiple sinus formation with added secondary infection – a condition described as scrofula and met with in emaciated, shrivelled-looking children who are always voraciously hungry, also in older subjects where tuberculosis is rife.

Urinary System
Violent pain may occur in the kidney region, aggravated on passing urine; the act of urination may be accompanied by rigor. A variety of bladder symptoms are noted, especially frequency with burnings and smarting; also anomalies in the appearance and consistence of the urine. It is well to consider the possible use of Sulphur in urinary complaints. The remedy may be effective with nocturnal enuresis, especially when the individual lies awake for a long time, and then wets the bed soon after dropping to sleep.

Genital System
Sulphur may be indicated with sterility. In connection with abortion it may be needed in sequence either to Belladonna or Sabina. Menstruation is apt to be irregularly irregular, the flow stopping abruptly on the third day and starting again on the fourth day. The period may be early or delayed and the flow scanty or abundant with black blood which excoriates the skin. Dysmenorrhoea is common. Shiverings precede hot flushes at the menopause, accompanied by 'all-gone' feelings owing to irregularities in blood distribution. Sensations of fullness and bearing-down are complained of in the pelvis, aggravated by standing. Burning and itching occur in the vulva, and such symptoms are often aggravated at the menopause when the auto-intoxications of the Sulphur diathesis are intensified by diminution in menstrual loss. The remedy may be called for in puerperal fever.

Locomotor System
The spine is extremely sensitive to any pressure or jar. There is marked weakness of the paraspinal muscles, resulting in a chronic stoop. Not only is the musculature weak but rheumatic-type pains occur in association with much stiffness, in which various joints are also involved. Low back pain, especially in the sacral region, causes disability in rising from a chair, the sufferer having to straighten up slowly. Pain in the knees is also worse on first rising from sitting. The limbs are apt to 'go to sleep' when recumbent. Pains are worse at night, especially on getting warm in bed. Cramp may also occur in the calves and soles at night. The remedy may be of value in synovitis, especially of the knee-joint. It has been used in ganglion, a condition in which Ruta may also be effective.

Skin
The skin affections of Sulphur are liable to be accompanied by much itching, with an uncontrollable desire to scratch; and scratching, although pleasant at first, gives rise to burning and smarting. Eruptions may be accompanied by much erythema, or there may be widespread pruritus without actual eruption. These conditions are typically aggravated by heat, especially the warmth of the bed, and also by contact with water or woollen clothing. There is a tendency for the skin eruptions to alternate with other manifestations, such as asthma. Wounds are slow to heal. Sepsis is common and tends to chronicity. Ulcers become indolent. Callosities form on pressure areas, notably palms and soles. Acne, pustular eruptions, soreness in flexures and contact areas, intertrigo, boils in crops, are conditions which may call for Sulphur, possibly in sequence to other indicated remedies.

MODALITIES

Heat, of course, aggravates, especially the warmth of the bed, but so does cold wet weather and severe cold. Another peculiarity is a strange sensitivity to water, which results in aggravation from washing or taking a bath. Feels worse after taking stimulants, even after eating. Staying for long in one position causes distress, and the standing posture even more so. Chronologically there is aggravation at 11 a.m. or noon, at night especially, and a tendency to feel worse on waking.

Amelioration or relief is noticed in dry, not too hot weather, and when lying on the right side.

CLINICAL NOTES

In Farrington's *Clinical Materia Medica* no less than eighty-nine conditions are mentioned in which Sulphur may be the indicated remedy. It will often be called for in patients who do not present the typical picture of the great unwashed or the great unwashable. Often the general modalities will be a strong guide to its use, or the fact that there is not the expected response to the apparently indicated remedy.

Sulphur has in fact been described as 'our mainstay in defective reaction'. It is often invaluable in intractable conditions which do not respond as expected, because of some deep-seated toxicosis which can only be reached and exteriorized by Sulphur. Such a state of affairs may be met with in acute disease which is hanging fire and slow in clearing up, or in chronic illness.

Again, the remedy may prove helpful in the absence of any very obvious indications for a particular remedy. It may in these circumstances bring to the surface more definite symptoms which can then be used as a guide to prescribing.

It is of value in illness resulting from suppression of eruptions or other symptoms, whether by drug action or by ointments or other means. It is to be considered in deep-seated sepsis, especially when associated with hectic fever and rigors.

Sulphur shares with Malandrinum and Thuja the ability to counter serious after-effects of vaccination.

When Aconite can deal with an acute exacerbation, Sulphur may be needed as the constitutional remedy to prevent recurrence. The remedy should not immediately precede Lycopodium, but be given in the sequence Sulphur→Calcarea Carb.→Lycopodium→Sulphur.

It is said not to be very effective below the 30c potency, but the 200c is a potency with a rather bad reputation for causing aggravations. It should never be given in high potency in advanced pulmonary tuberculosis.

Syphilinum (Lueticum)

SOURCE

Syphilis is a sexually-transmitted disease with an early infectious phase and later granulomatous developments. There is also a congenital form. The primary manifestation is muco-cutaneous, whilst the later lesions may involve any organ or system. The disease is spread by the spirochaete *Treponema pallidum*, whose natural host is man. Primary infection is almost always by sexual contact, though the passage of organisms in infected material through skin abrasions has been reported – notably in the case of John Hunter, the famous eighteenth-century surgeon.

Syphilis first appeared in Europe in the sixteenth century, and is thought to have been brought back from the Americas by early explorers. It spread rapidly, and at first was regarded as an acute, sometimes rapidly fatal disease. Only later did the extent of the chronic damage it could inflict become apparent. The classical treatments with mercury and arsenical preparations were almost as dangerous as the disease itself. In this century the discovery that *Treponema pallidum* was sensitive to penicillin gave rise to the hope that syphilis might be exterminated. This has not happened, and current sexual standards have led to an increase in its incidence.

Syphilis may be divided into three stages. In primary syphilis the whole body is invaded by organisms within a few hours of infection, but the primary lesions or chancre, a painless eroded ulcer with an indurated border, takes from ten to ninety days to develop. It occurs at the site of infection, and disappears after several weeks. The regional lymph nodes may become painlessly enlarged.

Secondary syphilis usually appears six to eight weeks after the disappearance of the chancre, and lasts for from two to six weeks. Most often it consists of a papulo-squamous eruption of the palms, soles and mucous membranes; but any area of the body may be affected, and the rash may take any form. Syphilis has been called 'the great imitator'. The rash is accompanied by headache and malaise, generalized shotty enlargement of the lymph nodes, and sore throat. There may also be a 'moth-eaten' type of alopecia.

Syphilinum (Lueticum)

During the primary and secondary stages of syphilis the patient is infectious, and diagnosis may be made by dark-ground microscopic examination of discharges, showing spirochaetes, or by serological tests. After this the disease becomes latent and non-infectious.

The third or late stage of syphilis manifests months or years later. The typical lesion is the gumma, a chronic granuloma which may occur in any tissue of the body, mimicking a number of other chronic conditions. The chief sites of late syphilis are the nervous system and the cardiovascular system.

Neurosyphilis appears insidiously, with gradually increasing disruption of nervous function. The chief forms are:

a) Meningo-vascular syphilis, where symptoms depend on the site and degree of involvement.

b) General paresis (dementia paralytica) involving the cerebral cortex and resulting in tremors, dysarthria, gradual loss of memory and concentration, personality changes (often delusions of grandeur) ending in total dementia.

c) Tabes dorsalis (locomotor ataxia) where there is chronic and usually progressive degeneration of the ascending sensory neurones in the posterior column of the spinal cord and the posterior sensory ganglia. The patient cannot feel his feet, walks on a broad base, and may eventually become paraplegic. He suffers from lightning pains in the legs and acute gastric crises. Pupillary changes (Argyll-Robertson pupil) may be present.

Cardiovascular syphilis attacks principally the aorta, large vessels and heart. Aneurysm of the ascending aorta can cause pressure in the mediastinum and hoarseness, or the patient may be symptom-free until death results from rupture of the aneurysm, myocardial failure or infarction.

Congenital Syphilis. Syphilis may be transmitted from the mother to a foetus in utero, and such an infant may show marasmus, bullous eruptions, hepatosplenomegaly and neurological involvement. Late congenital syphilis manifests in deformities of the nose and teeth, eighth nerve deafness and interstitial keratitis.

PROVINGS

The first suggestion that Syphilinum could be used as a nosode came from Lux in 1830, but the first proving was made by Swan in 1880. A clinico-therapeutic study was published by Wildes in 1891.

Syphilinum (Lueticum)

APPEARANCE

The stigmata of syphilis – saddle-shaped nose, Hutchinson's teeth, uneven pupils, sabre tibia – are well documented. The subject looks older than his years. This is particularly striking in the case of a baby who looks like a little old man.

PSYCHOLOGY

There is a great deal of fear: of the night, when everything is worse; of illness; of germs; of insanity; of financial ruin. Associated with fear is obsessional anxiety, expressed in the need to count railings, to wash the hands, and in repetition of words and phrases. There is loss of memory, for names, dates and recent events. Concentration is poor. Schoolchildren dread mathematics but do not fare much better with languages.

Apathy alternates with irritability, and even violence. There may be euphoria with delusions of grandeur, or paranoia and fear of persecution. The subject is undecided, disorderly and unstable.

Alcoholism and drug addiction are common.

PHYSIOLOGY

Insomnia is common, from midnight to 6 a.m. with consequent prostration in the morning. All symptoms are worse from sunset to sunrise, worse by the seaside and better in the mountains (cf. Medorrhinum).

Children may be undersized, and mentally and physically retarded.

There is a craving for alcohol, drugs and tobacco, and an aversion to meat.

SYMPTOMATOLOGY

Head
Bitemporal and occipital headaches. Sharp pains, worse at night. Right-sided facial neuralgia and facial palsy.

Eyes
Unilateral or bilateral ptosis. Pain in the eyeball with photophobia and watering. Vertical diplopia (one image above the other). Inflammation of the eyelids, with a feeling as of sand in the eyes on waking. Chronic phlyctenular conjunctivitis. Unequal pupils. Strabismus.

Ears
Chronic earache with purulent discharge. Deafness. Vertigo.

Nose

Anosmia. Burning irritation of the nostrils. Ozaena, with offensive crusty discharge.

Digestive System

Mouth and Pharynx. Crooked, carious teeth. Hutchinson's teeth. A feeling like a worm in the tooth. White-coated tongue with tooth-marks, or dry, fissured, burning tongue. Halitosis, with copious, dribbling saliva. Burning of the pharynx and gullet.

Abdomen. Nausea, with acid and burning sensations. Flatulence. Anal stricture, anal fissure, bleeding piles with burning, pricking pains. Perianal ulceration. Stubborn chronic constipation, alternating with crises of painless diarrhoea at 5 a.m. Rectal paresis.

Cardiovascular System

Sharp precordial pain at night. Pressure felt on the upper part of the sternum. A feeling of heat in the arteries.

Respiratory System.

Throat. Hypertrophy and chronic ulceration of the tonsils. Ulceration of the vocal chords. Hoarseness. Aphonia. The larynx is exquisitely painful to touch, especially at night, causing the patient to get up and walk about.

Lungs. Dry cough at 1 a.m. to 4 a.m., worse lying on the right side and at the approach of a storm. Chronic asthma, worse in summer and in warm humid weather.

Urogenital System.

Urinary. Micturition is slow and difficult, the meatus feels as if plugged in the morning. Nocturnal enuresis.

Genital – Men. Induration of the testicles and spermatic cord. Chronic inguinal lymphadenopathy.

Genital – Women. Induration of the cervix. Chronic vaginitis, painful to touch. Copious, thick, burning leucorrhoea, worse at night. Pruritus and ulceration of the vulva. Disorders of menstruation.

Musculo-Skeletal System

Cranial exostoses, which may be sensitive and even painful. Pain and stiffness of the dorsal muscles. Pain in the cervical spine, worse at night and from movement, relieved by heat. Pain in the shoulders and deltoids, better by day, better just after waking. Nocturnal pain in the tibia. Painful contraction of the leg muscles. Painful stiffness and coldness of the limbs.

Skin, Hair and Nails

Hair loss. 'Moth-eaten' patches of alopecia. Early whitening of the hair. Copper-coloured papulo-pustular rashes of the scalp and of the skin in general. Abscesses with foetid discharge. A variety of rashes, ulcers and induration of the skin.

MODALITIES

Worse: at night, from touch, beside the sea, from storms, from the cold of winter.
Better: from sunrise to sunset, from slow walking, in the mountains.
Laterality: Right.

CLINICAL NOTES

In chronic diseases where the appearance or history suggest a syphilitic background, and where other remedies do not quite cover the case or fail to act. Especially useful in neurotic and obsessional conditions, in varicose ulcers, and in certain cases of malabsorption.

Related remedies are: Mercurius, Arsenicum, Argentum Nit., Nitric Acid, Phytolacca, Aurum Met., Lycopodium, Lachesis, Lac Caninum.

Tarentula Hispanica

SOURCE

The spider from which this remedy is prepared is a species of wolf spider, *Lycosa tarentula*. It is found in Italy and Spain; in parts of Italy the phenomenon of tarentism still persists. This type of hysterical frenzied dancing stimulated by music, the tarantella, is by tradition said to result from a bite of the spider. It is, however, known that the bite of *Lycosa* can do little harm to man. *Lycosa* is a vicious-looking creature with large chelicerae or fangs; wolf-like it bounds along at high speed in pursuit of its prey. Whether actually bitten or not, contact with this brute, or indeed with other venomous creatures such as snakes or scorpions, may be the psychogenic factor responsible for these seizures of 'dancing mania' which occur at set seasons among the peasants of Apulia.

PHARMACOLOGY

The venom of this spider has an affinity with the motor and sensory functions of the nervous system, resulting in peculiarly bizarre motor restlessness and uncontrolled agitation. In the sensory sphere, there is an excessive sensitivity and excitability of all the perceptive senses; light and glaring colours irritate and aggravate; noises frighten and aggravate. An affinity with the lymphatic and circulatory systems can give rise to cellulitis, enlargement of lymph nodes, and intense vascular congestion, both faucial and cerebral, associated with facial pallor.

PROVING

A proving of Tarentula Hispanica was conducted and described by the Marquis Nunez, of Spain.

APPEARANCE

The face shows a pale, earthy hue. Eyes are wide, shining and staring, with a look almost of terror. Inflamed parts are dark red or purplish and swollen. Throbbing carotids are seen in the neck. Lymph nodes may be enlarged.

There is unceasing movement; constant jerking, twitching, running, dancing; the hands and fingers are never still.

Violent choreic movements involve especially the legs.

The patient may be rolling from side to side in distress, or appears about to choke.

Constantly picks at the fingers; screws up bits of paper and throws them away.

PSYCHOLOGY

Thought processes are in a state of turmoil and emotions are excessive. Extreme sexual excitement may manifest itself as lasciviousness, obscenity, nymphomania or exhibitionism.

Moods change abruptly; excessive gaiety with fits of laughing, singing, dancing and screaming may give place to deep depression with sombre fantasies, thoughts of death, or indifference and taciturnity bordering on stupor.

Is crafty and cunning, yet timid. Prone to acts of sudden violence; given to sly and furtive destructiveness. Shows incredible swiftness of action. Flies into a rage at least contradiction.

Feigns sickness, then looks round to see if observed.

Has indefinite fears of some intangible unknown.

Is physically affected by colour; may show an aversion to green.

Is phenomenally sensitive to music, but whether it is soothing, animating, exciting or irritating, whether ameliorating or aggravating, will depend on the kind of musical rhythms and on the emotional and imaginative susceptibility of the individual.

Visual impressions and images may attain such a degree of intensity that they appear as illusions and hallucinations – visions of ghostly shades, shapes, flashes, faces, frightening monsters, insects, strangers in the room, and the like.

Violent destructive mania may involve self-injury.

PHYSIOLOGY

There is a liability to coldness and chilliness with every complaint.

Appetite may be excessive or lacking. There may be a craving for raw food, and aversion to bread and roast meat. An intense burning thirst gives rise to a constant desire for large quantities of cold water.

Dream-filled sleep; perhaps sleepless before midnight.

Sweats are debilitating; may occur at night.

SYMPTOMATOLOGY

General

Symptoms are characterized by violence, torment, spasms and protean manifestations suggestive of hysteria. There is accompanying exhaustion and chilliness. Numerous and multifarious pains may occur as the result of peripheral nerve involvement. The body feels bruised all over, especially when in motion. A tendency to periodicity with annual recurrence of symptoms is claimed by some writers. Symptoms tend to be right-sided; involvement of the left arm and the right leg has been recorded (this is just the opposite to Agaricus).

Head

A great variety of headaches have been recorded, some associated with curious symptoms such as if 'a thousand needles were pricking the brain' or 'cold water was being poured on the head and over the body'. The headaches are made worse by stooping and by any contact; but some relief may be obtained by rubbing the head against the pillow.

Eyes

Photophobia accompanies headache. The right pupil may be enlarged and the left contracted. Pain is felt in the right eye. There may be a sensation of a foreign body in the eye – eyelash, splinter, sand. Vision may be dim.

Ears

Cracking may occur in the right ear, associated with pain and hiccough. Tinnitus is present at night, worse on waking.

Respiratory System

Chronic coryza is associated with frequent sneezing; it chiefly affects the right nostril. Epistaxis is profuse, with dark, quickly coagulating blood. A dry spasmodic cough is worse in the evening; it may be associated with enuresis. Smoking affords relief. Great oppression is felt in the chest, with panting respiration. The cough causes pain in head, chest and uterus. Attacks of suffocation occur with crying, screaming and restlessness.

Alimentary System

There is dryness of mouth and teeth. Toothache is throbbing in character and made worse by breathing in air. The fauces appear swollen and purple. There is a sensation of constriction when swallowing. Tonsils when inflamed may be so large as to obstruct breathing. Nausea and dizziness compel the patient to lie down. Acid vomiting is associated with burning in stomach and oesophagus; the stomach pain is aggravated by drinking water. There may be a sensation as if 'something alive was moving in or causing tingling in the stomach and rising up into the throat'. Various pains are recorded in the abdomen, mostly of a violent burning character. Pain as if parts were compressed is referred to hypogastrium, hips and pelvic organs. Profuse diarrhoea is accompanied by nausea, vomiting, fainting and prostration; the stools are dark and very offensive. Pain and burning occur in the anus after a stool.

Cardiovascular System
Precordial anxiety is associated with tumultuous palpitation. There is a feeling as if 'the heart was being squeezed or compressed' or 'was turning and twisting'. The sufferer cannot lie on the left side. The symptoms may be aggravated by putting the hands in cold water.

Lymphatic System
Involvement of cervical lymph nodes in association with tonsillitis may cause such severe swelling of the neck as to endanger life from obstruction to breathing.

Urinary System
Cystitis is accompanied by excruciating pain and acute retention. Dysuria occurs with frequent and very painful urination, worse at night. Enuresis is liable to occur when coughing, laughing, sneezing.

Genital System
Libido is increased in both sexes. Menses are early, profuse and followed by severe pruritus vulvae. During menstruation there is intolerable dryness of nose, throat, tongue and mouth. Uterine pain is accompanied by burning in hypogastrium and hips and a sensation of great weight in the pelvis.

Locomotor System
Rigidity and muscle cramps are accompanied by extreme weakness, numbness, trembling, even paresis of the legs, presumably due to involvement of the spinal cord. The least touch on the spine induces spasmodic pain in the chest and in the region of the heart. Pain and stiffness in the neck is made worse by attempts to move the head.

Skin

A variety of eruptions may be met with – purpuric spots, vesicular or miliary eruptions. Pruritis can be exteme; also sensations of formication, burning, scorching, numbness; hyperaesthesia is excessive, especially at the finger tips.

MODALITIES

The effects of music may aggravate or ameliorate, as mentioned above. Any strong emotion will cause aggravation.

Aggravating factors are cold, damp weather, exposure to cold air; feels worse when walking but nevertheless cannot keep still. Further aggravations are from noise, from light touch, by wetting hands in cold water, by bright light, when at rest, at night, after sleep, after coitus.

There is relief on dry sunny days and in the open air, though vertigo is aggravated out of doors. As already mentioned, music of the right tempo may soothe but may also excite. Is better in a warm room, from firm pressure and friction, and after a nosebleed.

CLINICAL NOTES

The chief indication for the remedy is the picture of perpetual motion coupled with psychological disturbance.

Tarentula cubensis, a spider rather larger and more hairy than *Lycosa hispanica*, also provides a most valuable remedy. It is indicated in conditions characterized by much blueness, for instance in boils or carbuncle, especially if accompanied by atrocious burning pains. It can also prove of value in moribund states, to soothe the final struggles.

Thuja Occidentalis

SOURCE

Thuja occidentalis, the so-called white cedar, or *Arbor vitae*, is an evergreen conifer, not a true cedar. It is a smallish tree found growing in cool, damp regions of North America. The wood is very resistant to decay; hence its use for outside purposes such as fences, poles and roof tiles – cedar shakes.

The tree with its tapered and somewhat twisted trunk may reach a height of forty-five feet. The wood is fragrant and light; hence its misnomer of cedar. The foliage is very suggestive of the cypress with its green, adpressed, flattened, imbricated scales. The tree, however, differs from the rather mournful cypress in its more cheerful, jaunty appearance with uptilted branches. The cones also are distinctive, being cylindrical in shape with out-curving scales, aligned in almost sessile rows like ranks of tiny penguins. Both foliage and cones give off an aromatic odour when crushed. A very fluid, light, transparent oil with a strong odour and a slightly acrid taste can be distilled from the foliage. The mother tincture is prepared from the fresh green twigs.

PHARMACOLOGY

This drug has a strong affinity with epithelial tissue, its irritant action leading to over-secretion by glandular cells and hyperplasia of epithelium with the formation of warty or condylomatous growths. Affinity with the mucous lining of the urinary tract causes acute inflammation accompanied by yellow discharge. It causes contraction of uterine muscle.

PROVING

The pathogenesis of Thuja was published by Hahnemann in the fifth volume of *Materia Medica Pura*.

APPEARANCE

A heavy trunk, short neck, thin limbs, waxy greasy skin and irregular teeth are listed as characteristic of the Thuja subject, and in general a sickly look.

512

The face is apt to be red with a prominent network of dilated capillaries, especially on the alae nasi. The hair is dry, often black, with a tendency to split at the tips, and dandruff is likely to be present. The nasolabial folds are well marked, the lips livid with a white transverse line across the lower lip which looks as if the subject had just taken a drink of milk. Pulsation of the temporal arteries may be obvious.

Excessive hairiness may be present in women, with the growth of a moustache and dark hair on the limbs. Obesity may be excessive. Movements tend to be unnaturally active and hurried. Hands are cold and clammy to touch. Speech is either hesitant or hurried.

Discharges are copious, foul-smelling, often greenish and thin. Peculiar odours may suggest fish-brine, garlic or honey.

PSYCHOLOGY

There is a tendency to feel dazed, confused, especially on waking from sleep. Inattention is due to the mind being preoccupied with persistent thoughts. The patient is apathetic, desiring to be left alone; is ill-humoured, peevish, lachrymose – music may provoke tears.

There is a proneness to excess – acts and talks hurriedly, is scrupulous over trifles and unduly touchy over minutiae.

Fixed ideas may obtrude – 'his soul is separated from his body' – strange people are standing beside the bed' – 'is pregnant' – 'something alive is moving around in the belly' – 'legs are made of wood'. One particular odd sensation is of brittleness and liability to shatter into little fragments. There is great sensitivity to people, 'atmosphere', and music.

PHYSIOLOGY

The Thuja subject is unduly chilly and may shiver all over on exposure of the body, even to warm air. Although the face may be hot, the rest of the body is cold with icy hands or fingertips, and notably cold feet and knees, even in bed.

Appetite is poor, with easy satiety after a few mouthfuls; often there is no desire for breakfast. There is a craving for salt and a preference for cold food; when eating must keep taking a drink to facilitate swallowing. There is a dislike of raw food and potatoes, and intolerance of onions.

Thirst is not marked; it is said that fluids when swallowed drop into the stomach with a gurgling sound.

Sleep is disturbed by anxious, amorous, sometimes frightful dreams, often of falling from a height. There is a tendency to wake about 4 a.m. and stay awake. Wakes later feeling unrefreshed.

Profuse sweats occur on uncovered parts only, or all over except on the head. Sweats tend to occur during sleep and cease on waking. The sweat is sweetish, strong-smelling, pungent.

SYMPTOMATOLOGY

General

All symptoms tend to be severe and excessive, but their onset is insidious. Emaciation and easy exhaustion are prominent features. Pains are described as shooting, burning or darting, and may drive the sufferer from bed. Joints crack, limbs jerk, muscles feel 'beaten', stiffness and heaviness are felt all over the body. When walking, however, the body may seem 'light'. Flushes of heat or pulsations occur in various sites, especially in the evening. Pain may be felt in small spots and in association with frequency of urination. Discharges tend to be very profuse. There is also a proneness to the formation of tumours, either benign or malignant. Laterality is left-sided.

Head

Vertigo is noticed on closing the eyes, and relieved by opening them. A severe stupefying headache is felt, especially in the left frontal region, like a 'nail being driven into the skull'; it is worse in the morning on waking or perhaps at bedtime, and is aggravated by stooping and by heat. It is relieved for the moment by touch or rubbing, and also in the open air. Severe neuralgia with stabbing pain is made worse by sitting up. A digging pain in the malar region is aggravated by lying on the affected side. The scalp is dry and scurfy and often excessively painful, especially on the left side, also extremely itchy. Alopecia is common on the vertex and the eyebrows tend to fall out. A chronic ulcer may occur on the scalp with indurated edges, a greyish base and a foetid discharge.

Eyes

Severe conjunctivitis occurs with much lachrymation; the lids are stuck together in the morning with formation of crusts. Shooting pains are felt in the eyes, relieved by warmth and by keeping the eyes covered. Vision may be dim, and objects looked at seem to tremble. Yellow flashes may be seen before the eyes. Warts on the lids, chalazion, styes may call for Thuja. A sensation as of cold air blowing onto the eyes may be noticed on opening the lids.

Ears
The ears crack on swallowing. Tearing jerks may be felt in the ears. Otorrhoea is very offensive. Aural polypi may be present. Ears may feel numb before the onset of an epileptic seizure.

Respiratory System
Acute fluent coryza is worse out of doors, accompanied by much sneezing and hoarseness. Chronic nasal catarrh occurs with thick, green, sanious mucopurulent discharge. Post-nasal discharge also tends to be present. There is a liability to the formation of nasal polypi. Left-sided sore throat, the pain being worse on breathing in air or on swallowing, is associated with hoarseness and a sensation as if a foreign body was lodged in the larynx or trachea. A violent convulsive cough is aggravated by inspiring cool air and is associated with yellow sputum. Thuja may be indicated in relation to asthma when the acute remedy is Arsenicum. A sense of oppression accompanied by throbbing and stitches may afflict the left side of the chest.

Alimentary System
Lips twitch. Small pustules occur on lips and bleed when touched. Teeth ache and are extremely sensitive to cold water. Marginal caries may be associated with pyorrhoea alveolaris. The tongue remains clean despite digestive upsets, but the tip of the tongue may be excessively sore. The mouth is very dry, feels as if full of blisters or as if burnt. Ulcers occur in the mouth. There is a raw feeling on the pharynx causing a constant desire to swallow for relief. Heartburn is associated with anorexia and foul rancid eructations. A sensation of weight in the stomach is noticed after a meal. There is soreness in the hypogastrium, and at times distinct throbbing in the right iliac fossa after walking. Much flatus is passed, especially in the morning; it is usually inodorous. Diarrhoea occurs with copious, pale, greasy stools, expelled forcibly with a gurgling sound; the stools are painless, and may occur regularly every morning after breakfast. A so-called bashful stool may be present, that is a stool that recedes into the rectum when partially extruded. This symptom is shared by Sanicula and Silica. Anal fissures, warts, condylomata may occur, associated with perianal moisture.

Cardiovascular System
The Thuja subject is liable to audible palpitation, especially when ascending stairs or when lying on the left side. The pulse, slow and of poor volume in the morning, tends to become full in the evening and increased in rate. Throbbing sensations may accompany this circulatory ebullition.

Urinary System

Urethritis occurs associated with a yellowish sticky discharge. Prostatitis is liable to become chronic and be accompanied by rheumatic pains. Frequency of urination is associated with acute cutting pain at the end of and after the passage of urine, which is dark in colour and pungent in odour.

Genital System

Balanitis occurs, associated with the presence of warty growths on the corona glandis, which bleed readily. Profuse sweating occurs on the external genitalia. Chancroid ulcer and condylomata may be present. In women a violent, stabbing, tearing pain may be felt in the left ovary during the menstrual period, made worse by walking. The pain extends into the left groin and thigh. Uterine polyps may occur, and pelvic peritonitis. Vaginal discharge is profuse, thick, green and irritating.

Locomotor System

Pain and stiffness occur in nape and back, associated with a bruised sensation. Rheumatic pains in various sites are accompanied by numbness; these are aggravated by warmth and worse before rain; they are also worse after midnight. They are relieved by cold, by sweating, and are better when rain actually starts. A severe backache may be relieved by walking. Jerkings and tremblings occur in the limbs. Thigh muscles feel weary and weak, and this may cause difficulty in going upstairs. Joints are involved, especially the knees, and pains may be felt in the Achilles tendon and the heels. The pain is often accompanied by a curious sensation when walking, as if the limbs were 'made of wood' or 'were brittle like glass, and would snap'. Fingertips may become swollen, red and numb. Thuja has been mentioned in relation to myositis ossificans.

Skin

Scaly patches occur on the skin, suggestive of psoriasis. Herpetic or pustular eruptions, warts on the dorsal aspect of the hands, condylomata of 'cauliflower' type with a fishy odour are all mentioned. Circular ulcers occur with broad indurated margins and a greyish base. Nails grow quickly, become easily deformed and tend to break easily. Widely distributed brownish spots may be present on the skin. Pruritus may be troublesome, especially in the evening and at night.

Thuja Occidentalis

MODALITIES

Aggravating factors are damp cold weather, heat of the bed, bright light and direct sun. The patient is also worse from movement, from drinking tea or coffee, or taking narcotics. Symptoms are aggravated during the menstrual period, at night, after breakfast, at 3 a.m. and 3 p.m.

Some relief is experienced in cool air, after sweating, by stretching the limbs, from scratching or being massaged.

CLINICAL NOTES

Thuja is a deeply-acting remedy and should not be repeated too frequently. It may be of service at times in acute conditions.

It should be considered when there is a history of gonorrhoea or shingles. Other aetiological factors pointing to the possible use of Thuja are vaccination with severe reaction, or repeated unsuccessful vaccination, serum injections, coccal infections, snakebite, excessive tea drinking.

Complementary remedies are Lachesis, Medorrhinum, Silica and Sycotic Co.

Tuberculinum

Tuberculosis was so prevalent early this century that eighty per cent of the population was infected before the age of twenty years. Today it is much rarer, due to improved standards of living and earlier diagnosis and treatment of this chronic illness.

Susceptibility to tuberculosis differs among the races. Caucasians and Mongolians have a higher natural immunity to the disease than Africans and American Indians, in whom the infection proceeds much more rapidly. Immunity to the disease is mediated by T-lymphocytes; the fact that TB recrudesces in old age may be due to reduced immune surveillance by T-lymphocytes.

PATHOGENESIS

The bacilli gain entry to the body via the lungs, gut or skin, but most early infections are in the lower two-thirds of the lungs, where there is maximum ventilation and therefore a high susceptibility to droplet deposition. They multiply freely and reach regional lymph nodes until their progress is stopped by the gradual development of immunity – a period of several weeks. At this stage caseous necrosis and epithelial granulomas develop, and slowly the primary site of the infection heals. However, the defences may fail, and in this case the disease may overwhelm the patient, or spread to the chronic stage.

PULMONARY TUBERCULOSIS

This may follow the initial infection, immediately or after a variable period of dormancy (even sixty years). The liquid caseous material in a cavity contains bacilli which may spread the disease to other parts of the lung. The onset of pulmonary TB is insidious, and the early symptoms are constitutional: fever in the evening or afternoon, night sweats, malaise, irritability and depression at the end of the day. Weight loss may or may not occur. A cough is commonly found, worse in the morning, and productive of yellow or green or blood-streaked sputum, which is usually odourless. The complications of pulmonary tuberculosis include haemoptysis, pleural effusion, TB meningitis, bronchopleural fistula and empyema.

TUBERCULOSIS OF OTHER ORGANS

a) Gastrointestinal tuberculosis: the symptoms are abdominal pain, cramping and diarrhoea.
b) Lymph nodes: most commonly enlarged are the hilar nodes related to the primary infection, but cervical lymphadenitis may occur, especially in black people.
c) The kidneys, spine (Pott's Disease), bones, genitals, peritoneum, pericardium, adrenals and meninges (TB meningitis), may all be involved. The disease may also be massively disseminated throughout the body (miliary TB) with the non-specific symptoms of weight loss, fever, sweats, weakness and gastrointestinal disturbance. Without specific treatment, death is inevitable.

SOURCE

The homoeopathic remedy Tuberculinum is a nosode prepared from tuberculous tissue. The original preparation known as Tuberculinum was introduced by Swan and prepared from a drop of pus obtained from a pulmonary tubercular abscess or sputum. Heath prepared a potency from a tuberculous lung in which the bacillus had been microscopically demonstrated, and this was known as Bacillinum. J. H. Clarke states, 'I do not find any appreciable difference between the action of Tuberculinum and that of Bacillinum. My own impression is that they are practically identical, and that one will answer to the indications of the other.' However, the literature often recommends one or the other in relation to a symptom or illness.

PROVING

Tuberculinum has not received a satisfactory proving, although fragmentary provings were conducted by Swan.

APPEARANCE

Subjects are often blonde, blue-eyed, tall and thin, with a narrow neck. They tend to be mentally active but physically weak. Frequently the body and limbs are covered with soft, fine hair.

PSYCHOLOGY

The patient may be depressed, anxious, irritable, sulky and complaining, or averse to work, especially mental work. Children are inclined to have temper tantrums. Fear of dogs has been described. There may be a desire for change, a love of travel, and a sensitivity to music.

PHYSIOLOGY

Symptoms are very changeable, moving from one part of the body to another and beginning and ending abruptly. There is a susceptibility to catching the common cold (Hepar Sulph.). Fatigue, faintness and general debility have been described. The circulation is disturbed, with alternating chills and flushes. There is a longing for the open air, and doors and windows are kept open. Rapid emaciation may occur in spite of eating well. There may be a craving for cold milk and sweets. In spite of being drowsy, the subject finds it difficult to fall asleep; his rest is broken by fearful dreams, during which he may cry out.

SYMPTOMATOLOGY

Head
Vertigo occurs, especially in the morning, and may be accompanied by headache, nausea and palpitation. Headaches are violent, felt 'deep in the head', and cause the patient to tear his hair or beat his head. He may have the sensation that the brain 'feels loose', or 'as if it were squeezed with an iron band'. Headaches of schoolgirls, worse for study and using the eyes for close work. Acute meningitis where the subject wakes frightened and screaming (Apis, Helleborus).

Eyes
Swollen lids may accompany the morning headache, and vision may be obscured during the attacks of vertigo.

Ears
Tinnitus is experienced, as well as a sticking pain from pharynx to ears.

Nose
Epistaxis or secretion of yellow-green thick mucus. Increased secretion of mucus may accompany frontal headache. Crops of small boils in the nostrils.

Neck
There may be cervical adenitis.

Respiratory System
The drug picture includes the symptoms of pulmonary tuberculosis: cough, fever, night sweats and general emaciation. A sensation of pressure is experienced in the chest. There may be pain through the left upper lung to the back, or a sticking pain in the chest and back, worse for movement. Haemoptysis can occur. Coughing fits with a chill and red face are worse in the morning, and aggravated by raising the arms. There is a mucous rattle in the chest.

Cardiovascular System
Early morning palpitations and a sensation of heaviness over the heart.

Digestive System
Loss of appetite is worse in the morning, but there may be extreme thirst. Nausea and vomiting may occur after every meal, with cramping pains in the stomach and aching in the splenic or hepatic regions. The subject may be constipated, with hard dry stools, or have diarrhoea with pricking and burning pains. Rectal pains and anal pruritus may occur.

Urinary System
Oliguria, but has to urinate often, especially during changes of weather.

Genital System
A burning sensation in the genitals, with pain in the testicles and spermatic cord, especially on the left side. The menstrual periods are early and profuse, and of long duration. There is severe dysmenorrhoea. Menstruation may return fourteen days after giving birth.

Reticulo-Endothelial System
Cervical, mesenteric and hilar lymph nodes are enlarged.

Locomotor System
Pains move from joint to joint and limb to limb. Joints tend to be stiff on initial movement, improving with continued motion (Rhus. Tox.). There is a sensation of fatigue and faintness in all the limbs.

Skin

The skin is dry, harsh, sensitive and easily tanned. There is itching all over the body, which changes its position when rubbed, and is worse in the evening in bed. The subject may have bronzed fingertips or great bronze patches on the forehead or temples. Erythematous eruptions may be present.

MODALITIES

Worse in a close atmosphere; for movement and exertion; in damp weather; on awakening; noise; mental excitement.

Better for cool wind and open air.

CLINICAL NOTES

This remedy is commonly used to treat patients with a 'tubercular taint', either a past personal history or a family history of the disease. Burnett recommended the use of a high potency when the taint was strong, but a 30c if it was not so obvious.

It is often used in children who are inclined to get catarrhal coryza and enlarged lymph nodes in response to infections, and those who are irritable and troublesome.

Related remedies are Psorinum, Sulphur, Phosphorus, Pulsatilla.

Veratrum Album

SOURCE

This remedy is prepared from the rootstocks of white hellebore, collected in early June before the flowers appear. The plant is a hardy perennial flowering from June to August; it is common in the mountains of Central and Southern Europe. The hairy stem grows to a height of two to five feet and bears a spike of greenish white small flowers having six petals. The leaves are large, ovoid-lanceolate in shape and prominently ribbed; they ensheath the stem at their base. The root is tuberous, brown on the surface, with long white fibres at the base. All parts of the plant are poisonous, even when dried; it was used in Roman times for poisoned daggers and arrows. It has an acrid taste and produces a sensation of burning in the mouth.

PHARMACOLOGY

A large number of alkaloids have been identified in the drug. There is an irritant affinity with mucous membrane; this causes violent sneezing, and in the alimentary tract burning pain, copious salivation, increased secretion of gastric and intestinal juices leading to vomiting and diarrhoea. The drug was used in ancient Greece as an 'evacuant'. The effect on the circulation is depressive, leading to pallor, slowing of pulse, fall in blood pressure, syncope, cold sweats and cramps. Involvement of the nervous system results in either stupor or mania.

PROVING

Veratrum Album was proved by Hahnemann and appears in the third volume of *Materia Medica Pura*.

APPEARANCE

The face is pale or bluish, eyes sunken, features drawn, with an expression of anguish or fear in anticipation of death. Jerking or twitching of facial muscles may be apparent.

The surface of the body is cold to the touch, and typically beads of cold sweat are obvious on the forehead. The skin generally has a bluish or livid hue. The skin of the palms is wrinkled; the hands and nails are blue. The skin remains puckered when pinched up.

The tongue is cold, as is the breath; the picture is one of collapse and dehydration; voice almost inaudible; pulse thready; watery saliva dribbling from mouth.

PSYCHOLOGY

Violent rage alternates with taciturnity; is unwilling to be left alone, but remains silent or talks to himself *sotto voce*.

Is unkindly, witty, loquacious, malicious – the dangerous dowager. May be inconsolable over some fancied misfortune. Tells outrageous lies.

There is restless, relentless activity; must be constantly occupied. If maniacal is destructive, wanting to cut up or tear to bits anything within reach; there is much wild talk, lewd, amorous or religious in slant.

Hallucinations are varied:

as if a lump of ice was on top of the head,

as if she had committed a crime,

as if she was pregnant or in the throes of childbirth,

as if something alive was rising up from the stomach,

as if the bowels were being cut up with sharp knives,

as if there were hot coals in the belly,

as if intestines were tied in a knot,

as if cold water was pouring through the veins,

as if the pain would drive him crazy.

A Veratrum Alb. condition may arise from fright, shock of injury, even from resentment.

PHYSIOLOGY

A creeping chilliness pervades the whole body; the coldness is persistent.

There is violent hunger and, rather curiously, a craving for cold dishes with a definite aversion to hot food. There is intolerance for fruit. Unquenchable thirst; desire for ice cold drinks. Craves ice to suck.

Sleep is much disturbed by dreams; coma vigil may supervene. Yawning is frequent.

Is bathed in cold sweats, which are especially evident on the forehead.

SYMPTOMATOLOGY

General
Pains are very severe, driving the sufferer frantic. Collapse and coldness are characteristic; prostration is extreme, with marked dehydration, icy coldness, possibly accompanied by shivering and rigors. Sweats and discharges are copious.

Head
Headache is accompanied by a sensation of weight or of a lump of ice on the vertex; it is aggravated by the least movement of the head. Firm pressure of the hand on the top of the head affords some relief. A severe type of headache is relieved by the onset of the menstrual period. A whirling type of vertigo is worse when attempting to walk.

Eyes
Eyeballs are painful and feel bruised. On rising from sitting or getting out of bed, sparks or black spots are seen before the eyes. Night-blindness precedes the menstrual period.

Ears
The ears feel alternatively hot and cold. Roaring tinnitus is noticed, especially when rising from the sitting posture.

Respiratory System
Violent sneezing occurs frequently. The nose feels icy cold. The nose becomes blocked at night in one nostril only. A loose, rattling cough such as is met with in elderly bronchitics who are too weak to bring up much sputum; a bout of coughing is followed by cold perspiration; there is a good deal of belching with the cough; it seems to come from low down and the patient tends to support the belly with both hands when coughing; the cough is worse in a warm room and aggravated when coming into a warm house from outside cold. There may be a tiresome tickle in the trachea or deep to the sternum, which is aggravated by breathing cold air. Moving about may result in a sensation of constriction and suffocation in the chest. Asthmatic respiration is eased by throwing the head back.

Alimentary System
The sense of taste may be lost, or a cool peppperminty taste may be noticed in the mouth. The throat is extremely dry. The tongue is pale and

cold and feels too heavy. Salivation is copious. Severe diarrhoea and vomiting is a prominent feature of this remedy. The vomiting is voluminous and the diarrhoea is violent, with copious green watery stools. Intense nausea precedes the vomiting, and concomitants are colic and cramps. The breath is cold and there is a sensation of either coldness or burning heat in the belly. The rapid dehydration induces faintness, feeble pulse, and the situation is further aggravated by the profuse accompanying sweats. The remedy may be called for in cholera when the profuse, gushing watery stools are accompanied by prostration and cramps in hands and feet, extending to the whole body. The diarrhoea may follow the drinking of cold water on a very hot day or eating raw fruit. A form of constipation occurs with frequent urge felt in the epigastrium and very difficult passage of large, hard, black balls; weakness and near fainting result from the effort required to pass the stool.

Cardiovascular System
A condition of cardiac asthenia results in easy fainting from slight emotion, from retching, from straining at stool. Violent palpitation may occur, the ribs being pushed outwards. Anginal pain may be present. A sensation of cold water coursing through the veins has been described.

Urinary System
Dysuria of various types may occur; also oliguria, even retention. There may be an urge to urinate even when the bladder is almost empty or when only very scanty amounts of dark-coloured urine are passed.

Genital System
Menstrual periods are early, profuse and prostrating. Dysmenorrhoea is accompanied by severe prostration, icy coldness, emotional disturbance and also, probably, vomiting and diarrhoea. Other indications for the remedy may be threatened abortion, nymphomania, puerperal mania.

Nervous System
Various neuralgias occur, accompanying vomiting and diarrhoea; the pain is aggravated by heat and relieved by cool applications.

Locomotor System
Rheumatic or neuralgic pains occur in the limbs in wet weather, made worse by the warmth of the bed, even driving the sufferer out of bed to walk up and down for relief. Legs feel painful and heavy, especially in

damp surroundings. Stiffness and paralytic weakness is felt in muscles of neck and back. A sensation of paralytic weakness, first in the right hip, then in the left, causes difficulty in walking.

Skin

A miliary eruption burns when scratched. Dry eruptions itch, especially at night. Desquamation may occur following erythema.

MODALITIES

Aggravating factors are cold damp weather, changes in weather, taking fluids, movement, touch, pressure, warmth, during a stool, perspiring, before and during menstruation, at night.

Amelioration derives from being at rest, lying down and from coolness.

CLINICAL NOTES

The alimentary syndrome provides a main indication for the use of the remedy. It is said to be of special value in childhood and old age, and in thin choleric nervy types. Emotional disturbance during menstruation, pregnancy or the puerperium calls for consideration of the remedy. Carbo Veg. is a complementary remedy.

Zincum Metallicum

SOURCE

Metallic zinc was smelted in China in A.D. 1637, where it was originally produced. The element occurs in zinc blende – a naturally-existing form of zinc sulphide – and in certain ores of lead and silver. Substantial quantities were formerly mined in Britain, but most of the world's supply comes now from the Americas and Australasia.

Zinc is described as a solid metal, of bluish white colour, scaly, ductile and possessing a feeble but perceptible odour and taste; the metal is very brittle and can be easily pulverized at a temperature of 250°C; it fuses at 360°C, losing its lustre as the result. When melted and very hot, it burns in the open air with a shining flame of a bright violet colour, diffusing small light flakes of zinc oxide into the surrounding air.

Today zinc is one of the most important metals in industry, notably in the production of alloys and in the process of galvanising, to give protection against rust.

It has been employed in medicine mainly in the form of the oxide, used externally in the treatment of ulcers and fissures and given internally in febrile states, hysteria, facial neuralgia, convulsions and tetanus.

PHARMACOLOGY

The metal has an affinity with the central nervous system, the heart, the muscular system and mucous membranes. Depression of the higher centres produces an increase in reflex irritability. Other effects are general weakness, ague-like attacks with prolonged rigors, muscular pains and aches, nausea, vomiting, diarrhoea and widespread formication. Extreme prostration or collapse is a feature of acute poisoning with salts of the metal.

PROVING

This was published by Hahnemann in the first edition of *Chronic Diseases*.

APPEARANCE

The Zinc subject presents a weak, weary, wasted appearance with pallor, sunken eyes and a countenance devoid of expression.

Muscular disturbance is evident in fine twitchings, awkward gait, a tendency to stagger in the dark or when walking with eyes closed, rolling the head from side to side on the pillow, and constant fidgety movements of the feet and legs, even in sleep.

Extreme asthenia may be manifest – the patient lies with eyes closed as if in coma and, when spoken to, hesitates, repeats the question to gain time and finally, speaking very slowly, gives a rational answer.

PSYCHOLOGY

The Zinc subject is likely to be brainy, hard-working, docile yet irritable; oversensitive, unable to throw things off and relax, either mentally or physically. Finally this over-activity gives place to slowness and extreme exhaustion.

The patient is then easily irritated by trifles, too tired to talk or listen to the conversation of other people, and apt to jump at the least noise.

He may appear preternaturally calm, especially in regard to death, of which he speaks with pleasure, though without any suicidal intent. Memory is impaired and a fear may obtrude that 'he is going to be arrested because he has committed an imaginary crime'.

The child is dictatorial, unsubdued by punishment.

Conditions calling for Zinc may be induced by overwork and overstress, or precipitated by a fright.

PHYSIOLOGY

Chilliness is a feature, especially when out of doors, or when touching some cold object. A sensation of coldness may be located in the abdomen or feet.

There may be a voracious appetite or complete anorexia. Eats and drinks with undue and unseemly haste. Often complains of a weak, all-gone sensation in the stomach at about 11 a.m. This peculiarity is shared by Natrum Carb., Phosphorus and Sulphur.

There is aversion to sugar, meat, fish and wine. The least quantity of the latter causes intense flushing. Thirst may be excessive, especially from noon to evening.

Sweats easily on slight pretext; at night perspiration may be profuse and continuous with a tendency to push back the bed-clothes.

Sleep is broken and unrefreshing, punctuated by vivid, usually distressing or terrifying, dreams. Liable to jerk awake in fear, or talk or walk in sleep. Complete inability to get to sleep may occur, with a tendency to hang the head down over the edge of the bed.

SYMPTOMATOLOGY

General

Illness or overwork, or in some cases night-watching, or drunkenness, results in a state of extreme exhaustion, evidenced by mental asthenia and muscular instability. The latter is particularly manifest in the constant fidgety movements of the feet and legs which accompany other symptoms. General weakness may also be accompanied by a tremulous vibration all through the body, associated with fainting spells, numbness of parts and deadly nausea. Suppression of eruptions, of menses, or of perspiration may give rise to symptoms.

Head

Vertigo is likely to be accompanied by pain, and may be preceded by a sensation of pressure at the root of the nose, or a feeling as if 'the eyes were being pulled together by a cord'. The head reels and there is a feeling as if 'he would fall over to the left'. The vertigo may be accompanied by nausea and fainting. Headache can be caused or made worse by taking even a small amount of wine; it is accompanied by soreness of scalp, photophobia and marked restlessness. Firm pressure gives relief, and also the menstrual flow. An occipital headache is described, associated with a sensation of weight on the vertex or at the root of the nose. Affections of the brain or meninges are accompanied by starting at least noise, jerking in sleep, sudden cries, rolling of the head from side to side, delirium and vomiting. Alopecia may be complete.

Eyes

Catarrhal conjunctivitis may occur, especially during the menstrual period; also pterygium at the inner canthus (at the lateral canthus suggests Graphites), with smarting, burning, itching, lachrymation, and sensation of sand under the eyelids. This tends to be worse in the evening and at night. Paretic ptosis may be present.

Ears

Earache in children, especially boys, with stabbing pains. Otitis media with foetid pus. Tinnitus of humming, whizzing, ringing noises, or crashing as of breaking glass.

Respiratory System

Nasal obstruction is accompanied by a sensation of pressure at the root of the nose, as if the nose is being pushed into the skull. A spasmodic cough, accompanied by burning and oppression in chest, is made worse at night on lying down, compelling the sufferer to sit up. There is great difficulty in expectorating, but the dyspnoea is relieved at once on bringing up phlegm. Spasmodic cough in children is accompanied by clutching of the external genitals. Asthma is worse in the evening after a meal, and is associated with a sensation of severe constriction in the chest; bringing up phlegm affords relief.

Alimentary System

Difficult dentition in children is accompanied by weakness, tendency to bore head into pillow, crying out in sleep, and fidgety feet. Teeth become loose and are sensitive when chewing; may feel elongated. Frequent toothache, especially in molars. Gums bleed at least touch; may show ulcers. There is complaint of a sweetish, metallic or bitter taste in the mouth, and much salivation. The tongue is coated at the base. Small yellow ulcers occur in the mouth on the inner aspect of the cheeks. Dryness or soreness of tongue may interfere with speech. Dryness and rawness of palate. Much mucus may accumulate at the back of the pharynx via the posterior nares. Globus hystericus may occur. Nausea is accompanied by much retching and vomiting of blood-streaked mucus; water is vomited as soon as swallowed. Flatulent colic is associated with the passage of hot flatus. Symptoms are aggravated by taking lemon or acid drinks, and by eating bread. Cramp-like pains occur in belly after meals, especially after breakfast. Constipation occurs with small hard stools expelled in fragments and with much straining. Diarrhoea is worse at night and associated with tenesmus, agitation, spasmodic twitching and head-rolling. Itching, crawling and burning sensations are felt at the anus after passage of stool.

Cardiovascular System

Irregular action of the heart may occur, associated with a sudden spasmodic bursting sensation in the cardiac region as if 'the heart would burst out of the chest', which feels 'constricted'. Accompaniments are dyspnoea and a slow, weak, irregular pulse. Varicose veins may be prominent in the lower limbs.

Genital System

There is a liability to priapism and premature ejaculation. Menses are likely to be too early, and associated with dysmenorrhoea and abdominal distension. The onset is preceded by extreme nervous agitation and back pains. These all disappear during the period, when there is a feeling of increased energy. The cough, however, is likely to recur during the menstrual flow. Left ovarian pain may occur, relieved by pressure and better during the menstrual period, but returning immediately after it is over. Pruritus vulvae is associated with hyperaesthesia of genitalia and increased libido.

Urinary System
Features to note are nervous retention of urine; also a tendency to enuresis when walking, coughing or sneezing. Again there may be paresis of the bladder with distension and overflow, or urination may only be possible in the sitting position or when leaning backwards.

Nervous System
Paralytic weakness occurs in the limbs, associated with trembling, stumbling and lightning pains, worse at rest and relieved by moving about. Chorea with constant movements, especially of feet, continuing in sleep, or irregular clonic spasms may be present (tonic spasms point to Cuprum). Other nervous affections which may suggest Zinc are encephalitis lethargica, Huntingdon's chorea, Korsakow's syndrome, G.P.I., exhaustion psychosis. Paraesthesias are common, especially formication of feet and legs; rubbing gives some relief. Concomitants are numbness and coldness.

Locomotor System
Severe shooting pains occur in the muscles of the back, notably in the lower thoracic and upper lumbar regions. These pains, which are also sometimes burning in character, are worse when sitting still or by drinking wine; walking about gives relief. Pain may be felt in the nape when writing.

Skin
Itching may occur in the flexures. A pruritic eruption is described on the dorsum of the hand, aggravated in cold weather. Tetters and herpetic ulcers are also mentioned.

MODALITIES

Aggravation is caused by any exertion, either physical or mental, from contact or jarring, by noise. Symptoms tend to be worse from 11 a.m. to noon, after dinner in the evening, and during the menstrual period.

There is relief from the appearance of eruptions (the patient is often too weak to bring out an exanthematous rash), from the flow of pent-up discharges, from diarrhoea.

CLINICAL NOTES

Among the many ailments suggested above, the main indications for Zinc are the exceptional degree of asthenia and the remarkable constancy of fidgety movements accompanying the illness. The remedy has been used with effect in post-morbillic encephalitis, and also in the early stages of smallpox.

Chamomilla and Nux Vomica are inimical to Zinc and should not be given in direct sequence.

Appendix

1. Ignatia; Nux Vomica
2. Argentum Nitricum; Gelsemium
3. Sepia; Silica
4. Sulphur; Phosphorus
5. Arsenicum Album; Lycopodium Clavatum
6. Lac Caninum; Lachesis
7. Stramonium; Belladonna; Hyoscyamus Niger
8. Helleborus Niger; Aconitum
9. Pulsatilla; Ranunculus Bulbosus
10. Apis Mellifica; Bryonia
11. Natrum Muriaticum; Kali Carbonicum
12. Rhus Toxicodendron; Ruta Graveolens
13. Ipecacuanha; Antimonium Tartaricum
14. Colchicum; Colocynthis
15. Carbo Vegetabilis; Calcarea Carbonica
16. Opium; Cannabis Indica
17. Chamomilla; Hepar Sulphuris Calcareum
18. Mercurius; Thuja
19. Causticum; Arum Triphyllum
20. Zincum; Conium
21. Cinchona; Phosphoricum Acidum
22. Phytolacca; Aurum Metallicum
23. Natrum Sulphuricum; Dulcamara
24. Baptisia; Pyrogenium
25. Graphites; Anacardium Orientale
26. Iodum; Bromium; Spongia Tosta
27. Psorinum; Baryta Carbonica
28. Calcarea Phosphorica; Calcarea Fluorica
29. Kali Bichromicum; Antimonium Crudum
30. Secale Cornutum; Veratrum Album
31. Cimicifuga Racemosa; Drosera
32. Cactus Grandiflora; Lilium Tigrinum
33. Mezereum; Kreosotum
34. Tarentula Hispanica; Lactrodectus Mactans
35. Plumbum Metallicum; Picricum Acidum
36. Rhododendron; Sanguinaria
37. Coffea Cruda; Cocculus Indica
38. Nitricum Acidum; Cantharis
39. Arnica; Hypericum
40. Cuprum Metallicum; Cicuta Virosa
41. Spigelia Anthelmia; Magnesia Phosphorica
42. Muriaticum Acidum; Ammonium Carbonicum
43. Sabina; Berberis
44. Ambra Grisea; Staphysagria
45. Platina; Alumina
46. Ledum; Agaricus Muscarius
47. Chelidonium; Cina

Index of Remedies